CLINICAL PSYCHOPHARMACOLOGY

A Practical Approach

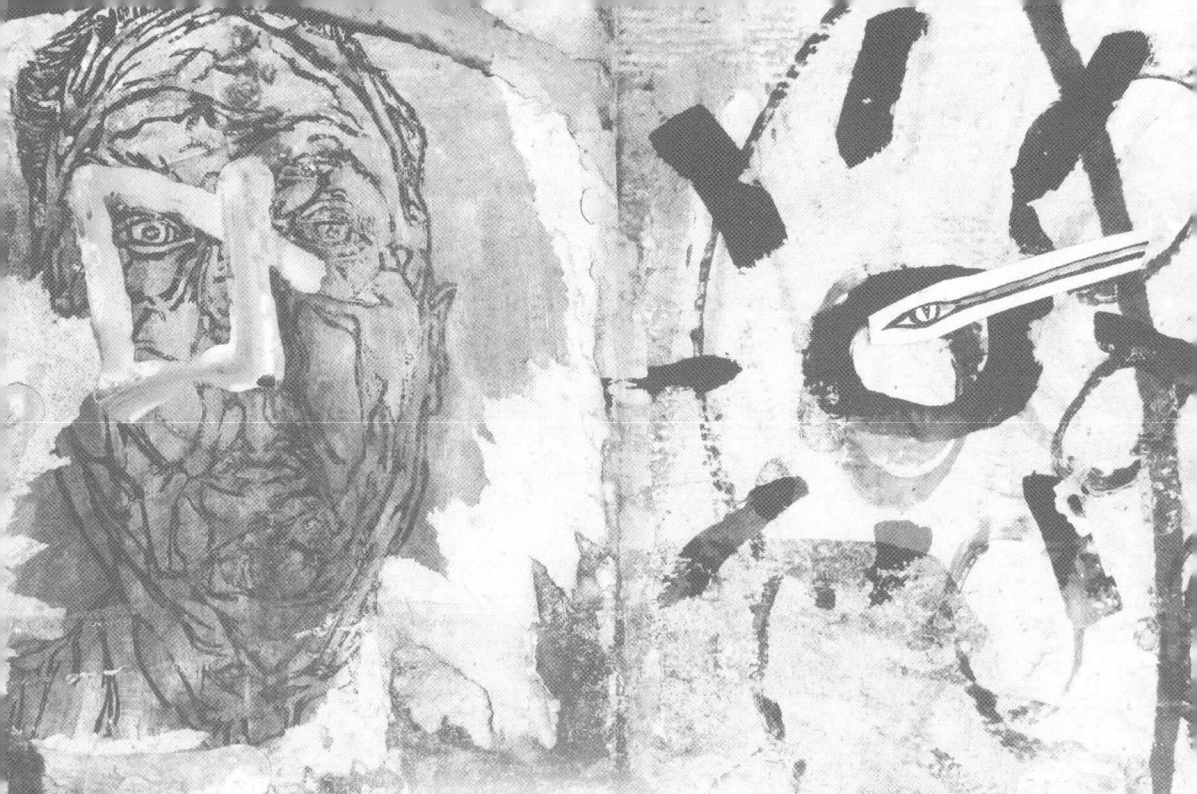

CLINICAL PSYCHOPHARMACOLOGY

A Practical Approach

Humberto Marin
Javier I Escobar
Rutgers University's Robert Wood Johnson Medical School, USA

World Scientific

NEW JERSEY • LONDON • SINGAPORE • BEIJING • SHANGHAI • HONG KONG • TAIPEI • CHENNAI

Published by

World Scientific Publishing Co. Pte. Ltd.

5 Toh Tuck Link, Singapore 596224

USA office: 27 Warren Street, Suite 401-402, Hackensack, NJ 07601

UK office: 57 Shelton Street, Covent Garden, London WC2H 9HE

Library of Congress Cataloging-in-Publication Data
Marin, Humberto.
Clinical psychopharmacology : a practical approach / Humberto Marin, Javier I. Escobar.
p. ; cm.
Includes bibliographical references and index.
ISBN 978-9814343657 (hardcover : alk. paper)
I. Escóbar, Javier. II. Title.
[DNLM: 1. Psychotropic Drugs--pharmacology. 2. Mental Disorders--drug therapy.
3. Psychopharmacology--methods. QV 77.2]
RM315
615.7'88--dc23

2013015751

British Library Cataloguing-in-Publication Data
A catalogue record for this book is available from the British Library.

Credit for Cover: Picture by Adam Olszewski, from his upcoming book *Fade Always*, depicting spontaneous drawings on the streets of New York City.

In-house Editor: Veronica Low

Typeset by Stallion Press
Email: enquiries@stallionpress.com

Printed in Singapore by B & Jo Enterprise Pte Ltd

Preface

This book aims not only to provide updated information on psychotropic drugs, but also to facilitate clinical decisions for drug management in mental health settings. To accomplish these goals, the book has three basic characteristics:

- it is evidence-based;
- it compares each individual drug with others in the same class and also those used for the same indications rather than describing them separately; and
- it steadily draws practical conclusions and makes recommendations about how to select and use medications in the treatment of specific mental disorders.

Clinical psychopharmacology, a field that began with the simultaneous discoveries of the first antidepressants, antipsychotics, and tranquilizers in the 1950s, expanded significantly in the following decades, thanks to large research investments, particularly from the pharmaceutical industry and the U.S. government. The promising trajectory of this research and the theoretical apparatus that nurtured it conferred a scientific aura to the process, bringing it to the public limelight. Active promotional efforts opened new clinical markets and drastically changed practice, moving beyond psychiatry into primary care, as evidenced by the broad prescription of SSRIs by primary care providers that has led to increased access to treatment of depression and anxiety disorders.

The development of new drugs brought significant profits and over time led to the proliferation of new, not really novel, drugs whose clinical use grew due to aggressive promotional efforts, more than therapeutic innovation. A number of authoritative textbooks on clinical psychopharmacology that describe medications side by side, have helped prescribers to view and handle psychotropic medications more objectively. However, a practical integrated approach to guide practitioners through this complex labyrinth of drugs with competing claims seems to be lacking.

This handbook aims at delivering integrated information on benefits and risks, and provides clues on the clinical use of psychiatric medications. It differs from traditional textbooks in that it uses a sequential approach to describe medications or medication groups, keeping the focus on important clinical areas, and providing specific recommendations to address a number of thorny issues in psychiatric practice. For example, how to choose a medication for initial treatment, what to do when the initial response is unsatisfactory, how to rank different types of medications for an indication, when or why to use low or high doses, when to use drug combinations, the risk of drug interactions with psychotropic medications, and several other drug management issues.

The target audience for this book are prescribers of psychotropic drugs, including psychiatrists, psychiatry residents, and primary care providers, but also other professionals working in the mental health field such as psychologists, nurses and social workers. The book is divided into 19 chapters. The first few chapters provide the general background for the use of psychiatric drugs in clinical practice. The chapters that follow focus on the large classes of drugs used for treating mental disorders with special emphasis in mood, anxiety, and psychotic disorders. At the end, there are brief chapters addressing punctual needs such as the treatment of dementia, attention disorders, or addictions in general psychiatry or primary care offices. Each of the clinical chapters or sections provides a comprehensive list of available medications, their comparative efficacy and safety profiles, as well as a "bottom line" with specific recommendations. A chapter on a critical but usually neglected subject, drug–drug interactions with psychotropic medications, closes the book.

Because of the potential conflict of interest in studies sponsored by the pharmaceutical industry, the National Institute of Mental Health of the USA (NIMH) launched independent, large-scale "effectiveness" studies designed to resemble "real-world" conditions, including patients with significant physical or mental comorbidities recruited in community and primary care settings. Other Western health authorities, for example, those in England and Germany, encouraged similar efforts. Relevant independent studies included CATIE, CUtLASS, and TEOSS for schizophrenia, STAR*D for depression, and STEP-BD for bipolar depression. Their findings figure prominently in the corresponding chapters of this book.

We aim at providing as much evidence-based data as possible. This is not an easy goal, as psychiatry lags behind other areas of medicine in the number and proportion of clinical decisions that can be based on sound evidence. For areas where this evidence is lacking, we make recommendations based on authoritative consensus or opinion and at times, on our own clinical experience (we clearly indicate when this is the case).

We want the use of this book to be an interactive enterprise. Questions, comments, criticisms, and suggestions are welcome. Please contact the authors at the following addresses: marinhu@rutgers.edu and escobaja@rutgers.edu

Humberto Marin
Javier I Escobar
New Brunswick, New Jersey
June 9, 2013

Contents

Chapter 1

Absorption, Transformation, and Elimination of Psychotropic Medications

The term 'pharmacokinetics' describes what happens to drugs after they are given to people. In the body, medications are **absorbed**, **distributed** to different body compartments, often **transformed** into inactive or active compounds, and finally **eliminated**. In the case of psychiatric medications, the target body compartment is the central nervous system (CNS), and this poses particular challenges.

1.1 Absorption

Drugs can be administered in a variety of ways. Most often, they are given orally, for intestinal absorption, but they can also be administered through the skin, the mucosal surfaces (eye, sublingual area, nose, and rectum), by injection (intramuscular, subcutaneous, intravenous, or in other locations), or by inhalation, for absorption in the lungs.

1.1.1 *Oral administration*

Oral administration is, in general, synonymous with gastrointestinal absorption. Medications that are meant to be absorbed in the mouth itself are not called 'oral,' but receive a more specific qualification, 'sublingual,' for example. These are discussed below. Oral forms are very diverse; they may be liquid or solid, or may be meant for the immediate or sustained release of the active substance(s), etc. The absorption of some psychotropic oral drugs may be affected by the presence, or absence, of food. For example, the absorption of the antipsychotic ziprasidone (Geodon) on an empty stomach can be 40% lower than that after a meal. It is important for patients to know what medications to take with or without food to guarantee optimal and stable levels. Besides this, some specific foods may also affect the intestinal absorption of medications. Naringin and other compounds present in citric juice, especially grapefruit, inactivate the oxidative enzyme CYP3A4 in the intestinal lining and the liver, and significantly increase the absorption and levels of medications metabolized by this enzyme, such as the antipsychotic quetiapine (Seroquel) as well as many benzodiazepines and hypnotics. A good rule of thumb is to always avoid taking medications with any sort of citric juice.

An important debate that applies mainly to oral medications is that of the difference between generic and brand drugs. In most cases, the discussion is probably irrelevant. For immediate-release oral preparations, both liquid and solid, which disintegrate/dissolve shortly after ingestion, the main determinant of the absorbed amount and the peak serum values is the amount of active compound in the preparation. Given good manufacturing practices, like those followed in developed countries, controlling the amount of compound per manufacturing unit is easily done, and immediate-release generics, in general, do not show significant pharmacokinetic differences with brand compounds. For slow-release oral forms, however, mimicking the rate of release over time is more difficult and, even if the total amount of absorbed drug is the same, the curve of serum concentrations may show differences and some patients may notice them.

1.1.2 *Sublingual administration ("under the tongue")*

Some drugs are meant to be absorbed in the mouth, seeking either to have a faster onset of action (such as nitrates used for angina attacks, or nicotine replacement therapies), or to avoid "first-pass elimination": the process by which drugs absorbed in the gastrointestinal tract are mostly inactivated in the intestinal lining and the liver, and may not reach the general circulation in effective amounts, such as the antipsychotic asenapine. Let us keep in mind that the intestinal lining carries metabolic enzymes such as CYP3A4, and transport proteins that pump medications out of the body. Contrary to what happens in the case of gastric, enteric, and colonic veins, those in the mouth and rectum do not pour into the portal vein, and thus avoid the first-pass effect. It is important to emphasize that sublingual administration is completely different from the soluble tablets that dissolve in the mouth, a formulation offered for many psychotropic medications. These soluble preparations do not need to be placed under the tongue, because they are well absorbed in the intestinal lumen. Rather than pharmacokinetic reasons, these are addressing patient-related reasons, such as patients who have difficulty swallowing solid forms or patients with adherence problems who may "cheek" the medication.

1.1.3 *Transdermal administration*

Major reasons to administer a drug through the skin include avoidance of "first-pass elimination" or trying to attain a more controlled release of the drug (or both). Usually, a skin patch is used that releases a predictable amount of medication per unit of time. Examples of this include the stimulant patch Daytrana (containing methylphenidate) or the antidepressant patch EMSAM (containing the monoamine oxidase inhibitor selegiline).

1.1.4 *Respiratory administration, intranasal or inhalation*

The nose and respiratory tract offer a large area of fast absorption, giving "immediate" peaks in serum concentration. In psychiatric patients, this way of administration is mainly used for addictive substances, both illegal (cocaine, opiates, solvents, etc.) and legal (tobacco and nicotine inhalers for smoking cessation). An inhaler form of the typical antipsychotic loxapine, under the name Adasuve, was recently approved in the USA for the treatment of agitation in patients with schizophrenia and bipolar disorder, and a haloperidol inhaler is currently under study.

1.1.5 *Short-acting injectable forms*

Medications available in this form include typical and atypical antipsychotics, benzodiazepines, and anticholinergic agents, for the management of acute extrapyramidal symptoms (EPS).

1.1.6 *Long-acting injectable preparations*

These are given by intramuscular injection and the active medication is slowly released. In psychiatry, these forms are mainly depot antipsychotics that tend to be used in patients with treatment adherence problems. They include Haldol Depot (haloperidol decanoate), Prolixin Depot (fluphenazine decanoate), Risperdal Consta (risperidone micropellets), Invega Sustenna (paliperidone palmitate), Zyprexa Relprevv (olanzapine pamoate), and Abilify Maintena (aripiprazole). Due to their slow absorption, long-acting preparations may take days or weeks to build adequate therapeutic levels. For that reason, it is recommended that a patient be started on an oral preparation long before they are scheduled to start the depot form. This also allows checking for adverse effects of individual agents prior to committing to a long-term injectable regime. If a patient experiences severe adverse effects to a long-acting preparation, these are likely to stay for a long period of time. The oral form is tapered down some weeks after onset of the depot antipsychotic, and the dose of the injectable form titrated up if there is indication of insufficient effect.

1.2 Distribution: Differences Between Serum and Cerebrospinal Fluid/Brain Concentrations

When we assess the pharmacokinetics of psychiatric medications, we generally apply the same measures used for systemic drugs employed in other areas of medicine. These include serum concentration, serum half-life, serum peak concentration, and area under the curve (AUC). This indirect measuring is done due to the difficulty of making direct measurements in the brain and cerebrospinal fluid (CSF). However, we must keep in mind that what really counts for the clinical effect of psychotropic medications is not the serum concentration but their concentration in the brain and CSF, and that these can be very different from those in serum.

Thus, even though there is some proportionality between serum and CSF/brain drug concentrations, these are usually different. Most drugs do not enter the brain by simple diffusion, but by active transport at the blood–brain barrier (BBB). The BBB also contains mechanisms that pump drugs out of the brain. Besides this, some drugs can be transformed or metabolized at the brain. Finally, to add to the complexity, the permeability of the BBB changes with inflammatory processes and age. The actual levels of drugs in the CSF and brain are only a weak reflection of the serum levels, as we take into account all these dynamic processes. As a result of this, the relationship between dose/serum levels and response is more difficult to establish for psychiatric than systemic medications. Usually, psychotropic drugs have a wider dosing range than other types of drugs and, with some exceptions, serum levels in clinical psychopharmacology are significantly less useful than in other areas of medicine.

1.3 Metabolism and Elimination

Drugs are metabolized (transformed) in many organs of the body and in many different ways. Psychiatric medications and their metabolites can be eliminated through different organ systems and their outflows (the urine, the bile, the skin, and the lungs). For practical reasons, in this chapter, we will discuss in detail only the two most relevant metabolic systems in humans: the cytochrome system (or CYP450 enzyme system) and the conjugation system (UGTs). Most medications, and sometimes also their metabolites, are chemically transformed inside the body. This transformation is called phase I metabolism. Some unchanged drugs, as well as a good number of metabolites produced in phase I metabolism, are conjugated — this means bound to a more water-soluble molecule — to facilitate excretion. This conjugation is called phase II metabolism.

1.3.1 *Phase I metabolism*

Phase I metabolism is an enzyme-driven mechanism that chemically transforms drugs. It involves mainly, but not exclusively, the process of oxidation.

Examples of oxidative systems of clinical importance in humans include:

(1) CYP450 (or cytochrome P450) system;
(2) alcohol dehydrogenase and aldehyde dehydrogenase (aldehyde oxidase);
(3) xantine oxidase;
(4) monoamine oxidases (MAOs);
(5) aromatases; and
(6) alkylhydrazine oxidase.

Among the metabolic oxidative systems in the body, the CYP450 is by far the dominant one, and our discussion of oxidation will focus on this system. The cytochromes are fairly abundant in nature, and close to 700 of these enzymes have been identified in different species. They are heme-containing microsomal enzymes, located in the endoplasmic reticulum; they convert most lipid-soluble compounds to more easily excreted water-soluble polar forms. Despite the high number of cytochromes, less than a dozen of them (located in families 1, 2, and 3) are important when discussing drug metabolism in humans. The most important CYP450 in all of medicine is CYP3A4. Reportedly, approximately half of the medications currently available in the USA are metabolized by CYP3A4. The second most important CYP enzyme in medicine, and the most important in psychiatry, is CYP2D6 (to avoid duplications, we present the tables of CYP450 enzymes and their main substrates in Chapter 19 on drug–drug interactions). Some CYP450 enzymes exhibit genetic polymorphisms, meaning that different individuals may carry different variants of the gene and therefore may show differences in the activity of the respective enzyme. Individuals with decreased enzymatic activity are called 'slow' or 'poor' metabolizers, and those with increased activity 'fast metabolizers.' Among the cytochrome enzymes that concern us, genetic polymorphisms with clinical implications have been described for CYP1A2, 2C9, 2C19, 2D6, and 3A4. Recently, some experts have started recommending the massive genetic screening of people receiving psychotropic medications metabolized by polymorphic CYP450 genes, mainly to detect the poor or slow metabolizers who would be at higher risk of toxicity, or the fast metabolizers who could become treatment-resistant. However, we must keep in mind that the number of poor metabolizers for these cytochromes for most populations, at least in the USA, is low (under 10%), and that the degree of enzymatic activity is also affected by other medical and environmental factors. Thus, huge differences in enzyme activity have been reported between individuals with the same gene variant (up to 60-fold). In our view, a safer approach to this problem is simply to start psychotropic medications at doses at the low end of the therapeutic spectrum and increasing them gradually, so that response and/or side effects will be noticed early. Genetic screening could be used in problem cases to confirm a suspicion of genetically based abnormal metabolism, or in populations requiring special care, such as the prescription of the anticonvulsant carbamazepine (Tegretol) to populations from the Far East, for which the FDA has issued a black box warning associated with a variant of the HLA-B gene (HLA-B*1502).

1.3.1.1 *Inhibition and induction of CYP450 enzymes*

As mentioned above, although genetic polymorphism is an important determinant of cytochrome activity, it is not the only one. *In vivo*, the activity of CYP450 enzymes is also influenced by medical and environmental factors such as, for example, hepatic or renal illness, some foods, smoking, and use of some medications, supplements, and illegal substances. Numerous drugs and exogenous substances have the potential to inhibit (decrease) or induce (enhance) the activity of different CYP450 enzymes. Inhibition of a specific cytochrome leads to decreased metabolism and increased levels and activity of the enzyme substrates. Induction of a cytochrome leads to increased metabolism and decreased levels and activity of its substrates (we present the tables of CYP450 substrates, inhibitors, and inducers in Chapter 19).

1.3.2 *Phase II metabolism (conjugation)*

Conjugation enzymes catalyze the transfer of sugars, especially glucuronic acid, to a variety of molecules, both endogenous and xenobiotics, to make them more hydrophilic and more easily excreted. Many of the substances conjugated to sugars by this system are the products of the oxidative enzymes, so very often it is seen as just a continuation of the oxidative metabolic reactions. However, conjugation is the main elimination pathway for numerous active drugs that are not oxidized, or for active metabolites of oxidized drugs.

The conjugation enzymes, uridine-5′-diphospho-glycosyltransferases, also called uridine-5′-diphospho-glucuronosyltransferases, or UGTs, are expressed in many tissues, but the most relevant are those in the intestine, liver, and kidneys. For conjugation, UGTs require a cofactor, uridine-5′-diphospho-glucuronic acid (UDPGA), to provide glucuronic acid.

As with the cytochromes, there are multiple UGTs relevant to drug metabolism in humans. However, the selectivity of conjugation enzymes for their substrates is lower than that of oxidative enzymes. Once a substrate has saturated the preferred UGT enzyme, it may be taken up by other UGTs. This way, a substrate may saturate, and decrease the activity of practically the whole system. Another process by which conjugation substrates may decrease the activity of the whole system is by exhausting the required cofactor, UDPGA.

1.3.2.1 *Inhibition and induction of conjugation enzymes*

As with the CYP450 oxidative enzymes, some medical conditions and medications, foods, supplements, illegal substances, and other environmental compounds may inhibit (decrease) or induce (increase) the activity of conjugation enzymes, and in this way increase or decrease the levels and activity of the enzyme substrates. Among psychotropic medications, the most frequent conjugation inhibitor causing toxicity is divalproex (valproate, or valproic acid), but alcohol, NSAIDs, and acetaminophen are also risky, especially at high doses. On the other hand, the most frequent conjugation inducer causing decreased effects is carbamazepine. In Chapter 19 on drug–drug interactions, the reader may find a list of substrates, inhibitors, and inducers for the most relevant conjugation enzymes.

1.4 Additional Concepts in Pharmacokinetics

1.4.1 *Steady state*

Steady state is an important concept for all medications, but especially for those administered with the aim of reaching a certain “target level” in serum. After starting a medication, the serum levels go up for a while, until a balance is reached between absorption and elimination and the levels stabilize ("plateau"). This is the "steady state." An approximate but reliable estimate of the time to reach steady state is four or five times the elimination half-life. This means, for example, that in healthy young adults, levels of lithium are steady after just two and a half days (12 h × 5), while in the elderly, reaching steady levels of lithium can take up to one week (36 h × 5).

1.4.2 *Dose–response relationship*

For most psychotropic medications, the dose–response curve has typically the form of an elongated S ("sigmoidal"). Thus, if we use the horizontal axis for dose and the vertical axis for response, when we start a medication at a low dose, we have a "flat" segment in which the drug shows no significant effect. After a threshold dose, the effect appears and the curve starts going up with subsequent increases in the dose. Then, at a certain optimal dose value, the effect "plateaus." This means that the curve becomes horizontal again, and additional dose increases do not produce a substantial increase in the effect of the drug, though they significantly increase the risk of toxicity, side effects, and adverse reactions. For some psychotropic medications, such as antipsychotics, it is not even desirable to reach the upper part of the vertical segment of the curve, as it is in this part that the most significant side effects appear, including EPS.

1.4.3 *Therapeutic margin*

There are significant differences in safety across all psychotropic medications. One of the most widely used ways to measure safety is calculating how far apart are therapeutic doses from "dangerous" or "lethal" doses (therapeutic margin). The "median effective dose 50" refers to the dose that produces the expected response in 50% of the subjects. In a similar way, we may calculate the "median lethal dose 50," the dose that causes the death of 50% of the subjects. Along the same line, when we examine a harmful effect of a drug, we can calculate the "median toxic dose 50," and so on. The relationship between the effective and the toxic or lethal doses is the therapeutic margin of a medication. In psychiatry, most of the medications prescribed today have therapeutic margins in the three-digit range (higher than 100:1), such as SSRIs (selective serotonin reuptake inhibitors), which means they are generally safe or very safe medications. However, some useful medications, such as lithium, have therapeutic margins in the single digits.

Chapter 2

Neurotransmitters, Receptors, and Transporters

Most of the available psychiatric medications are believed to work, directly or indirectly, by activating or inhibiting neurotransmitter receptors in the brain. Some drugs directly bind receptors and activate or inactivate them (**agonists** and **antagonists**, respectively). Other drugs change the amount of neurotransmitter available to bind the receptors. They may, for example, inhibit the pumps that remove neurotransmitters from the synaptic space, decrease the metabolism of neurotransmitters, or increase neurotransmitter release. A few medications may decrease the amount of neurotransmitter in the synapses that is available for release. Psychiatric medications can also cause side effects and adverse reactions by affecting receptors different from those involved in their therapeutic actions, in some cases, outside the central nervous system (CNS).

2.1 Main Types of Receptors in the Brain

Receptors are the main target sites for the action of psychotropic drugs. They are key elements in synaptic transmission from neuron to neuron. The basic function of receptors is the recognition of a signaling molecule resulting in signal transduction. This latter property distinguishes a receptor from the simpler "binding site," which may exist independently from a receptor. Below, we discuss the main types of receptors present in the nervous system.

2.1.1 *Division of receptors according to the processes they trigger*

2.1.1.1 *Ionotropic receptors*

These receptors are coupled with an ionic channel. The neurotransmitter and other ligands open or close the channel. The entry of the electrically charged ion affects the polarity of the cell membrane and with it the excitability of the cell.

2.1.1.2 *Metabotropic receptors*

Metabotropics, or G protein-coupled receptors, are receptors connected to intracellular messenger systems, the G proteins. Activation or blocking of the receptors starts or impedes a series of intracellular events that lead to an "effector" being activated.

2.1.1.3 *Receptor tyrosine kinases*

These are proteins usually activated by neurotrophins such as brain-derived neurotrophic factor (BDNF), other neurotrophic factors, and cytokines. They govern the trophic state (growth) of the target cell, including sometimes the production of other messengers, and triggering "cascades" of events.

2.1.1.4 *Nuclear receptors*

These are transcription factors that regulate the expression of specific genes. The transmitters for these receptors are usually hormones, such as adrenal, thyroid, or sexual hormones. Once activated, the hormone–receptor complex is transported to the nucleus, where, with cofactors, it activates or represses gene expression.

2.1.1.5 *Receptors associated with neurotransmitter pumps*

These receptors govern the action of the pumps that capture molecules of neurotransmitter in the extracellular space and transport them back into the cell to be stored and reused. The most relevant neurotransmitter pumps are the reuptake transporters for serotonin, norepinephrine, and dopamine, described in detail at the end of this chapter.

2.1.2 *Division of receptors according to their localization in pre- or post-synaptic neurons*

Receptors may also be classified according to their localization in the neurons that release the neurotransmitter (pre-synaptic neuron) or in the neurons that are the target of the neurotransmitter (post-synaptic neurons). According to this, receptors are divided into autoreceptors and heteroreceptors.

2.1.2.1 *Autoreceptors*

These are receptors located in neurons containing the ligand (pre-synaptic neuron). They can be located at the synapse (in the axon or "nerve terminal"), or on the neuronal body (soma) and dendrites. Synaptic autoreceptors are usually part of a feedback mechanism to regulate the release of neurotransmitter. When stimulated by the neurotransmitter released into the synapse, they exert a negative feedback on the release of more neurotransmitter. Somatic and dendritic autoreceptors work in the way same as receptors located in post-synaptic target cells, usually controlling the firing rate of neurons.

2.1.2.2 *Heteroreceptors*

These are receptors located in post-synaptic neurons that do not contain the specific ligand (post-synaptic neurons). Thus, they are stimulated only in neuron-to-neuron transmission (for example, serotonin receptors on GABA or dopamine neurons).

2.2 Neurotransmitters

Reportedly, over 200 neurotransmitters have been identified in the human brain. Besides this, the receptors for the most important neurotransmitters show multiple subtypes, and are present in multiple brain circuits, which often exert different and even opposite effects. However, a working knowledge of the main neurotransmitters and their receptors/transporters is a pre-condition for the study of psychopharmacology these days. We hope that the synthetic review that follows may help place many of the theoretical postulates of psychopharmacology in a clinical/practical perspective, and guide the reader in understanding the actions, both therapeutic and adverse, of our current psychiatric medications.

The main neurotransmitters of relevance to psychopharmacology are:

(1) monoamines (serotonin, norepinephrine, dopamine, and histamine);
(2) amino acids (glutamate, GABA, and others);
(3) acetylcholine;
(4) neuropeptides (opioid, pituitary, hypothalamic-releasing factors, and others); and
(5) neurotrophins (BDNF and other trophic factors).

2.2.1 *Serotonin*

Serotonin is abundant in the body, particularly in the gastrointestinal system, but also in immune cells, the respiratory system, bone, and platelets. However, in the brain, serotonin is not as widely disseminated as other neurotransmitters such as glutamate, GABA, dopamine, and norepinephrine. Serotonin is mainly found in the midline raphe nuclei of the brainstem. Despite this relative concentration in a few brain areas, serotonin is active in multiple brain circuits and is involved in the modulation of some of the most important brain functions, including emotions, pain perception, motor behavior, sleep, feeding, sexuality, and social cognition. Serotonin does not cross the blood–brain barrier and it is synthesized locally in the nervous system. Serotonin's precursor is the dietary amino acid L-tryptophan, which enters the nervous system via a carrier mechanism with limited capacity. Thus, dietary L-tryptophan depletion is a proven way to decrease serotonin synthesis in the brain, and has shown to induce depression relapse in patients treated with serotonin reuptake inhibitors. The first step in the production of serotonin from tryptophan is the addition of a hydroxyl group, catalyzed by tryptophan hydroxylase, which is the rate-limiting enzyme in the process. The first step in the metabolism of serotonin is oxidation by monoamine oxidase (MAO)-A, which also oxidizes norepinephrine.

2.2.1.1 *Types of serotonin receptors*

Fourteen 5-HT receptor subtypes have been identified so far. They have been grouped in seven families, numbered 1 through 7. These receptors are detailed below.

5-HT$_{1A}$. In serotonergic neurons, the 5-HT$_{1A}$ receptor functions as an inhibitory autoreceptor. It seems to be centrally involved in depression and anxiety, and also in sexual behavior, cognition, motor behavior, and pain perception. Serotonergic medications may exert their delayed antidepressant effect and improve hippocampal neurogenesis through the downregulation of these receptors. Also, buspirone, an anti-anxiety medication, is a partial agonist for 5-HT$_{1A}$. This subtype may also mediate serotonergic antidepressant-induced sexual dysfunction.

5-HT$_{1B}$. This receptor, highly expressed in the basal ganglia, appears to be implicated in drug addictions and anxiety, and has been related to the modulation of impulsivity, aggressive behaviors, and locomotion activity. This receptor, together with **5-HT$_{1C}$** and **5-HT$_{1D}$**, seem to be present in blood vessels and play a role in the action of the triptans, which are effective serotonergic antimigraine drugs.

5-HT$_{1E}$. Little is known about this receptor due to lack of selective agonists/antagonists.

5-HT$_{1F}$ has been suggested as a brain target to control neurogenic inflammation as a cause of migraine (triptans show high affinity for this receptor).

5-HT$_{2A}$ is present, besides in the brain, in peripheral locations such as platelets and smooth muscle. In the brain, 5-HT$_{2A}$ has been implicated in cognition, specifically memory processes.

5-HT$_{2B}$ seems to be expressed mainly in the heart and intestine, and apparently plays a role in the cardiac effects of the serotonergic appetite-suppressing drug dexfenfluramine.

5-HT$_{2C}$ is ubiquitous in the brain, and seems to be related to anxiety, cognition, and appetite. Stimulation of this receptor subtype has anxiogenic and appetite-suppressing effects.

5-HT$_3$ is different from other serotonergic receptors in that it is associated with an ion channel, rather than G protein activation. Its activation increases the entry of anions Na^+ and K^+, causing neuronal excitation. 5-HT$_3$ antagonists, such as ondansetron, are antiemetic and may also have anti-anxiety and positive effects on cognitive functions.

5-HT$_4$ receptor agonists increase colonic motility. In the brain, this receptor seems to be associated with anticonvulsant activity and stress response.

5-HT$_5$ receptors are believed to have similar roles to those described for 5-HT$_{1A}$ receptors in conditions/functions such as anxiety, sleep, incontinence, food intake, learning, memory, pain, and chemoreceptor pathways.

2.2.2 *Dopamine*

Three dopaminergic systems are important for the purposes of this book: (1) the mesocorticolimbic system, (2) the nigrostriatal system, and (3) the tuberohyposphyseal system. The *mesocorticolimbic* system is usually subdivided into the *mesolimbic* and *mesocortical* pathways. The mesolimbic pathway plays a central role in emotions and reward/addictions; it is believed that excessive dopaminergic stimulation in this system causes the positive symptoms of schizophrenia. The mesocortical pathway involves functions such as attention, working memory, and initiative; it is believed that low dopaminergic activity in this system causes or contributes to the negative symptoms of schizophrenia. The *nigrostriatal* system is involved in the control of voluntary movements, but also, as has been learned more recently, in reward and addictions. The blockade of dopaminergic neurons in this system produces extrapyramidal symptoms (EPS). The *tuberohypophysial* (tuberoinfundibular) system controls the release of prolactin produced in the pituitary. The blockade of dopaminergic neurons in this system produces hyperprolactinemia.

In the CNS, dopamine is more widely distributed than serotonin. The precursor for dopamine is the amino acid L-tyrosine, which enters the brain via active transport. The rate-limiting enzyme in dopamine synthesis is L-tyrosine hydroxylase that catalyzes the addition of a hydroxyl group to L-tyrosine to form L-deoxyphenyl alanine (L-DOPA). L-DOPA is then converted to dopamine by DOPA decarboxylase. Dopamine is metabolized by MAOs and, secondarily, catechol-O-methyltransferase (COMT).

2.2.2.1 *Types of dopamine receptors*

So far, five dopamine D receptor subtypes have been identified and grouped into two families: D_1 and D_2.

D_1 family includes the D_1 and D_5 receptors. The D_1 is the most widespread dopamine receptor in the brain, and the most prevalent dopamine receptor in the frontal cortex. This receptor may then be associated with the cognitive functions of dopamine, such as the control of working memory and attention. The D_1 agonist apomorphin is an emetic. Other D_1 agonists have cardiovascular effects. The D_5 receptor has a more restricted distribution and is mainly located in the limbic system and the striatum. Its expression in the thalamus suggests a role in the perception of painful stimuli.

D_2 family contains the D_2 receptor (with two subtypes: short, D_{2S}, and long, D_{2L}), the D_3, and the D_4 receptors. Blockade of D_2 receptors seems to be central to the therapeutic action and side effects of all currently available antipsychotic drugs. D_2 receptors are involved in voluntary movements, and D_2 blockers may induce EPS, while some agonists are useful in the treatment of Parkinson's disease. D_2 receptors also control the release of prolactin by the pituitary, and D_2 blockers cause hyperprolactinemia while agonists inhibit the release of prolactin and are used in the treatment of prolactinoma. D_2 antagonists are also useful in the treatment of gastric motility disorders. The D_3 receptor may be associated with the control of locomotion, and also may be a target for BDNF. The D_4 receptor is expressed in the frontal cortex and the limbic system. Clozapine has relatively high affinity for this receptor and this could be related to its unique antipsychotic effect. The D_4 receptor has also been associated with novelty-seeking ("thrill-seeking").

2.2.3 *Norepinephrine*

Noradrenergic neurons project from two major places in the brainstem: the locus ceruleus and the lateral tegmental nuclei, throughout the nervous system. The main functions these neurons appear to be involved in include arousal, attention/vigilance, and stress response. Norepinephrine is formed by the addition of a hydroxyl group to dopamine, a reaction catalyzed by dopamine-β-hydroxylase. The first step in the metabolism of norepinephrine is oxidation by MAO-A, which also degrades serotonin. Norepinephrine is also metabolized by COMT, an enzyme with a wide variety of substrates but with less affinity for norepinephrine than MAO-A.

2.2.3.1 *Types of norepinephrine receptors*

Adrenergic receptors include the α receptors (divided into α_1 and α_2 types) and β receptors (divided into β_1, β_2, and β_3 types).

α_1 receptors include the A, B, and D subtypes. The α_1 receptors seem to be more relevant to smooth muscle than the nervous system. Stimulation of α_1 receptors leads mainly to vasoconstriction in many areas of the body. This is important in psychopharmacology, as many psychiatric medications block these receptors, and may induce hypotension and syncope.

α_2 receptors include the A, B, and C subtypes. The α_2 receptors seem to be more relevant to the CNS than the α_1 type.They function as autoreceptors in adrenergic neurons, inhibiting the release of norepinephrine. Thus, blockade of α_2 receptors results in increased norepinephrine release in the CNS. The α_2 receptors also inhibit the release of insulin and increase the release of glucagon at the pancreas, and cause contraction of the sphincters in the gastrointestinal tract.

β_1 receptors have important cardiovascular effects. Their stimulation increases cardiac output and renin secretion by the kidney. They seem to be related to both depression and, especially, anxiety. In animals, antidepressants seem to induce a downregulation or desensitization of these receptors in the brain. Also, cardiovascular medications blocking β_1 receptors have an anti-anxiety effect.

β_2 receptors dilate arteries in the skeletal muscle, relax smooth muscle in the bronchi and other systems, and increase glycogenolysis and gluconeogenesis. These receptors seem to influence the modulation of emotional memory (they are abundant in the amygdala), and thus they are likely involved in post-traumatic stress disorder and other chronic mood disorders.

β_3 receptors appear to play a role in metabolism, especially in lypolisis and thermoregulation. They are more abundant in fat tissue and seem to be absent in the nervous system.

2.2.4 *Acetylcholine*

Acetylcholine is widely distributed throughout the body, as part of the autonomic nervous system. In the brain, there are two large clusters of cholinergic neurons, the basal forebrain and the mesopontine complexes, that send projections to distant areas, including the cortex and the limbic system. The forebrain complex is significantly affected in Alzheimer's disease, especially the nucleus basalis. Mesopontine fibers go to the thalamus and the brainstem, including, interestingly, dopaminergic areas such as the substantia nigra and the striatum. Likely related to the above, anticholinergic medications exert an antiparkinsonian action. Acetylcholine is produced from choline, by the transfer of an acetyl group from acetyl coenzyme A, a reaction catalyzed by choline acetyltransferase. Acetylcholine is broken down mainly by acetylcholinesterase.

2.2.4.1 *Types of cholinergic receptors*

Receptors binding acetylcholine (cholinergic receptors) are involved in important cognitive functions such as sleep, alertness, perception, and voluntary movements. There are two main classes of cholinergic receptors: *muscarinic* and *nicotinic*.

Cholinergic muscarinic (M) receptors. Five subtypes of M receptors have been identified (M_1 through M_5). M_1 is the most prevalent muscarinic receptor in the forebrain, including the cortex, limbic system, and striatum. M_1 seems to be centrally involved in memory and synaptic plasticity. M_2 receptors are widely distributed in the brain, and their activation seems to be associated with analgesia and hypothermia. So far, M_3 receptors seem to be more important in other body systems, such as the gastrointestinal or genitourinary tracts, than in the CNS. M_4 receptors in the striatum appear to counterbalance dopamine effects and M_4 blockers are being considered as antiparkinson medications. The M_5 receptors seem to be more relevant in the circulatory than in the nervous system.

Nicotinic receptors. Nicotinic receptors are difficult to classify into subtypes, as they are composed of variable numbers and combinations of different protein subunits. From the functional point of view, there are two main classes of nicotinic receptors relevant to pharmacology: those present in skeletal muscle and those in the neurons. Skeletal muscle nicotinic receptors are the target of muscle relaxants, such as curare derivatives. In the brain, nicotinic receptors are widely distributed. They seem to play an important role in cognitive functions such as attention, working memory, and processing speed. Some pre-synaptic nicotinic receptors have been identified that seem to modulate the release of acetylcholine and other neurotransmitters, including dopamine, norepinephrine, serotonin, glutamate, and GABA. Because of this, nicotinic receptors could play a significant role in disorders apparently due to changes in other receptors/neurotransmitters, such as schizophrenia or attention deficit disorders. Tobacco dependence seems to develop through the continued stimulation of nicotinic receptors by nicotine in the dopaminergic reward pathways of the mesolimbic system.

2.2.5 *Glutamate*

Glutamate is the main excitatory neurotransmitter, widely distributed in the brain, and present in up to 70%–80% of synapses. Interestingly, and different from most other neurotransmitters, glutamate receptors exist almost only in the nervous system. Glutamate seems to be associated with several critical functions and processes, including learning, memory, and neuroplasticity. On the other hand, glutamatergic excitotoxicity causes neuronal damage or death. Glutamate receptors are numerous and very diverse. Besides neurons, glutamate receptors are expressed in developing astrocytes and oligodendrocytes, suggesting that they are relevant to glial cell development and function.

2.2.5.1 *Glutamate activity and neuroplasticity*

It is generally accepted that processes such as learning and memory involve changes in synapses. Glutamate is central to the regulation of synaptic plasticity. Laboratory studies have shown that brief and intense glutamatergic stimulation leads to increased synaptic efficacy (long-term potentiation, LTP). On the other hand, stable low-frequency glutamatergic stimulation leads to decreased synaptic efficacy (long-term depression, LTD). These processes seem to be important in regions like the hippocampus, involved in the acquisition of new memories. However, excessive glutamatergic signaling leads to neuronal toxicity and death. Cellular stress (for example, hypoxia following stroke) leads to the increased entry of Ca^{2+} through NMDA receptor channels (see below). Among other phenomena, this causes a massive release of glutamate to the extracellular space, with the activation of AMPA receptors that leads to excessive excitation and damage.

2.2.5.2 *Types of glutamate receptors*

Glutamate receptors are grossly divided, according to their mechanism, into *ionotropic* and *metabotropic*. Glutamate receptors are less specific than those for other important neurotransmitters. They may accept or even require other agonists to become activated.

Ionotropic glutamate receptor subtypes are defined by chemicals that bind each of them more selectively than glutamate. So far, three subtypes are recognized, according to the analogs of glutamate they bind: *AMPA* receptors (α-amino-3-hydroxy-5-methyl-4-isoxazole propionic acid); *KA* receptors (kainic acid), and *NMDA* receptors (*N*-methyl-D-aspartic acid).

(1) AMPA receptors mediate the excitatory post-synaptic currents in most of the CNS. There are some indications that enhancing AMPA relative to NMDA output may be an important mechanism of the action of antidepressants.
(2) KA receptors seem to have a pre-synaptic localization, meaning that they may reduce glutamatergic neurotransmission when activated. KA receptors are observed to be associated with synaptic plasticity in areas of the brain involved in mood regulation. Abnormalities of KA receptors could be associated with mania.
(3) NMDA receptors exhibit a complex activation process. First, it is necessary for AMPA receptors to depolarize the membrane, as NMDA receptors have a blocking binding site for an anion (Mg^{2+}) that has to be removed by membrane depolarization. Second, NMDA receptor activation requires, besides glutamate, the simultaneous binding of another ligand, glycine or D-cycloserine, before the channel opens. Thus, the activation of NMDA receptors means the confluence or "coordination" of several events: release of glutamate, release of glycine or D-cycloserine, and depolarization of the membrane by AMPA receptors.

Metabotropic glutamate receptors (mGluRs) are associated with intracellular messenger systems. mGluRs seem to play mainly an inhibitory role. They are G protein-coupled receptors, and include eight types of receptors (numbered 1 through 8), organized in three subgroups. Group I includes mGluR1 and 5; group II includes mGluR2 and 3; and group III includes mGluR4, 6, 7, and 8. Group I receptors are found in pre- and post-synaptic neurons.

Groups II and III receptors seem to be "extra-synaptic" and have a negative, inhibitory effect on the release of glutamate itself and GABA. These group II and III receptors, located far from the synapses, would only be activated in cases of excessive glutamate release, probably in toxic and pathologic conditions. Agonism of some glutamatergic group II receptors seems to have anti-anxiety, antipsychotic, and neuroprotective effects.

2.2.6 *GABA*

Gamma-aminobutyric acid (GABA) is the main inhibitory neurotransmitter. It is widely distributed in the brain and is involved in multiple functions and disorders, including mood, sleep, alertness, memory, muscle relaxation, anxiety, schizophrenia, and convulsive and addictive disorders.

2.2.6.1 *Types of GABA receptors*

Two main classes of GABA receptors have been identified: $GABA_A$ and $GABA_B$.

$GABA_A$. This is, by far, the more abundant of the two GABA receptors. It is an ionotropic receptor that controls a cation (Cl^-) channel. Activation of the $GABA_A$ receptor induces the opening of the Cl^- channel, and the entry of this negative ion contributes to the polarization and stabilization of the cell membrane. The $GABA_A$ receptor is a large one, composed of five subunits. There are five subunit types, with multiple variations, for a total of at least 18 identified subunits. The high number of combinations makes $GABA_A$ receptors very heterogeneous. This heterogeneity is likely necessary for the many separate important functions that GABA performs in the brain. $GABA_A$ receptors also have a number of different "allosteric" binding sites for substances that modulate the activity of the receptor. These substances include benzodiazepines, alcohol, anesthetics, anticonvulsants, and toxic proconvulsant substances such as picrotoxin. Different subunits may mediate the different effects of drugs. Thus, the α_2 subunit seems to be related to anxiolysis, while α_1 would be important for sedation/amnesia. This has triggered intensive pharmacological research for more selective GABAergic drugs. The first of these to reach the market have been hypnotic medications such as zolpidem, zaleplon, and zopiclone, and the search continues for more specific anti-anxiety, anticonvulsive, alerting, or memory-improving drugs.

$GABA_B$. These are metabotropic, G protein-coupled receptors. Pharmacologically, they are identified by binding the agonist baclofen, which does not affect $GABA_A$ receptors. They are present in pre- and post-synaptic neurons, acting to stabilize the neuronal membrane and inhibit neurotransmitter release. $GABA_B$ receptors are composed of seven subunits, and the combination of two of these seven-subunit complexes (dimerization) seems to be necessary for them to become functional. Besides the muscle relaxation induced by substances such as baclofen, $GABA_B$ receptors appear to be associated with pain perception/analgesia and the behavioral effects of alcohol.

2.2.7 *Histamine*

Histamine, a critical compound for inflammatory and allergic processes, is relevant in psychopharmacology mainly due to the ability of a significant number of psychotropic medications to induce sedation and weight gain by blocking histamine receptors in the brain. In some cases, antihistamines are used as hypnotic and anti-anxiety medications. Histamine is produced by decarboxilation of the amino acid histidine. In the brain, it is primarily metabolized by histamine-*N*-methyltransferase.

2.2.7.1 *Types of histamine receptors*

Four types of histamine receptors have been identified.

H_1 receptors are the most abundant histamine receptors in the body. Among other responses, they induce vasodilation, increase endothelial permeability of the blood vessels, and trigger bronchoconstriction. They are the main histamine receptors involved in allergic reactions. In the nervous system, H_1 receptors are associated with motion sickness and tend to increase neuronal excitation, increasing arousal and reducing appetite.

H_2 receptors are found mainly in the parietal cells of the stomach, where they increase acid secretion. In the CNS, their role is unclear; it has been hypothesized that they decrease pain perception. H_2 receptors are associated with sexual function; H_2 antagonists may induce erectile dysfunction and decrease libido, and local histamine administration may improve erection ability.

H_3 receptors seem to inhibit the release of histamine and other important neurotransmitters: acetylcholine, dopamine, norepinephrine, and serotonin. Antagonism of these receptors appears to increase wakefulness, decrease appetite, and enhance cognition.

H_4 receptors are found mainly in the white blood cells, thymus, spleen, and colon. They seem to play a role in chemotaxis.

2.3 Neurotransmitter Reuptake Transporters

Neurotransmitter reuptake transporters are proteins located in the cell membrane. They pump neurotransmitters released to the extracellular space back into the cell, to be stored and utilized again. Transporter mechanisms have been identified for practically any important neurotransmitter, including glutamate, GABA, glycine, adenosine, serotonin, dopamine, norepinephrine, and histamine. Important psychiatric medications, such as SSRIs (selective serotonin reuptake inhibitors), SNRIs (serotonin–norepinephrine reuptake inhibitors), and TCAs (tricyclic antidepressants), work by inhibiting the reuptake pumps for the monoamines involved in mood, this way increasing the levels of free serotonin, norepinephrine, and dopamine in the extracellular space. Because of their pharmacological importance, we will review only the reuptake transporters for these three monoamines.

Monoamine transporters both limit the duration of action of the released monoamines and replenish again the intracellular monoamine store. In general, reuptake transporters are specific for each monoamine, but in conditions of deficit (inhibition) for one of the transporters, other transporters may pump the affected monoamine. Monoamine transporter proteins are coded by polymorphic alleles, meaning that several variants of the gene, and the protein, may exist with different levels of activity. From this, it has been hypothesized that different alleles for these proteins may confer different risks for psychiatric disorders, such as depression, anxiety, attention deficit, psychosis, or stress disorders. Perhaps the most widely publicized of these association studies is the one suggesting that individuals carrying the so-called short variant for the serotonin transporter are more likely than those carrying the so-called long variant to develop depression following significant life stress. However, despite the growing number of studies, this association has not been conclusively proven. In other studies, variations in the serotonin transporter alleles have been associated with differences in social cognition. Other studies suggest an association of some norepinephrine and, especially, dopamine transporter allele variants with ADHD (attention deficit hyperactivity disorder).

Neurotransmitter reuptake is an active, energy-consuming process that can be inhibited by some medications. Besides depression, anxiety, and psychosis, monoamine reuptake proteins are important also for the action of some substances of abuse, such as cocaine, amphetamines, and MDMA. Stimulating and rewarding properties of cocaine are likely associated with the inhibition of dopamine and also, to some extent, serotonin and norepinephrine reuptake.

References

Berger M, Honig G, Wade JM, Tecott LH. Monoamine neurotransmitters. In: Sadock BJ, Sadock VA, Ruiz P, eds. *Kaplan and Sadock's Comprehensive Textbook of Psychiatry*. 6th ed. Lippincott Williams & Wilkins, New York, 2009, pp. 65–76.

Coyle JT. Amino acid neurotransmitters. In: Sadock BJ, Sadock VA, Ruiz P, eds. *Kaplan and Saddock's Comprehensive Textbook of Psychiatry*. 6th ed. Lippincott Williams & Wilkins, New York, 2009, pp. 76–84.

Filip M, Bader M. Overview on 5-HT receptors and their role in physiology and pathology of the central nervous system. *Pharm Rep* 2009;61:761–777.

Iversen L. Neurotransmitter transporters and their impact in the development of psychopharmacology. *Br J Pharm* 2006;147:S82–S88.

Risch N, Herrell R, Lehner T, *et al.* Interaction between the serotonin transporter gene (5-HTTLPR), stressful life events, and risk of depression — a meta-analysis. *JAMA* 2009;301(23):2462–2471.

Chapter 3

Antipsychotics: A General View of Therapeutic and Adverse Effects

In this chapter, we review the characteristics shared by all currently marketed antipsychotics, old and new, or, as some call them, 'typical' and 'atypical.' This includes their common antipsychotic mechanism, their clinical effects in psychotic patients, and the risk for side effects and adverse reactions such as extrapyramidal symptoms (EPS), weight gain and metabolic syndrome, hyperprolactinemia, malignant arrhythmia, increased mortality in patients with dementia, and other risky or undesirable effects. For the discussion of individual characteristics of currently or recently available antipsychotic drugs, we refer the reader to the next chapter.

3.1 Classic Antipsychotics

The first antipsychotic drug, chlorpromazine (Thorazine, Largactil), still in use worldwide, was introduced in the USA in 1952. It was originally produced at Rhône-Poulenc laboratories in Paris, by the addition of a chlorine atom in position 2 of the promazine molecule, and clinical studies by Jean Delay and Pierre Deniker showed its remarkable clinical effects on psychoses. Similar drugs soon followed which, despite differences in dopamine-blocking potency, and consequently in dosing, shared the same general mechanism of action and clinical efficacy of chlorpromazine. The impact of these medications in the treatment of severe mental disorders was huge, and psychopharmacological research flourished. In his 1968 presidential address to the newly created American College of Neuropsychopharmacology, Nathan S. Kline stated that "*the single most dramatic effect of what psychopharmaceuticals have done is their effect on mental hospital population.*" Thus, the number of patients hospitalized in mental institutions in the USA, which had climbed steadily to a peak of 558,900 patients in 1954, declined to 426,700 in 1968, less than two decades after the advent of chlorpromazine. Of course, other treatments, such as antidepressants, and non-pharmacological factors (e.g., changes in social policies) may have played a role as well, but the pivotal factor appeared to be the introduction of antipsychotics.

An important fact to remember, especially when comparing old and new antipsychotics, is that initially, the old antipsychotics were used in high dosages, up to 10-fold the doses recommended today. Because of this, the reported incidence of toxicity and adverse reactions with old antipsychotics needs to be re-examined with particular care. This prescription of high doses derived from the belief that a complete "saturation" of the dopamine receptors was necessary for the optimal effect of antipsychotic drugs on psychotic symptoms. To make sure dopamine receptors were "saturated," the antipsychotic dose was pushed up until patients showed EPS (extrapyramidal symptoms), especially parkinsonism (this was the so-called neuroleptic threshold). The Prescribing Information for haloperidol in the USA, that has not been reviewed for several decades (available only electronically, as none of the old antipsychotics is described in detail in the current printed edition of the Physicians Desk Reference), still recommends the following doses: "***Adults:*** *1 to 2 mg 2 or 3 times daily, initially, followed by upward adjustment as tolerated until the desired effect is achieved or limiting side effects appear. Clinical experience has shown that it is seldom necessary to employ dosages greater than 4 to 6 mg 3 times daily. However, 30 to 40 mg/day may be required in severely disturbed patients who remain inadequately controlled by lower doses. Up to 100 mg/day has been used occasionally in particularly resistant patients.*" Even by the year 2000, after several new or "atypical" antipsychotics have been in the market for almost a decade, psychiatric publications still recommended, for the old antipsychotics, upper daily dosage limits as high as 2,000 mg for chlorpromazine, 100 mg for haloperidol, 64 mg for perphenazine, 40 mg for trifluoperazine, 60 mg for thiotixene, and 40 mg for fluphenazine. The reader can compare these doses with the recent recommendations of an International Consensus Panel that we present in Table 3.1.

3.2 New Antipsychotics

Against this backdrop of old antipsychotics used at high doses that "tranquilized" and "immobilized" patients (the so-called chemical restraint), the new or "atypical" antipsychotics made their entrance in the early 1990s. The first of these "atypicals" to be introduced to the market was clozapine

Table 3.1 Recommended doses of old and new antipsychotics.

Drug	**Starting dose (mg/day)**	**Target dose (mg/day)**	**Maximum dose (mg/day)**
Chlorpromazine	100	300–600	800
Droperidol	3.0	4.5–8.8	12.0
Fluphenazine	3.0	5–15	20
Haloperidol	3.0	5–10	20
Loxapine	17.5	20–100	200
Mesoridazine	25	100–250	400
Molindone	22.5	50–188	225
Perphenazine	8.0	12–24	42
Pimozide	2.0	4.0–6.0	10
Prochlorperazine	15	15–48	90
Thioridazine	88	200–500	800
Thiothixene	6.0	15–30	40
Trifluoperazine	5.0	10–20	35
Aripiprazole	10	15–30	30
Clozapine	25	200–500	800
Olanzapine	5	10–20	30
Paliperidone	3	6–9	12
Quetiapine	100	400–800	1000
Risperidone	2.0	4.0–6.0	8.5
Ziprasidone	40	120–160	200
Amisulpride	100	400–800	1000
Benperidol	0.5	1.0–3.0	3.5
Clopenthixol	17.5	22–90	138
Clorprothixene	50	200–40	600
Clotiapine	40	10–120	240
Flupenthixol	3.0	5.0–12	18
Levomepromazine	50	150–400	500
Oxypertine	40	80–150	200
Pericyazine	20	20–50	60
Remoxipride	75	112–225	225
Sertindole	4.0	12–20	22
Sulpiride	100	300–600	1000
Trifluperidol	1.0	1.0–3.0	3.0

(*Continued*)

Table 3.1 (*Continued*)

Drug	Starting dose (mg/day)	Target dose (mg/day)	Maximum dose (mg/day)
Triflupromazine	10	22–125	150
Zotepine	50	100–300	400
Zuclopenthixol	20	20–60	80

Upper group, old antipsychotics available or recently available in the USA. Middle group, new antipsychotics available in the USA (asenapine, iloperidone, and lurasidone not included). Lower group, other antipsychotics available worldwide (adapted from Gartner *et al.*, 2010).

(Clozaril, Leponex), a drug whose development started in Europe back in the 1950s. Since the prevailing belief at the time was that the capacity of a drug to induce EPS paralleled its clinical efficacy on psychotic symptoms, clozapine's lower propensity to cause EPS was initially interpreted as meaning lower efficacy. Thus, the medication was shelved until the early 1970s, when it was introduced in Europe. Soon thereafter, reports on the apparition of agranuloctytosis in clozapine-treated patients began to surface, and clozapine was withdrawn from the market in 1975. However, the unique response that some patients had shown to clozapine and the fact that this improvement could not be maintained when the patient was switched back to "typical" neuroleptics, kept alive the interest in this drug. A seminal study in the USA, coordinated by Gil Honigfeld at Sandoz (Kane *et al.*, 1988), demonstrated clozapine's efficacy in patients resistant to other neuroleptics, and clozapine was then approved for clinical use in the USA in 1990, with stipulated guidelines that monitored and restricted its clinical use.

The superior efficacy and low propensity for EPS seen with clozapine fueled the expectation that a new generation of antipsychotics, more effective and safer than the existing "typical" ones, would soon become available. Risperidone (Risperdal) was approved in the USA in 1993, and quickly thereafter, a number of drugs appeared, including olanzapine (Zyprexa), quetiapine (Seroquel), and ziprasidone (Geodon). Less than a decade later, we saw the arrival of aripiprazole (Abilify), and more recently paliperidone (Invega, a risperidone metabolite), asenapine (Saphris), iloperidone (Fanapt), and, in 2011, lurasidone (Latuda). Because of its demonstrated efficacy (and perhaps to emphasize the relatively low risk of EPS for the new agents), the usual comparator chosen for clinical trials with the new medications was the potent conventional antipsychotic, haloperidol, used at relatively high doses, likely to cause EPS. A recent large examination of the haloperidol doses used in comparisons with the new antipsychotics points out that "*in all of the included studies (N = 49), the midpoint of the required doses were above the midpoint of the official recommended doses in the United States and United Kingdom for moderately ill patients. In 94% (U.S.) and 80% (UK) of the studies, they were above the upper border of the recommended doses.*" (Hugenholtz *et al.*, 2006)

The proposition that, as a group, the "atypical" antipsychotics had a significantly lower risk for EPS than the "typical" ones, was the key difference emphasized from these early clinical trials with the new agents. However, other claims were also made (supported by isolated laboratory or clinical observations rather than sound clinical trials), including a better effect of the new agents on cognition and negative symptoms, a lower cardiac risk (for at least some of the new drugs), and a better quality of life. Because these comparisons were based on the studies sponsored by the pharmaceutical industry, large, independent, and publicly funded studies were considered necessary to avoid conflicts of interest and take a fresh look at the issues of clinical efficacy and safety. The most relevant of these studies were the Clinical Antipsychotic Trial of Intervention Effectiveness (CATIE), sponsored by the U.S. National Institute of Mental Health (NIMH), and the Cost Utility of the Latest Antipsychotic Drugs in Schizophrenia Study (CUtLASS 1), sponsored by the UK National Health Service. Another important study was the Treatment of Early-Onset Schizophrenia Spectrum Disorders (TEOSS) study that focused on early-onset schizophrenia, and compared two new (atypical) to one old (typical) antipsychotic. This study was also supported by NIMH grants.

3.3 Are the New Antipsychotics Clinically Different from the Old Ones?

Since the introduction of the first antipsychotic, chlorpromazine, in 1952, over 50 old or "typical" antipsychotics, and close to a dozen new or "atypical" antipsychotics have been introduced and, in some cases, withdrawn from the market, worldwide. However, we continue to obtain basically the same clinical results as we did half a century ago on symptoms and course of psychotic disorders. In light of the results from recent independent and large clinical studies such as CATIE and CUtLASS, the clear demarcation between "typical" and "atypical," or "first-" and "second-generation" antipsychotics (FGAs and SGAs), has blurred. With the exception of clozapine, for which there is strong evidence of superior efficacy in treatment-resistant schizophrenia, the rest of the atypical drugs appear to have similar efficacy, improve the same type of symptoms, and carry a side-effect risk as significant as the old (typical) neuroleptics, albeit of a different nature (see Table 3.2).

Table 3.2 Overlaps between "old" and "new" (or "typical" and "atypical") antipsychotics.

Efficacy	Except for clozapine, large and independent studies (CATIE, CUtLASS, TEOSS) have shown comparable efficacy for old and new antipsychotics in the treatment of schizophrenia and related disorders, including early psychosis. Both old and new antipsychotics show efficacy in the treatment and prevention of mania.
Symptomatic domains improved in schizophrenia	Both old and new antipsychotics have particular efficacy for positive symptoms. The effect on negative symptoms is not as clear.
Effects on cognition	Large and independent clinical studies (CATIE, CUtLASS) have shown a similar modest effect on cognition for old and new antipsychotics.
Side effects/adverse reactions	Both old and new antipsychotics, including clozapine, have potential for acute EPS, chronic EPS (such as tardive dyskinesia), and catastrophic motor effects (such as NMS). The risk seems to vary across individual antipsychotics rather than between "old" and "new" as groups. Both "old" and "new" antipsychotics have the potential for serious metabolic side effects (such as weight gain and diabetes). Risk seems to vary between individual antipsychotics rather than between "old" and "new" as groups. Both old and new antipsychotics have potential for serious adverse reactions such as QT prolongation and malignant arrhythmia, increased risk of death in the demented elderly, and hyperprolactinemia.
Acute toxicity	The "new" antipsychotic agents are not safer than the "old" antipsychotics still in the market. Actually, people who overdose on "new" agents seem to be at higher risk for outcomes like death, respiratory depression, coma, and hypotension than those who overdose on "old" agents.
Lack of clinical relevance of partial D_2 agonism of new antipsychotics	The partial agonism of aripiprazole at the D_2 receptor has not translated in clinical advantages. EPS, especially akathisia, are fairly common with aripiprazole. In Parkinson's disease (PD) patients, aripiprazole has proven riskier than quetiapine and clozapine, which continue to be the standard treatment for the psychosis induced by dopaminergic agents in PD patients.
Cost-effectiveness	According to effectiveness trials, "old" antipsychotics seem to be more "cost-effective" than the "new" ones.

With each passing day, the differentiation of antipsychotics into "typical" and "atypical" classes appears to be less justified. In clinical practice, these days, we have come to accept that both antipsychotic groups are a "mixed bag," with some drugs resembling those in the other class more closely than some in their own. In the words of a prominent psychopharmacologist: "*Efficacy variations within SGAs and FGAs result in overlaps between the two groups. Regarding safety, FGAs elicit more extrapyramidal side effects and tardive dyskinesia as well as prolactin elevations than SGAs, whereas some SGAs tend to be associated with more weight gain and disturbances in lipid and glucose regulation than FGAs. However, there are again considerable differences between individual agents and overlaps between the two groups in terms of side effects. The classification of antipsychotics into the two groups is no longer useful. The treatment selection for an individual patient should focus on the suitability of an individual antipsychotic for that patient rather than on the group membership of the drug.*" (Volavka *et al.*, 2009) We share the above opinion, and agree that there is little support these days for the concept of "atypicality" of antipsychotic drugs. A caveat is necessary here: in order to make a fair comparison between "old" and "new" antipsychotics, we must first reconsider the doses used in the original studies of the old antipsychotics, and then recommended for clinical use, decades ago. To this effect, in Table 3.1, we offer the recommendations of a recent consensus panel, on the dosing of old and new antipsychotics currently in use worldwide (Gardner *et al.*, 2010). We also refer the reader interested in updated antipsychotic equivalents to a recent publication showing the chlorpromazine and haloperidol equivalents for old and new antipsychotics, calculated using regression to compare each drug to these two agents (Andreasen *et al.*, 2010).

3.4 Current Concepts Regarding Antipsychotic Action and the D_2 Receptor

All clinically effective antipsychotics ("old" and "new") share as a common characteristic their potent antagonism of striatal dopamine D_2 receptors. This antidopaminergic effect remains the central tenet for the neurobiological basis of antipsychotic treatment. However, the way we view D_2 receptor blockade in schizophrenia has changed in recent years. As mentioned above, the initial clinical goal in the treatment of schizophrenia was a "saturation" of the dopamine D_2 receptors, defined clinically by parkinsonian symptoms. More recently, however, with techniques such as PET and SPECT, we have been able to examine *in vivo* the relationship between D_2 receptor occupancy on the one hand, and antipsychotic efficacy and side effects, on the other. A "threshold" has thus been established for efficacy in the range of 65%–70% D_2 receptor occupancy. Administering a dose that pushes D_2 receptor occupancy over this threshold seems to optimize the chances of clinical response (Waddington *et al.*, 2003).

Complementing this information, there are data indicating that a D_2 receptor occupancy over 80% markedly increases the risk of EPS. Thus, there appears to be a narrow therapeutic window for efficacy plus tolerability, in the treatment of schizophrenia, which is in the range of 65%–80% of D_2 receptor occupancy. To use an example, for haloperidol, a 2 mg/day dose has been reported to cause a D_2 receptor occupancy of 67%, while a 5 mg/day dose approaches 80% D_2 occupancy. Thus, 2 mg/day would be the approximate minimal dose necessary for clinical efficacy, and doses beyond 5 mg would be increasingly more likely to cause EPS. These general rules, however, are subject to individual variance; some individuals may respond to lower D_2 occupancy levels, and treatment-resistant individuals may fail to respond to occupancy values exceeding the 70% threshold (Waddington *et al.*, 2003). A sensible application of this concept of a D_2 occupancy therapeutic window with both old and new antipsychotics is to start a drug at the low end of the therapeutic dose range, and to increase it gradually. This should significantly decrease the incidence of EPS and the need for anticholinergic medications or medication changes. In the sections devoted to the adverse effects of antipsychotics in this chapter, and to individual antipsychotics in the next one, we will discuss this issue in more detail.

3.5 Comparison Between Typical and Atypical Antipsychotics

3.5.1 *Are there differences in the general efficacy and effectiveness of typical and atypical antipsychotics?*

The bottom line is that, with the exception of clozapine, there appears to be no significant differences between old and new antipsychotics in clinical efficacy (usually measured as symptom change), or clinical effectiveness (measured as enhancing quality of life, functioning, and other "real-life" outcomes). In the text that follows, we will provide some details on each of the most recent independent studies comparing old and new antipsychotics.

(1) The initial phase of the publicly funded CATIE in the USA, compared four new antipsychotics (olanzapine, quetiapine, risperidone, and ziprasidone) with an old antipsychotic, perphenazine, using discontinuation of treatment as the primary outcome measure. Time to discontinuation of treatment for any reason was longer in the olanzapine group. However, the differences did not reach statistical significance with the perphenazine or ziprasidone groups, though they did with the quetiapine or risperidone groups (Lieberman *et al.*, 2005). In any case, the number of patients abandoning treatment was high for all the antipsychotics, including olanzapine, thus rendering any observed difference meaningless.

(2) Regarding "family burden," another measure of treatment effectiveness in schizophrenia, the CATIE study found similar effects for the old and new antipsychotics: "Despite significant reductions of the problem behavior and resource demands/disruption factors, there were no significant differences between perphenazine and any of the second-generation medications." (Perlick *et al.*, 2010)

(3) The large non-commercially funded European study CUtLASS 1, compared the effect on quality of life for a large number of old or "first generation" antipsychotics (with most patients being on sulpiride, trifluoperazine, chlorpromazine, and haloperidol) versus four new or "second generation" antipsychotics (amisulpride, olanzapine, quetiapine, and risperidone). The authors of this study concluded that there was "no disadvantage in terms of quality of life, symptoms, or associated costs of care across 1 year in commencing treatment with FGAs rather than atypical SGAs in people with schizophrenia whose medication is being changed because of intolerance or inadequate response." (Jones *et al.*, 2006)

(4) In China, a 12-month open-label trial compared the old antipsychotic chlorpromazine and six new antipsychotics in 1,133 subjects with schizophrenia or schizophreniform disorder, with treatment discontinuation for any reason as the primary measure. Discontinuation rates within 12 months were 41.4% for chlorpromazine, 39.5% for sulpiride, 36.7% for clozapine, 40.2% for risperidone, 39.6% for olanzapine, 46.9% for quetiapine, and 40.2% for aripiprazole, with no significant statistical difference on discontinuation due to relapse, intolerability, patient decision, or non-adherence. EPS were more common with chlorpromazine and sulpiride; anticholinergic side effects were more common with clozapine and chlorpromazine; and weight gain was more common with clozapine and olanzapine (Guo *et al.*, 2011).

(5) The publicly funded TEOSS study compared the efficacy and safety of an FGA, molindone, with two SGAs, olanzapine and risperidone, in the treatment of early-onset schizophrenia and schizoaffective disorder. It concludes: "Risperidone and olanzapine did not demonstrate superior efficacy over molindone for treating early onset schizophrenia and schizoaffective disorder. Adverse effects were frequent but differed between medications. The results question the nearly exclusive use of second-generation antipsychotics to treat early-onset schizophrenia and schizoaffective disorder. The safety findings related to weight gain and metabolic problems raise important public health concerns, given the widespread use of second-generation antipsychotics in youth for nonpsychotic disorders." (Sikich *et al.*, 2008)

(6) Another study on first-episode schizophrenia, funded by the German government through the German Research Network on Schizophrenia, compared two antipsychotics, risperidone and low-dose haloperidol. They reported that "both antipsychotics were equally effective regarding significant symptom restriction and improvement in quality of life. Extrapyramidal symptoms were slightly higher with haloperidol. The overall dropout rate of 68%, however, was not significantly different between the 2 drug groups." (Gaebel *et al.*, 2007)

(7) A meta-analysis of 15 randomized clinical trials (RCTs) on early psychosis worldwide, that included 2,522 patients, led to the following conclusion: "This meta-analysis revealed no significant differences between typical and atypical antipsychotics in discontinuation rates or in short-term improvement in individuals with first-episode psychosis. However, treatment with atypical antipsychotics was associated with relatively more weight gain, whereas treatment with typicals was associated with a greater incidence of extrapyramidal side effects." (Crosley *et al.*, 2010)

3.5.2 *Are there differences in the cognitive effects of typical and atypical antipsychotics?*

Results of the various studies that have examined this issue showed no substantive differences between old and new antipsychotics on cognitive function in patients with schizophrenia. This included results from the CATIE study, reporting no differences between olanzapine, quetiapine, risperidone, and ziprasidone, and the old antipsychotic perphenazine, with regard to cognition: "After 2 months of antipsychotic treatment, all groups had a small but significant improvement in neurocognition. There were no differences between any pair of agents, including the typical drug perphenazine." (Keefe *et al.*, 2007)

The CATIE study did not find any differences between old and new antipsychotics in their effects on other areas related to cognition, such as psychosocial functioning or emotional perception:

(1) "All antipsychotic treatment groups in all phases made modest improvements in psychosocial functioning. There were no differences among them after 6, 12, or 18 months." (Swartz *et al.*, 2007)

(2) "Most treatments were associated with a small, non-statistically significant improvement in emotion perception at two months, although they did not differ from one another." (Penn *et al.*, 2009)

The European First Episode Schizophrenia Trial (EUFEST), a randomized, open-label trial sponsored by AstraZeneca, Pfizer, United States Pharmaceutical Group, and Sanofi, compared the cognitive effects of haloperidol with those of four SGAs: amisulpride, olanzapine, quetiapine, and ziprasidone. A major conclusion of this study was that "treatment with antipsychotic medication is associated with moderate improvement in the cognitive test performance of patients who have schizophreniform disorder or who are in their first episode of schizophrenia. The magnitude of improvement does not differ between treatment with haloperidol and treatment with second-generation antipsychotics. Moreover, cognitive improvement is weakly related to symptom change." (Davidson *et al.*, 2009)

3.5.3 *Are there differences in the acute toxicity of typical and atypical antipsychotics?*

In acute overdose, the new antipsychotics are not safer than the old ones and, in fact, the opposite may be true. A 10-year retrospective cohort study examining this issue found that patients taking new antipsychotics were at higher risk for a serious adverse outcome or death than those taking old agents. They calculated that for the new agents, the odds ratio (OR) and 95% confidence interval (CI) for adverse outcomes, compared to the old ones, were: respiratory depression 2.39 (1.09–5.26), coma 2.18 (1.30–3.65), and hypotension 1.80 (1.23–2.63). The only significant area favoring the new agents was their having lower odds of dystonia 0.12 (0.08–0.19) or rigidity 0.30 (0.10–0.90) versus the old ones. They concluded that "SGAs appear no safer than FGAs in acute overdose. While neuromuscular symptoms appear less frequently with SGAs compared to FGAs, the relatively greater rates of central nervous system depression associated with SGA overdose may be more dangerous." (Ciranni *et al.*, 2009)

3.6 Metabolic Side Effects of Antipsychotic Drugs

It has been known for decades that cardiovascular risk factors and disorders (obesity, diabetes, dyslipidemia, coronary artery disease, hypertension, and the like) are more prevalent among people with schizophrenia compared to the general population. Recent studies have confirmed this. A 2005 publication analyzed the prevalence of metabolic syndrome, comparing CATIE's baseline observations with general population data from the third National Health and Nutrition Survey (NHANES III). The authors estimated that the ORs for metabolic syndrome among CATIE's chronic schizophrenic patients, relative to NHANES III, was 2.38 for males and 3.51 for females (McEvoy *et al.*, 2005). A British comparison of metabolic disease and cardiovascular risk found that people treated with antipsychotics in the community had an OR for metabolic syndrome of 3.68 (95% CI: 1.71–7.93) compared to age- and gender-matched controls (Mackin *et al.*, 2007). A Spanish study with

1,452 outpatients with schizophrenia treated with antipsychotics found that their risk for coronary heart disease and metabolic syndrome were in the same range as those of members of the general population who were on average 10 to 15 years older (Bobes *et al.*, 2007).

Because of this elevated cardiometabolic risk in chronic schizophrenic patients, it was hypothesized that schizophrenia in itself was a liability for cardiovascular risk factors. This belief led to a complacent attitude, minimizing the risk of medications. However, systematic observations in patients given the new drugs have altered the former perception. The observed high frequency of diabetes and other metabolic disorders in patients treated with "atypical" antipsychotics has generated significant concern and stimulated new research. Recent studies in never-treated and first-episode schizophrenic patients show that the incidence of diabetes and metabolic syndrome in this population is no different from that of the general population, and that metabolic disturbances seem to develop rather quickly following the initiation of treatment with SGAs (De Hert *et al.*, 2008; Graham *et al.*, 2008; Verma *et al.*, 2009; Nielsen *et al.*, 2010; Padmavati *et al.*, 2010). Significant changes in parameters as critical as body mass index (BMI) and mean waist circumference have been observed after just one month of treatment with antipsychotics (Tarricone *et al.*, 2008). Further proof of the critical importance of antipsychotics in the development of metabolic syndrome is the observation that patients with bipolar disorder and schizophrenia treated with SGAs have similarly high rates of metabolic syndrome. This suggests that metabolic dysregulation is not primarily linked to diagnosis (Correll *et al.*, 2008). A recent review of cardiometabolic outcomes in the first treated episode of psychosis states: "Two key hypotheses were identified based on this review: (1) in general, there is no difference in cardiovascular risk assessed by weight or metabolic indices between individuals with an untreated first episode of psychosis and healthy controls and (2) cardiovascular risk increases after first exposure to any antipsychotic drug. A rank order of drugs can be derived but there is no evidence of significant class differences." (Foley *et al.*, 2011)

This worsening of cardiometabolic risk factors also occurs in patients previously exposed to treatment with antipsychotic drugs. In the CATIE study, in patients with chronic schizophrenia, the percentage of patients gaining more than 7% of body weight during antipsychotic treatment were, in descending order, 30% for olanzapine, 16% for quetiapine, 14% for risperidone, 12% for perphenazine, and 7% for ziprasidone (Lieberman *et al.*, 2005).

As mentioned before, the risk for diabetes and metabolic syndrome seems to vary among individual antipsychotics, but not between antipsychotic classes. It seems to be the highest for clozapine and olanzapine, intermediate for risperidone and quetiapine (and, probably, asenapine and paliperidone), and low for haloperidol and other high-potency old and new antipsychotics such as perphenazine, trifluoperazine, molindone, ziprasidone, and aripiprazole (and, probably, iloperidone and lurasidone).

In any case, the emergence of metabolic side effects following the introduction of the new antipsychotics is alarming. Since the introduction of the new antipsychotics in the USA, the obesity rate among schizophrenic patients is growing even faster than the exploding national rate for obesity. Within 14 years (1988–2002), the net difference in the prevalence of obesity between inpatients with schizophrenia and "controls" grew from +4.7% to +14.7%. A similar significant increase in the rates of diabetes and diabetic ketoacidosis has been also reported in schizophrenic patients, compared to national rates (see Table 3.3 and Reist *et al.*, 2007).

3.6.1 *Weight gain risk with antipsychotics*

Perhaps the most comprehensive and reliable examination of antipsychotic-induced weight gain is the meta-analysis published by Allison *et al.*, in 1999. They calculated that, after a 10-week treatment, placebo induced a mean weight reduction of 0.74 kg. Among the old antipsychotics included, weight change ranged from an increase of 3.19 kg with thioridazine to a reduction of 0.39 kg with molindone. Among new antipsychotics, it ranged from an increase of 4.45 kg with clozapine and 4.15 kg with olanzapine, to 0.04 kg with ziprasidone (Allison *et al.*, 1999).

The risk for antipsychotic-induced weight gain seems to have a significant negative association with age; the younger the patient, the higher the risk (Smith *et al.*, 2008). In a study with 338 youths aged 4 to 19 years, after a median of 10.8 weeks of treatment, weight gain was 8.5 kg with olanzapine, 6.1 kg with quetiapine, 5.3 kg with risperidone, and 4.4 kg with aripiprazole (Correll *et al.*, 2009).

Table 3.3 New antipsychotics and metabolic disorders in inpatients with schizophrenia (controls were inpatients without diagnosis of schizophrenia or schizoaffective disorder) (adapted from Reist *et al.*, 2007).

Metabolic disorder	Prevalence 1988, before introduction of new antipsychotics	Prevalence 2002, when new antipsychotics had 86% of the market
Obesity	5.9% (controls 1.2%)	18.5% (controls 3.8%)
Diabetes mellitus	6.1 % (controls 7.5%)	17.4% (controls 15.3%)
Diabetic ketoacidosis	0.20% (controls 0.26%)	0.47% (controls 0.41%)

Gender also seems to influence the magnitude of weight gain in patients treated with antipsychotics. A retrospective analysis of patients receiving clozapine, olanzapine, and risperidone reports that increased BMI in the parents, premorbid BMI in the patient, female gender, and a younger age were all predictors for antipsychotic-induced weight gain during treatment with atypical antipsychotics (Gebhardt *et al.*, 2009).

In Table 3.4, we present the estimated weight change with antipsychotics over a 10-week period. In this table, we can see there is no clear separation between old and new classes of antipsychotics, with regard to weight gain.

We have included in the table antipsychotics introduced after the publication of the original analysis, estimating their position in the list from the published clinical information and, especially, their relative affinity for histamine H_1 and dopamine D_2 receptors. The antipsychotic with the highest

Table 3.4 Estimated weight gain with individual antipsychotics, in descending order.

Antipsychotic	Weight change at 10 weeks/kg (95% CI)[a]
Clozapine	4.45 (3.02–5.88)
Olanzapine	4.15 (3.82–4.48)
Thioridazine/mesoridazine	3.19 (1.39–4.99)
Sertindole	2.92 (1.76–4.08)
Chlorpromazine	2.58 (0.91–4.25)
Quetiapine[b]	
Risperidone	2.10 (1.69–2.51)
Paliperidone	
Asenapine	
Iloperidone	
Haloperidol	1.08 (0.35–1.81)
Fluphenazine	0.43 (-0.65–1.51)
Ziprasidone	0.04 (-0.49–0.57)
Aripiprazole	
Lurasidone	
Molindone	-0.39 (-2.43–1.65)
Placebo	-0.74 (-1.60–0.12)

[a]Figures are from Allison *et al.*, 1999.

[b]In italics, we have included newer medications, calculating their approximate position in the list from the published clinical data and, especially, receptor affinity (affinity for H_1 relative to affinity for D_2).

risk for weight gain, clozapine, has an affinity for H_1 300 times higher than that for D_2, while the antipsychotic with the lowest risk, molindone, has an affinity for H_1 that is less than one-hundredth of that for D_2 (for receptor affinity of antipsychotics, see Table 3.5).

3.6.2 *Antipsychotic-induced diabetes mellitus and metabolic syndrome*

Antipsychotic-associated diabetes mellitus is a well-established reality in current clinical practice. Now, we are becoming aware that the emergence of diabetes mellitus in patients treated with antipsychotics is just part of

Table 3.5 Old and new antipsychotics: comparison of affinity for relevant receptors[a].

Drug	D_2	α_1	α_2	H_1	M_1
Old Antipsychotics					
Haloperidol	2.6	17	600	260	>10,000
Loxapine	9.8	28	250	5	
Molindone	120	2,500	625	>10,000	>10,000
Perphenazine	1.4	10	500	8	1,500
New Antipsychotics[b]					
Aripiprazole	0.34	57	74	61	6,780
Asenapine	1.3	1.2	1.2	1.0	8128
Clozapine	229	24	159	0.78	33
Iloperidone	6.3	36	3	473	4,898
Lurasidone	0.994	47.9	10.8 (2c) 40.7 (2a)	>1,000	>1,000
Olanzapine	20	19	170	7	73
Paliperidone	2.8	10	80	3.4	>10,000
Risperidone	2.2	2.4	7.5	2.1	>10,000
Quetiapine (*N*-quetiapine)	626 (489)	14.6 (46.4)	617 (1290)	4.41 (1.15)	1086 (38.3)
Ziprasidone	4.8	10	310	47	300

[a]Data are for the equilibrium constant (K_i) in nM, the concentration necessary to block 50% of receptors. The lower the K_i, the more potent the drug.

[b]Figures for the newer antipsychotics are taken from the current U.S. Prescribing Information, except when it gives a range, a word estimate ("high," "low," etc.), or no information. Other figures are mainly, but not only, from Correll *et al.*, 2010.

Based on several sources, mainly Correll *et al.*, 2010 and Miyamoto *et al.*, 2003.

antipsychotic-induced metabolic syndrome. A recent cross-sectional study in Denmark compared the prevalence of metabolic syndrome in outpatients on antipsychotic drug treatment with a general population group of 3,303 randomly selected people. Of the antipsychotic-treated patients, 48.2% fulfilled criteria for metabolic syndrome, compared with 29.6% of the general population. Also, compared with the general population, after adjustment for age and gender, the OR of metabolic syndrome among antipsychotic-treated patients was 2.7 (Krane-Gartiser *et al.*, 2011). What remains to be determined is the precise relative risk of each individual antipsychotic drug to induce metabolic disturbances. A study published in 2005, compared the incidence of drug-treated diabetes in about 3,000 patients taking haloperidol, olanzapine, risperidone, and quetiapine with that of about 6,000 controls. It showed risk ratios (95% CI), in descending order, of 33.7 (9.2–123.6) for quetiapine, 20.4 (6.9–60.3) for olanzapine, 18.7 (8.2–42.8) for risperidone, and 12.4 (6.3–24.5) for haloperidol, respectively (Sacchetti *et al.*, 2005). A recent Bayesian signal detection analysis of the FDA Adverse Event Database for diabetes-related adverse events found these adjusted, reporting ratios (90% CI) for diabetes mellitus, in descending order: olanzapine 9.69 (9.2–10.0), risperidone 3.8 (3.5–4.1), quetiapine 3.5 (3.2–3.9), clozapine 3.1 (2.9–3.3), ziprasidone 2.4 (2.0–2.9), aripiprazole 2.4 (1.9–2.9), and haloperidol 2.0 (1.7–2.3) (Baker *et al.*, 2009).

The mechanisms for antipsychotic-associated diabetes mellitus are most probably multifactorial. Weight gain is surely one of these factors, and antipsychotics with the greatest risk for weight gain seem to have also the highest risk for diabetes. However, it has also been reported that half the cases of antipsychotic-associated new-onset diabetes mellitus show no weight gain at the time of presentation, supporting the existence of other, more direct antipsychotic effects on glucose metabolism or regulation, independently of adiposity. Experimental studies have shown that the two antipsychotics with the higher risk for diabetes, clozapine and olanzapine, impair glucose regulation, and this effect appears to be independent of adiposity. There is also some evidence that these drugs can impair pancreatic beta-cell function. Several potential mechanisms for this glucose dysregulation have been highlighted. For example, administration of a potent 5-HT_2 receptor antagonist to healthy volunteers significantly decreased insulin sensitivity. This shows the potential of antipsychotics, especially the new ones, to suppress 5-HT_{2A} receptor-mediated glucose uptake in muscle or adipose tissue (Buchholz *et al.*, 2008). Other postulated mechanisms include antipsychotic activity at the cholinergic M_3 receptor, which control secretory processes at adrenergic α_1 receptors; or at serotonergic 5-HT_{2c} receptors, which influence weight gain, or effects on the ATP-sensitive K^+ ion channels.

Metabolic syndrome is characterized by insulin resistance, central obesity, dyslipidemia, and hypertension. It is a condition highly predictive of type 2 diabetes mellitus and cardiovascular disease. Metabolic syndrome has been reported to be two to four times more common in antipsychotic-treated schizophrenics than in an appropriate reference population. The development of metabolic syndrome is closely, but not exclusively, associated with weight gain. In an eight-year cohort study with clozapine, the authors conclude: "For patients treated with clozapine, metabolic syndrome and most metabolic parameters were related to weight gain; however, glucose dysregulation was associated with treatment duration independently of weight gain." (Bai *et al.*, 2010) A direct effect on dyslipidemia, independent of obesity, has also been reported for clozapine and olanzapine: "...independently of body mass, dyslipidemia was significantly associated with AP treatment, in particular with OLZ and CLZ. These findings indicate a primary effect of APs on lipid regulation, important in understanding their mechanism of action, and with clinical implications." (Birkenaes *et al.*, 2008)

3.7 Extrapyramidal Symptoms of Antipsychotics

EPS resulting from treatment with antipsychotic drugs are routinely divided into acute (parkinsonism, akathisia, acute dystonia), and delayed (tardive dyskinesia). Neuroleptic malignant syndrome (NMS), a catastrophic muscular adverse effect related to dopaminergic blockade, and catatonia (a contradictorily defined motor syndrome) will also be considered briefly in this section.

3.7.1 *Are there any differences in the risk for EPS among typical and atypical antipsychotics?*

Perhaps one of the greatest surprises emerging from the CATIE study was the lack of statistically significant differences between the "old" antipsychotic perphenazine and the "new" antipsychotics olanzapine, quetiapine, risperidone, and ziprasidone in any of the scales used to measure EPS (AIMS, Barnes Akathisia Rating Scale, Simpson Angus EPS), although perhenazine had a higher rate of discontinuation due to EPS. Moreover, even though the number of cases was too low in order to reach statistical significance, ziprasidone appeared to induce more akathisia and dystonia events than perphenazine (see Table 3.6). The large independent British study, CUtLASS 1, also failed to show any difference between FGAs and SGAs in the three EPS rating scales used (Simpson-Angus, Barnes Akathisia Rating Scale, and AIMS) or in their total (Jones *et al.*, 2006).

Table 3.6 Motor outcomes in the CATIE study (from Lieberman *et al.*, 2005 and Caroff *et al.*, 2011).

Outcome	Olanzapine	Perphenazine	Quetiapine	Risperidone	Ziprasidone	*p*-value
Discontinuation due to EPS[a]	2% (8/336)	8% (22/261)	3% (10/337)	3% (11/341)	4% (7/185)	0.002
Anticholinergic medication added[a]	7% (25/336)	10% (26/261)	3% (11/337)	9% 32(341)	8% (14/185)	0.01
Parkinsonism[a]	7% (16/240)	6% (15/243)	4% (10/247)	8% (20/238)	5% (6/129)	0.50
Akathisia[a]	5% (12/234)	7% (16/241)	5% (12/248)	6% (12/240)	10% (13/132)	0.19
Acute dystonia[b]	0	1	1	1	3	
Tardive dyskinesia[a]	14% (32/236)	17% (41/237)	13% (30/236)	16% (38/238)	14% (18/126)	0.23

[a]Percentage (number/total number of patients).
[b]Number of cases.

The similarity in EPS outcomes for old and new antipsychotics seen in the CATIE study was an utterly unexpected finding, as the strongest marketing point during the introduction of the atypical antipsychotics was their reportedly significantly lower risk for EPS. At the time, an intense discussion was stimulated, intent on finding a serotonergic explanation (especially in the receptor 5-HT_{2a}) for this reportedly lower liability of "atypicals" to produce EPS. However, when we compare any antipsychotic agents regarding risk for EPS, we must take into account their individual D_2-blocking potency, and in both groups of antipsychotics, we find drugs with high and low affinity for D_2, meaning high and low risk for EPS. A meta-analysis of 31 RCTs with 2,320 patients, published in the *Lancet* in 2003, concludes: "Optimum doses of low potency conventional antipsychotics might not induce more EPS than new generation drugs." (Leucht *et al.*, 2003)

Thus, the blanket statement that "typical" antipsychotics induce more EPS than all the "atypical" ones is no longer tenable. Surely, the highly potent "old" antipsychotics still in use (haloperidol, fluphenazine, perphenazine, trifluoperazine, molindone, etc.) are more likely to induce EPS than the low- or middle-potency "new" antipsychotics (clozapine, quetiapine, and olanzapine), as they also induce more EPS than middle-potency old antipsychotics such as chlorpromazine. When we compare high-potency "typicals" with the recent high-potency "atypicals," the differences start to vanish. Since the introduction of the new antipsychotics, the EPS liability figures for them have been rising, especially for the most potent dopamine D_2-blocking agents such as risperidone, ziprasidone, and aripiprazole. The most recent ones (paliperidone, iloperidone, lurasidone, and asenapine) are also potent dopaminergic D_2 blockers and therefore likely to induce a significant number of EPS, both acute and chronic. Even though reliable prospective independent "hand-to-hand" comparisons between old and new antipsychotics are limited practically to CATIE and CUtLASS, other types of analysis confirm this. A 2009 meta-analysis compared patients on SGAs and haloperidol at doses <12 mg/day, in terms of the relative risk to need antiparkinsonian medication. The percentage having antiparkinsonian medication added ranged from 7% for clozapine-treated patients to 79% for those treated with ziprasidone (see Table 3.7 and Leucht *et al.*, 2009). In any case, all the new antipsychotics (including clozapine) may induce not only acute EPS (acute dystonia, parkinsonism, and akathisia), but also tardive dyskinesia and NMS.

An important general consideration regarding antipsychotic-induced EPS is that, though acute EPS are generally reversible, they are not benign and their appearance should be seen as a bad omen, as they seem to predict late EPS, such as tardive dyskinesia (Tenback *et al.*, 2006). For this reason, in patients experiencing acute EPS, the authors recommend, whenever possible, decreasing the antipsychotic dose or switching medications rather than using adjunctive medication to control the adverse effects.

Regarding the association of antipsychotic-induced EPS and diagnosis, the conventional wisdom has been that patients with mood disorders treated with antipsychotics are at even higher risk for EPS than schizophrenia spectrum patients. This belief seems to be confirmed by recent publications showing that patients with non-schizophreniform disorders, such as unipolar depression or bipolar disorder, seem to be at higher risk of antipsychotic-induced EPS than schizophrenic patients (Gao *et al.*, 2008).

Table 3.7. New antipsychotics: Risk for use of antiparkinsonian medication, relative to a haloperidol dose <12 mg/day (from Leucht *et al.*, 2009).

Medication	Relative risk (95% CI)
Aripiprazole	0.48 (0.32–0.72)
Clozapine	0.07 (0.01–0.49)
Olanzapine	0.47 (0.34–0.65)
Quetiapine	0.33 (0.20–0.55)
Risperidone	0.74 (0.67–0.81)
Ziprasidone	0.79 (0.62–1.02)

Before discussing individual antipsychotic-induced EPS, we want to discuss the practice of starting anticholinergic medications simultaneously with antipsychotic agents, to prevent EPS. We strongly disagree with this approach, for several reasons: (1) most patients are not going to experience EPS with judicious dosing; (2) anticholinergic agents carry a significant side effect burden, including urinary retention, constipation, glaucoma exacerbation, and cognitive impairment; and (3) considering that acute EPS can predict late EPS, we prefer to identify the patients at risk.

In the following section, we will discuss separately the main types of antipsychotic-induced EPS.

3.7.2 *Acute dystonia*

Acute dystonias are sudden spasms of voluntary muscles that very often involve the face, neck, eyes, or throat, causing frightening experiences such as extreme arching of the neck, uncontrollable turning of the eyes, and difficulty swallowing or breathing. They occur in the very first hours or days of antipsychotic treatment. In recent years, possibly due to more careful prescribing and an acknowledgment of the expert recommendation to start all antipsychotic agents, "typical" and "atypical," at low doses, acute dystonia has become a relatively rare occurrence. The few instances of acute dystonia happen mainly in patients receiving parenteral antipsychotics at hospital wards and emergency departments, or patients receiving depot injectable antipsychotics. Patient risk factors for dystonia include young age, male gender, African-American ethnicity, history of dystonia, cocaine/stimulant use, mood disorders (versus schizophrenia), and electrolytic/endocrine disturbances (Caroff *et al.*, 2011). The risk of an individual antipsychotic to induce acute dystonia is directly related to both the dose given and the potency of the drug at blocking the D_2 receptor, and this applies to both old and new antipsychotics. Thus, we may expect that the less potent new antipsychotics (clozapine, quetiapine, and olanzapine) show low rates of dystonia. Meanwhile, the rates of dystonia for the potent new agents (risperidone/paliperidone, ziprasidone, aripiprazole, iloperidone, asenapine, and lurasidone) should be close to those of old agents such as haloperidol or perphenazine.

The best approach to prevent dystonia, as well as any other EPS, is to prescribe antipsychotic drugs judiciously, starting at the low end of the therapeutic dose range, and going up gradually, according to clinical response. Once dystonia makes an appearance, the administration of an oral or parenteral (in emergency situations) anticholinergic agent (benztropine, trihexyphenidyl, biperiden, etc.) usually works well. However, the prolonged use of anticholinergic agents needs to be avoided whenever possible, since they carry their own risk for adverse reactions. Because of this, and because of the axiom that acute EPS predicts late EPS, in the presence of dystonia one should consider stopping the antipsychotic, decreasing the dose, or switching to an agent with lower liability for EPS.

3.7.3 *Parkinsonism (slowness, tremor, and rigidity)*

Parkinsonism mimics the external symptoms of Parkinson's disease: tremor, muscular rigidity, and psychomotor slowness. Formerly a characteristic feature of patients treated with antipsychotics, parkinsonism is on the wane, even among patients taking old agents, thanks to prescribers' compliance in using lower dose ranges. Similarly to what was described in the case of dystonia, the propensity for an individual antipsychotic to induce parkinsonian symptoms depends mainly on the drug's potency at blocking the D_2 receptor and the dose utilized. As a corollary of this, there are significant differences among the new antipsychotic drugs in their propensity to induce parkinsonism. The most potent D_2 blockers among the new drugs, such as aripiprazole and ziprasidone, seem to have a significantly higher risk for parkinsonian signs, including stiffness and tremor than, for example, olanzapine (Edwards *et al.*, 2009).

The ideal management of antipsychotic-induced parkinsonian reactions is the discontinuation or dose reduction of the offending agent, or the switch to an agent with lower EPS liability. Parkinsonism may respond to anticholinergic medications. However, often, the response to these agents is not as good as that seen in acute dystonia. As discussed before, an additional reason to try discontinuing/switching/decreasing the dose, instead of adding anticholinergic agents, is the evidence pointing at acute EPS as predictors of late EPS, such as tardive dystonia/dyskinesias.

3.7.4 *Akathisia*

The word 'akathisia' comes from a Greek term meaning "unable to remain seated." It is an uncontrollable urge to move, usually starting in the legs but often generalized. For some patients, the psychic experience of restlessness is very disturbing, and any report of "anxiety" in patients taking antipsychotics or other EPS-inducing medications should trigger the suspicion of akathisia. Akathisia may happen at the beginning of treatment or any time the D_2-blocking activity goes up (due to dose increases, antipsychotic polypharmacy, or addition of medications that inhibit antipsychotic metabolism).

Following the decrease in the incidence of antipsychotic-induced acute dystonias and parkinsonian reactions, akathisia is the most frequently observed acute EPS nowadays. An important reason for this is the high incidence of akathisia with the most potent "atypical" antipsychotics, such as aripiprazole and ziprasidone. In the CATIE study, there were no statistically significant differences in the incidence of akathisia between the old antipsychotic perphenazine and the four new antipsychotics included (Lieberman *et al.*, 2005; Caroff *et al.*, 2011). Regarding individual antipsychotics, the incidence of akathisia for potent old agents, such as haloperidol or perphenazine, has been usually put at around 20% to 35% in routine practice. However, the highest propensity for akathisia has been historically attributed to molindone. Below, we comment on the incidence of akathisia seen with "atypical" antipsychotics. This will be based primarily on two recent reviews (Kane *et al.*, 2009; Kumar *et al.*, 2009).

3.7.4.1 *Clozapine*

Most studies show low rates of akathisia for clozapine; however, some of them show comparable rates with old antipsychotics. Two factors confuse the issue of akathisia with clozapine: (1) there are no placebo-controlled studies where akathisia is an outcome, and (2) patients on clozapine have usually received multiple previous antipsychotics and may have persistent EPS attributable to these drugs.

3.7.4.2 *Risperidone*

Risperidone seems to show higher rates of akathisia than clozapine, olanzapine, and quetiapine, and at least one study showed higher rates of akathisia with risperidone than haloperidol. For risperidone, dose seems to be a big variable for akathisia risk (and likely for the incidence of other EPS), with the risk for high dose risperidone being comparable to that of potent old antipsychotics.

3.7.4.3 *Olanzapine*

Some studies show an akathisia rate similar to placebo. Oral olanzapine has, in general, shown a lower rate of akathisia than haloperidol and other old antipsychotics. Studies comparing olanzapine to more potent new antipsychotics show either comparable rates of akathisia or an advantage for olanzapine. Thus, olanzapine likely has higher rates of akathisia than clozapine or quetiapine, but lower rates than risperidone, paliperidone, aripiprazole, or ziprasidone.

3.7.4.4 *Quetiapine*

This drug has shown either comparable or slightly elevated akathisia rates compared to placebo, and lower rates compared to old antipsychotics and risperidone. In synthesis, quetiapine seems to have a low risk for akathisia in relation to other antipsychotics.

3.7.4.5 *Ziprasidone*

In most studies comparing it to placebo, ziprasidone has had the higher akathisia rate; compared to haloperidol, it has shown usually a lower rate. One study has shown similar rates to aripiprazole; another, a lower rate than risperidone. As mentioned, ziprasidone had the highest akathisia incidence in the CATIE study, higher than even perphenazine (though the differences were not statistically significant). In synthesis, patients on ziprasidone seem to be at high risk for akathisia.

3.7.4.6 *Aripiprazole*

Several early studies with aripiprazole revealed akathisia rates comparable to placebo. However, recent studies and clinical reports suggest a risk of akathisia in the same range of the potent old antipsychotics. As mentioned, over one-third of patients on aripiprazole in studies of the drug as adjunct treatment in depression showed akathisia/restlessness (U.S. Prescribing Information).

3.7.4.7 *Recently introduced new antipsychotics (paliperidone, iloperidone, asenapine, and lurasidone)*

All of these are potent dopaminergic blockers, some with structural resemblance to risperidone or ziprasidone. Thus, though we have to wait for clinical information to start trickling in, we are not optimistic about their EPS profile in general.

3.7.4.8 *Management of akathisia*

Discontinuing the offending drug, decreasing the dose, or switching to a less risky agent is the ideal management of akathisia. Again, keep in mind that acute EPS predict late EPS. Medication treatments of antipsychotic-induced akathisia, with moderate strength of evidence and, usually, moderate clinical effect, include anticholinergic drugs, lipophilic beta-blockers (with all the concomitant cardiovascular side effects), benzodiazepines, and, recently, mirtazapine.

3.7.5 *Tardive dyskinesia*

Tardive dyskinesia (TD) consists in frequent unintentional, or even unconscious, contractions of voluntary muscles. It usually starts in the fine muscles of the face and the hands, causing for example the "rabbit syndrome," when the perioral muscles are involved, or the "rolling pill syndrome," when the hands are involved. Even in mild cases, manifestations of TD in the face and hands cause a social suffering that is far in excess of the motor dysfunction itself. TD may progress to affect critical functions such as speech, swallowing, breathing, writing, or ambulating. The adjective 'tardive' alludes to the relatively late appearance of this syndrome during antipsychotic treatment, and the increased risk with increased duration of treatment. However, in some cases, irreversible EPS such as TD may appear just after a few weeks of antipsychotic treatment. Usually, three months of treatment is considered the divider between acute and tardive EPS. In contrast to acute EPS, TD is frequently irreversible, even when antipsychotic treatment is stopped. Another feature distinguishing TD from acute EPS is that TD often gets worse when the antipsychotic is stopped or the dose decreased (neuroleptic withdrawal dyskinesia). The risk for TD has been reported as higher in the elderly, especially in females, but it can be observed in patients of any age.

TD appeared to have a high prevalence in the past, when high antipsychotic doses were the rule, and surely the prevalence today is lower. However, the decrease in TD rates after the introduction of the "atypical" antipsychotics does not seem to be as significant as once believed. An analysis evaluating the cost-effectiveness of reduced TD with the new antipsychotics comments: "It is thus likely that the reduction in risk of extrapyramidal symptoms as well as of tardive dyskinesia with second-generation antipsychotics has been overstated." (Rosenheck, 2007) A recent prospective cohort study in Connecticut found that, compared to the users of "typical" antipsychotics, the adjusted TD incidence rate for subjects treated with "atypical" antipsychotics alone was 68% (Woods *et al.*, 2010). This is a far cry from the 10% of the risk for TD with the new agents, compared to old antipsychotics, proclaimed during marketing campaigns for the new medications. The Connecticut study observes that, among patients who had been recently exposed to atypical antipsychotics alone, TD appeared at a rate "more similar to that for conventional antipsychotics than in most previous studies." They conclude, "Despite high penetration of atypical antipsychotics into clinical practice, the incidence and prevalence of tardive dyskinesia appeared relatively unchanged since the 1980s." In the CATIE results, there was no statistical difference between the TD rates for perphenazine and the four new antipsychotics included in the study (Lieberman *et al.*, 2005; Caroff *et al.*, 2011).

Risk for TD with any individual antipsychotic seems to be related to dose, duration of treatment, and potency of dopamine D_2 blockade, rather than with being a "typical" or "atypical" agent. This means that, among the new antipsychotics, probably aripiprazole, asenapine, iloperidone, lurasidone, paliperidone, risperidone, and ziprasidone have a higher risk than clozapine, olanzapine, and quetiapine. For example, the frequency of aripiprazole-associated TD was high enough to trigger a case review that concludes, "This largest reported series draws attention to the growing incidence of TD and other drug-induced movement disorders associated with 'atypical antipsychotics.'" (Sierra Pena *et al.*, 2011)

One widely accepted theory is that TD is caused by a reactive hyperactivity of dopamine receptors (due to increased number or sensitivity, or both) that finally overcomes the antipsychotic dopamine blockade. This is supported by the fact, mentioned above, that discontinuation of the antipsychotic is followed by a sudden worsening of TD in up to half the patients. Also congruent with this theory is the fact that TD can be controlled, at least temporarily, by increasing the antipsychotic dose or switching to a more potent agent. Thus, frequently, we see reports on the efficacy of the most potent new antipsychotics in the "treatment" of TD. The main objection to this practice is the possibility that, after some time, the TD reappears with added force to overcome that higher level of dopamine blockade. Many medications have been proposed for the treatment of TD, starting with clozapine, and including GABAergic medications and several anticonvulsants. The clinical results have been disappointing. The monoamine depletor tetrabenazine (Xenazine), which also has antipsychotic properties, has long been used overseas in the treatment of TD. In the USA, it was recently approved for the treatment of Huntington's chorea. Tetrabenazine reversibly depletes monoamine vesicles (such as dopamine, serotonin, norepinephrine, and histamine) in nerve terminals. The principal drawbacks are a steep price and the risk of depression, sedation, fatigue, anxiety, and/or akathisia.

3.8 Neuroleptic Malignant Syndrome

NMS is not an unequivocal concept. The name itself is likely a misnomer. Syndromes resembling NMS have been reported in association not only with antipsychotic drugs but antidepressants, anticonvulsants, anesthetics, drugs of abuse, and non-psychiatric medications such as statins. The reported triggers include severe systemic or neurological illness such as malignancy, dehydration, hyperosmolar diabetic coma, brain lesions, or neuropsychiatric lupus erythematosus. "There are controversies associated with virtually all important aspects of NMS. At the moment, it is not clear if this drug reaction is idiosyncratic or not, what diagnostic criteria are the most appropriate for usual clinical practice, and it seems that the estimated incidence is not in accordance with the number of treated patients. There are rather different approaches to the pathophysiological mechanisms, differential diagnosis, and treatment." (Margetic *et al.*, 2010)

In any case, the "classical" definition of NMS includes hyperthermia, slowness, rigidity, delirium, and autonomic instability. It is generally considered to be a catastrophic form of EPS with high lethality. Fully fledged NMS is considered the last stage in a progression of severity starting with antipsychotic-induced parkinsonism (Strawn *et al.*, 2007). Regarding its frequency, recent new information has pointed to flaws in the calculations of incidence that have produced substantial overestimates, mainly related to study size. A recent review points out that large samples consistently indicate a lower incidence of NMS than small ones: "…the range varied from 30 per 1,000 in the smallest studies, to as low as 0.17 to 0.2 per 1,000 in the largest studies." On the other hand, very likely we are diagnosing only the severest cases, and proposed changes in the definition, especially related to the need for hyperthermia to be present, would increase the number of cases (Gillman, 2010).

NMS has been reported for all the antipsychotics that have been in the market for at least some time, both "old" and "new," including clozapine and even the recently introduced asenapine and iloperidone (Singh *et al.*, 2010; Guanci *et al.*, 2012). The risk of NMS with individual antipsychotics seems to be related to potency of dopamine D_2 blockade and dose. Thus, NMS was relatively frequent in the first decades of antipsychotic use, surely due not only to the prescription of potent agents, but also dosing schedules that we consider unjustifiable these days. However, with the market shift to the "atypical" antipsychotics, most of the reports of NMS in recent years, for both adult and children, refer to them (Ananth *et al.*, 2004; Croarkin *et al.*, 2008; Neuhut *et al.*, 2009). The new antipsychotics most recently introduced in the USA (ziprasidone, aripiprazole, paliperidone, iloperidone, asenapine, and lurasidone) are on the high-potency end of the spectrum. Thus, if any change can be foreseen in the incidence of NMS cases in the USA in coming years, it should be upward. There is debate regarding practically every aspect of the specific treatment of NMS. The need for prompt and intensive supportive treatment is, however, universally accepted, but its details exceed the scope of this textbook, aimed at psychiatrists rather than emergency and ICU practitioners.

3.9 Catatonia

Catatonia is a syndrome that periodically waxes and wanes in Western psychiatry, especially in the European school. It was described before antipsychotics were available, and comprises a group of parkinsonian features (immobility, mutism, withdrawal, "negativism," and rigidity) plus other heterogeneous and even contradictory motor characteristics, such as manic agitation, or "waxy flexibility" (patients keeping the position in which they are passively placed). It is said that catatonia can be observed in patients with schizophrenia, mood disorders, other psychiatric conditions, withdrawal from benzodiazepines and other drugs, as well as in a wide range of neurological and medical conditions. In our opinion, many cases of catatonia diagnosed in patients receiving antipsychotic therapy may be symptoms of pervasive parkinsonism. This would probably place these patients at high risk for other complications such as NMS. The fact that schizophrenic patients labeled as 'catatonic' respond poorly to benzodiazepines, which, according to catatonia experts, would induce rapid improvements in catatonia associated with other conditions, may support the above supposition (Rosebush *et al.*, 2010).

3.10 Antipsychotic-Induced Hyperprolactinemia

Antipsychotic-induced hyperprolactinemia is a common occurrence with worrisome long-term effects, which tends to receive little attention. Prolactin secretion in the pituitary gland is under the control of different neurotransmitters, hormones, and peptides. In humans, dopamine is the main prolactin-inhibiting factor. Dopamine released by the tuberoinfundibular neurons in the hypothalamus is transported to the pituitary gland by the portal hypophyseal circulation. Stimulation of D_2 receptors in the membrane of pituitary lactotroph cells decreases the gene transcription, synthesis, and release of prolactin. Thus, D_2 receptor blockade increases prolactin release. In general, the higher the D_2-blocking properties of an antipsychotic, the higher the risk for hyperprolactinemia. However, the correlation is not perfect, as we will discuss below, indicating that other factors are also in play. Elevated serum prolactin may lead to serious consequences, both in the short and long terms, from sexual dysfunction to osteoporosis and infertility (see Table 3.8).

Table 3.8 Potential risks of sustained hyperprolactinemia (partially based on Madhusoodanan *et al.*, 2010).

Female	Male
Reproductive function: Amenorrhea, oligomenorrhea, anovulation, habitual abortion (increased risk for breast and endometrial cancer?)	Hypogonadotrophic hypogonadism: Decreased libido, decreased mass muscle and body hair, infertility
Breast: Engorgement, galactorrhea, dysplasia	Breast: Galactorrhea, gynecomastia
Sexual dysfunction	Sexual dysfunction: Decreased libido, erectile dysfunction, ejaculatory dysfunction
Behavioral and mood changes	Behavioral and mood changes
Osteoporosis	Osteoporosis
Prolactinoma	Prolactinoma
Increased platelet aggregation?	

A new troublesome feature is the likely association of prolactin-increasing antipsychotics with pituitary prolactinoma. An analysis of the U.S. FDA Adverse Event Reporting System mentions "higher than expected post marketing reports of pituitary tumors associated with risperidone, a potent dopamine D_2-receptor antagonist antipsychotic." In a more general sense, this analysis also confirms the special vulnerability of women and children to the adverse effects of hyperprolactinemia. Thus, nearly 82% of all reports of adverse events related to increases in prolactin were seen in women, and several cases of prolactinoma were reported in children (three associated with risperidone and one with olanzapine) (Szarfman *et al.*, 2006).

In the publicly funded TEOSS study of early-onset schizophrenia, prolactin levels showed an increase of about 80% in patients taking risperidone, and a net decrease in patients taking the "typical" antipsychotic molindone and the "atypical" olanzapine (Sikich *et al.*, 2008). Levels of prolactin were apparently not measured in the CATIE study. However, in CATIE, the incidence of outcome measures closely associated with hyperprolactinemia (gynecomastia/galactorrhea and menstrual irregularities) seemed to be higher for risperidone and then ziprasidone than for the "old" antipsychotic perphenazine and the new antipsychotics olanzapine and quetiapine, although the differences did not reach statistical significance (Lieberman *et al.*, 2005). In summary, regarding risk for hyperprolactinemia with individual antipsychotics, risperidone, its metabolite paliperidone, and sulpiride (an "atypical" antipsychotic never introduced in the USA) are clearly outliers on the high side, while quetiapine, aripiprazole, and clozapine seem to have the lowest risk. In the middle between these extremes are haloperidol, ziprasidone, olanzapine, and possibly the most recently introduced antipsychotic drugs. Regarding monitoring prolactin increases, it is probably safer to monitor patients on risperidone, paliperidone, and sulpiride once they have been on a stable dose for several weeks. For other antipsychotics, clinical monitoring of symptoms such as menstrual irregularities, breast engorgement, decreased libido, and other types of sexual dysfunction should be done regularly, and prolactin levels measured if there is any clinical suspicion of hyperprolactinemia. Of course, the best intervention for hyperprolactinemia is prevention, a statement that is also true for practically every adverse effect mentioned in this chapter, since the risk for hyperprolactinemia is dose-related. Thus, judicious dosing, starting at the low end of the efficacy spectrum, and going up gradually according to response, is the best way to protect our patients.

3.11 Sexual Side Effects of Antipsychotics

Patients with schizophrenia show a high baseline prevalence of sexual dysfunction. On top of this, antipsychotic drugs interfere with sexual function through multiple mechanisms, significantly lessening quality of life and, in some cases, creating immediate and/or long-term medical risks (see Table 3.9). Thus, sexual side effects need to be actively monitored, as most patients will be reluctant to report them spontaneously. Above, we have discussed hyperprolactinemia, an important mechanism for antipsychotic-induced sexual dysfunction. In the paragraph below, we will discuss in some detail a disturbing sexual side effect of antipsychotics: priapism.

Table 3.9 Mechanisms of antipsychotic induced sexual dysfunction (partially based on Baggaley *et al.*, 2008).

Drug effect	Physiological effect	Sexual function effect
H receptor antagonism	Sedation	Impaired arousal
D receptor antagonism (basal ganglia)	Inhibition of motivation/reward	Decreased libido
D_2 receptor antagonism (hypophysis)	Hyperprolactinemia	Decreased libido, impaired arousal, impaired orgasm
Cholinergic receptor antagonism	Parasympathetic dysfunction, reduced peripheral vasodilation	Erectile dysfunction
α-adrenergic receptor antagonism	Sympathetic dysfunction, abnormal peripheral vasodilation	Priapism, and abnormal ejaculation and lubrication

Priapism is a prolonged, usually painful, unprovoked erection that is not alleviated through sexual activity and which, if uncontrolled, may lead to erectile dysfunction (in approximately 50% of cases) or even penile necrosis. Priapism may be due to medical diseases affecting nervous tissue, or surrounding tissues (including blood conditions). For example, priapism is relatively frequent in males with sickle cell anemia, who may suffer from repeated episodes ("stuttering priapism"). Priapism may be caused by several types of medications, usually through interference with α-adrenergic receptors in the vasculature. Practically any antipsychotic may induce priapism, and α_1 blockade has been blamed in this case (Andersohn *et al.*, 2010). This is supported by the fact that antipsychotics with a clearly higher D_2 than α_1 affinity seem to be reported less often as a cause of priapism. Among the "old" antipsychotics, chlorpromazine and thioridazine seem to have the most reports, while potent D_2 blockers with relatively low α_1 activity (such as haloperidol, perphenazine, and molindone) seem to be low risk. Among the new antipsychotics, risperidone appears to have the most reports, though we must acknowledge that this could be related to its being the atypical antipsychotic drug that has been the longest in the market, second only to clozapine. In any case, medications like risperidone, olanzapine, and asenapine (which have a comparable affinity at D_2 and α_1), and also quetiapine and clozapine (which have even higher affinity for α_1 than for D_2) should be the antipsychotic agents with the highest risk to induce priapism. A case of a female condition related to priapism, "clitoral priapism," has been reported with olanzapine (Bucur *et al.*, 2004).

3.12 Antihistamine Adverse Effects of Antipsychotics

Blockade of histamine H_1 receptors produces both increased appetite and sedation. Because of this, the risk of an individual antipsychotic to induce weight gain is closely associated with its sedation potential. Thus, excessive sedation is a very common problem with clozapine, which also has the highest potential for weight gain. Regarding the incidence of sedation with "atypical" antipsychotics with high potential for weight gain, according to the U.S. Prescribing Information, the incidence of sedation during treatment with olanzapine (Zyprexa) is 29% (compared to 13% with placebo). For quetiapine, the U.S. Prescribing Information reports an incidence of somnolence of 18% (compared to 11% with placebo) in schizophrenia trials and 57% (compared to 15% with placebo) in bipolar depression trials. Antipsychotics marketed in the USA with high potential for sedation include thioridazine, chlorpromazine, clozapine, olanzapine, and quetiapine. Antipsychotics with moderate potential include risperidone, paliperidone, and asenapine. Antipsychotics with low risk for sedation include haloperidol, fluphenazine, molindone, ziprasidone, aripiprazole, lurasidone, and iloperidone. Antipsychotics with potential to cause sedation can be useful in agitated patients with psychosis or bipolar disorder. However, they should be avoided in patients with already impaired cognition, such as patients with delirium or in the cognitively impaired elderly.

3.13 Anticholinergic Adverse Effects of Antipsychotics: Cognitive and Peripheral

Drugs that decrease the effects of acetylcholine by blocking muscarinic M_1 receptors cause both cognitive impairment and autonomic side effects such as constipation, urinary retention, dry mouth, and sexual dysfunction. Antipsychotics with significant anticholinergic M_1-blocking action include chlorpromazine and thioridazine among the "old" antipsychotics, and clozapine, olanzapine, and quetiapine among the "new" ones. Antipsychotics with little or negligible anticholinergic effects include haloperidol, molindone, and perphenazine among the "old" antipsychotics, and aripiprazole, asenapine, iloperidone, lurasidone, paliperidone, risperidone, and ziprasidone among the "new" ones (Chew *et al.*, 2008). Before examining in more detail the anticholinergic side effects of antipsychotic drugs, we want to remind the reader that patients on anticholinergic antipsychotics, especially the elderly, are often exposed to antidepressants and non-psychotropic drugs with anticholinergic properties that may potentiate the adverse effects of antipsychotics. Among antidepressants, the tricyclic antidepressants and mirtazapine appear to have the highest propensity for anticholinergic effects. Also, a large number of non-psychotropic medications may induce or worsen anticholinergic effects, including antihistamines, antispasmodic drugs, or medications that reduce urinary frequency such as oxybutinin and tolterodine. A combination with high potential for serious side effects is that of anticholinergic antipsychotics and anticholinergic medications used to treat EPS. Urinary retention is commonly seen during treatment with anticholinergic antipsychotic drugs, especially in the elderly. However, this may affect people of any age. There is a report of enlarged urinary bladder (megacystis) in a fetus, possibly caused by transplacental exposure to antipsychotic drugs. The size of the bladder returned to normal two weeks after the mother stopped taking the drugs (Okuno *et al.*, 1999). Constipation is also a common anticholinergic effect from antipsychotic drugs that may entail unexpected severity, including reports of paralytic ileus (Rondla *et al.*, 2007). A recent retrospective study in 273 patients with schizophrenia who were prescribed antipsychotics (2/3 atypicals and 1/3 typicals) showed that 36.6% of them had at least one new pharmacological intervention for the problem of constipation. About half of the affected patients (16%) required enemas for constipation unresponsive to oral treatments. The authors remind us also of the additional risk factors for constipation in patients with schizophrenia, including diet and lack of exercise (De Hert *et al.*, 2011). One of the most troubling and, unfortunately, often overlooked anticholinergic side effect of antipsychotics is their negative effect on cognition and global function. A study of cognitive training in 55 schizophrenic patients treated with antipsychotics found a significant negative association between serum anticholinergic activity and performance in MATRICS-based measures of verbal working memory and verbal learning and memory. "These findings underscore the cognitive cost of medications that carry a high anticholinergic burden. The findings also have implications for the design and evaluation of cognitive treatments for schizophrenia." (Vinogradov *et al.*, 2009) A prospective cohort study in an elderly population living in the community, using physical performance tests (four-meter walking speed, balance, and chair stand test), found that users of antipsychotic drugs showed a higher deterioration than users of benzodiazepine drugs only, another psychotropic group known to cause cognitive impairment (Landi *et al.*, 2007). These findings are all the more worrisome considering the increasing use of anticholinergic antipsychotics, such as olanzapine or quetiapine, in the elderly. A very disturbing fact is the use of anticholinergic antipsychotics in patients at risk for, or suffering from delirium. In the authors' view, the use of sedating or anticholinergic antipsychotics in the treatment of delirium cannot be justified.

3.14 Antipsychotics and the Risk of Seizures

All antipsychotics seem to have the potential to lower the seizure threshold, and should be used with care in patients with a history of seizures, or those taking other medications known to decrease the seizure threshold, or having other risk factors for seizures. However, the risk appears to be smaller than reported in past decades. Some of the likely factors for this decrease are the use of lower antipsychotic doses, and a more gradual titration schedule for antipsychotic drugs. Medications reportedly having a higher risk for seizures than other antipsychotics are chlorpromazine and thioridazine among the "old" antipsychotics, and clozapine among the "new" (Hedges *et al.*, 2003). In the next chapter, on individual antipsychotics, we will discuss the risk for seizures with clozapine in more detail.

3.15 Vascular Side Effects of Antipsychotics

In this section, we will briefly discuss vascular adverse effects of antipsychotics caused by blockade of α-adrenergic receptors in the vascular system. This refers mainly to orthostatic hypotension and reflex tachycardia. Orthostatic hypotension is a sudden drop in systolic blood pressure upon standing from a seating or lying position. It induces reflex tachycardia which worsens the cardiac ischemia. Clinical features may progress to dizziness or syncope, falls, seizures, stroke, cardiac ischemia with arrhythmias, and sudden death. Antipsychotics show this effect early in treatment, usually with the first doses, but patients gradually develop tolerance and the reaction generally subsides. Orthostasis (postural hypotension) is particularly risky in the elderly or in patients with preexistent vascular and cardiac illness. Currently marketed "old" antipsychotics with significant risk for orthostatic hypotension include mainly chlorpromazine and thioridazine. Among the "new" antipsychotics, clozapine and iloperidone (Fanapt) have the highest risk to induce syncope, requiring a careful titration process (discussed in the next chapter). Quetiapine also shows an affinity for α_1 receptors that is larger than that for D_2 receptors, and presents significant risk of orthostasis. The U.S. Prescribing Information for quetiapine (Seroquel) reports an incidence of syncope of 1% (compared to 0.2% with placebo). Other new antipsychotics with clear risk for orthostasis include asenapine, olanzapine, and risperidone/paliperidone.

3.16 Antipsychotics and the Risk of Malignant Arrythmia and Sudden Cardiac Death

The first report of sudden cardiac deaths associated with high doses of antipsychotics came in 1963. This report included two patients who died while taking very high doses of thioridazine (1,500 and 3,600 mg/day) (Kelly *et al.*, 1963). Besides thioridazine, other "old" or "typical" antipsychotics associated with a high risk of arrhythmia included pimozide and droperidol. In the case of other phenothiazines and, especially, for the butyrophenone haloperidol, it was concluded that they were associated with malignant arrhythmia but that the risk was low. The issue of malignant arrhythmia with antipsychotics came to the forefront again following the premarketing trials of the "atypical" antipsychotic sertindole, which showed a high incidence of sudden death and syncope. Sertindole was never approved in the USA, but it was introduced in Europe, where it was eventually withdrawn in the late 1990s. In 2000, at the requirement of the FDA,

Pfizer Laboratories, the makers of the new antipsychotic ziprasidone (Geodon), submitted information — that in our opinion is the best to date — on the arrhythmogenic potential of the new antipsychotics, compared to thioridazine and haloperidol (FDA Psychopharmacological Drugs Advisory Committee, 19 July 2000). This information is also offered in the publication by Glassman *et al.* (2001) (see Table 3.10). Here, we can see that, regarding changes in the QT interval, thioridazine is clearly an outlier on the high side, but also that haloperidol looks relatively safe in this regard compared to the "atypical" antipsychotics risperidone, olanzapine, quetiapine, and ziprasidone. The above-mentioned publication states: "At this point in time, an atypical antipsychotic without concern does not exist. In order to balance the risks and benefits of these drugs, the psychiatrist will have to add torsades de pointes, QTc interval, potassium rectifier current, hypertriglyceridemia, serum insulin, and person-years of observation to his or her vocabulary." (Glassman *et al.*, 2001) More recently, a retrospective cohort study of Medicaid enrollees in Tennessee compared users of antipsychotics (44,128 on typical and 46,089 on atypical antipsychotics) with 186,600 nonusers. It was found that both groups of antipsychotic users had higher rates of sudden death than nonusers. The adjusted incidence rate ratios were 1.99 (95% CI: 1.68–2.34) for typical antipsychotics and 2.26 (1.88–2.72) for atypical antipsychotics (Ray *et al.*, 2009).

In England, a population case-control study looked at sudden death associated with drugs having a propensity to prolong the QT interval in subjects 20–85 years of age (from a community with an estimated population of 2.1 million), who had a post-mortem examination ruling common causes of death and no evidence of drug overdose. They found adjusted ORs for death

Table 3.10 Effect of new antipsychotics on the QTc, compared to thioridazine and haloperidol, in descending order of effect (adapted from Glassman *et al.*, 2001).

Drug	Baseline mean QTc (Bazett correction)	Steady-state mean change	95% CI
Thioridazine	395.9	35.6	30.5–40.7
Ziprasidone	402.1	20.3	14.2–26.4
Quetiapine	398.0	14.5	9.5–19.5
Risperidone	396.3	11.6	7.4–15.8
Olanzapine	397.9	6.8	0.8–12.7
Haloperidol	394.7	4.7	-2.0–11.3

(0–30 days) of 3.35 (95% CI: 1.64–6.83) for typical antipsychotics, and 4.97 (2.78–8.90) for atypical antipsychotics (Jolly *et al.*, 2009).

Thus, the potential for most antipsychotics to induce cardiac arrhythmia and the risk of sudden death appear to be well established even though this occurrence is rare. However, some experts continue to insist that this risk remains unproved, particularly for the new antipsychotics (Lieberman *et al.*, 2009).

3.17 Antipsychotics and Increased Morbidity and Mortality in Patients with Dementia

In a Public Health Advisory report dated 11 April 2005, the U.S. FDA issued this warning: "The Food and Drug Administration has determined that the treatment of behavioral disorders in elderly patients with dementia with atypical (second generation) antipsychotic medications is associated with increased mortality." Of a total of 17 placebo-controlled trials performed with olanzapine (Zyprexa), aripiprazole (Abilify), risperidone (Risperdal), and quetiapine (Seroquel) in demented elderly patients with behavioral disorders, 15 showed numerical increases in mortality in the drug-treated group compared to the placebo-treated patients. These studies enrolled a total of 5,106 patients, and several analyses have demonstrated an approximately 1.6–1.7-fold increase in mortality in these studies. Examination of the specific causes of these deaths revealed that most were either due to heart-related events (e.g., heart failure, sudden death) or infections (mostly pneumonia). On 16 June 2008, the FDA issued another alert, including both types of antipsychotics: "Both conventional and atypical antipsychotics are associated with an increased risk of mortality in elderly patients treated for dementia-related psychosis." This 2008 FDA alert includes an explicit contraindication: "Antipsychotics are not indicated for the treatment of dementia-related psychosis." Looking at the evidence for these warnings, it has been observed that the body of information supporting them comes in large part from secondary data analyses that are mainly retrospective (Wang *et al.*, 2005; Schneider *et al.*, 2005). This is understandable, as it is difficult to conduct prospective studies with numbers sufficient for statistical certainty while exposing patients to potentially negative outcomes. However, recent information from prospective studies is confirming the retrospective information regarding the elevated incidence of serious events or death in dementia patients treated with antipsychotics, both typical and atypical. In the prospective DART-AD study, sponsored by the UK Alzheimer's Research Trust, 165 Alzheimer's disease patients on antipsychotics were randomized to either continue antipsychotics ($N = 64$) or receive placebo ($N = 64$). Results showed a decrease in survival for patients who continued to receive antipsychotic drug compared with those who received placebo. Thus, at 12 months, the cumulative probability of survival was 70% (95% CI: 58%–80%) in the continued treatment group versus 77% (64%–85%) in the placebo group. More pronounced differences were observed at longer follow-up periods: 24-month survival 46% *vs.* 71%; 36-month survival 30% *vs.* 59% (Ballard *et al.*, 2009).

The increased risk for serious adverse events or death in dementia patients undergoing antipsychotic treatment seems to be independent from place of living (community versus nursing home), or the general effect of psychiatric medications. A retrospective cohort study, sponsored by the Canadian Institutes of Health Research, identified 20,682 older adults with dementia living in the community. This study found that, relative to those patients who did not receive antipsychotic treatment, community-dwelling older adults who had a newly dispensed "atypical" antipsychotic were 3.2 times more likely (95% CI: 2.77–3.68), and those who received "typical" antipsychotic therapy 3.8 times more likely (95% CI: 3.31–4.39), to develop any serious event during the 30 days of follow-up. The pattern of serious events was similar but less pronounced among older adults living in a nursing home (Rochon *et al.*, 2008). Another retrospective cohort study, drawing data from the U.S. Veterans Administration, found that all groups taking antipsychotic drugs had significantly higher mortality rates (22.6%–29.1%) than patients taking other psychiatric medications (14.6%). Adjusted mortality risks were similar for atypical, combined atypical–conventional, and conventional antipsychotics. Except for anticonvulsants, the adjusted risks for all individual classes of non-antipsychotic drugs were significantly lower than the risk for antipsychotics (Kales *et al.*, 2007). Very recently, a retrospective study of 33,604 outpatients with dementia from the U.S. Veterans Administration found a somewhat higher risk of death with the use of haloperidol than the "atypical" antipsychotics in this population. The 180-day hazard ratio was 1.59 for haloperidol compared to 1.00 with risperidone (the reference), and 0.74 with quetiapine (Kales *et al.*, 2012). However, this study exemplifies the problems with most comparisons of "typical" and "atypical" antipsychotics, regarding how comparable different populations really are, as patients receiving haloperidol were more likely to have the medication prescribed by non-psychiatrists, exhibited more medical problems, and included a higher percentage of African-Americans. Finally, we want to discuss the possibility that factors playing a role in the excess mortality of antipsychotic-treated demented patients may also affect other at-risk populations taking antipsychotics. Some studies have shown that while specific risks of antipsychotic medications (for example, risk of stroke) are higher in dementia populations, they are also present in non-demented subjects treated with antipsychotic drugs. A self-controlled study estimated the risk for stroke associated to treatment with antipsychotic in patients with and without dementia. Comparing the ratios (95% CI) for the event during periods of exposure to medication to periods of non-exposure, they found an increased risk in both groups, though higher in the dementia group. "In patients receiving any antipsychotic drug, the rate ratios were 3.50 (2.97–4.2) for those with dementia and 1.41 (1.29–1.55) for those without dementia." (Douglas *et al.*, 2008) Recently, a study in patients with parkinsonism, including 5,391 patients who died during the study, and a matched comparison group of 25,937 who were still alive, found that individuals exposed to atypical antipsychotics had an adjusted OR of death twice that of non-exposed controls. Interestingly, the results for quetiapine were similar to those of other atypicals (Marras *et al.*, 2012). In summary, (1) the evidence strongly supports that there is an increased risk of death attached to antipsychotic treatment in demented patients; (2) the beneficial effect of antipsychotics in the treatment of behavioral and psychotic symptoms of dementia seems highly questionable (Gentile, 2010); and (3) the FDA categorically recommends to avoid antipsychotics in psychotic patients with dementia. Therefore, it is our opinion that physicians who continue to prescribe antipsychotic drugs in this population are taking an unreasonable risk and that this may lead to significant professional liability.

3.18 Antipsychotics and Suicide

Completed suicide in schizophrenia tends to appear most frequently early in the course of the disease. A Finnish cohort study of young subjects with schizophrenia (16–39 years), found that suicide accounted for 50% of all deaths. They report an overall suicide rate of 7%, with a large gender difference (2.9% for women and 9.2% for men) (Alaraisanen *et al.*, 2009). In view of this, it has been postulated that early antipsychotic treatment may reduce suicide. Results from a retrospective national cohort study in Finland appeared to support this view by showing that, in a population of schizophrenic patients with suicidal ideation or behavior, treatment was associated with lower mortality from suicide and from other causes (Haukka *et al.*, 2008). The problem with this latter study is its retrospective design. In hindsight, it is difficult to assign causality for an outcome that could be influenced by myriad factors. For example, schizophrenics who stay in treatment are more likely to have superior social support, better functioning, and better physical health than those who do not. In prospective studies, which should be the gold standard in the field, only clozapine has been associated with a decrease in suicide rates of patients with schizophrenia (Meltzer *et al.*, 2003).

3.19 Antipsychotics and the Risk of Cancer

The possible association of schizophrenia, as a disease, and antipsychotic drug treatment with the appearance of cancer has been raised periodically for decades. However, the quality of the data has not allowed for any conclusive judgment. A large, prospective study of a cohort of 3,470 patients with schizophrenia followed for 11 years, examined predictors of cancer-related mortality. A major finding in this study was that the cancer-related mortality in patients with schizophrenia was significantly elevated for breast cancer in women and lung cancer in men (Tran *et al.*, 2009). Obviously, the high prevalence of smoking among schizophrenic patients is a key factor for lung cancer. However, establishing an association between antipsychotics and mortality from breast cancer (through hyperprolactinemia) is difficult, since several other factors prevalent in schizophrenic patients, such as obesity, less access to care, and being nulliparous, may also play a role.

References

Alaraisanen A, Miettunen J, Rasanen P, *et al.* Suicide rate in schizophrenia in the Northern Finland 1966 birth cohort. *Soc Psychiat Epidemiol* 2009;44:1107–1110.

Allison DB, Mentore JL, Moonseong H, *et al.* Antipsychotic-induced weight gain: A comprehensive research synthesis. *Am J Psychiatry* 1999;156:1686–1696.

Ananth J, Parameswaran S, Gunatilake S, *et al.* Neuroleptic malignant syndrome and atypical antipsychotic drugs. *J Clin Psychiatry* 2004;65(4):464–470.

Andersohn F, Schmedt N, Weinmann S, *et al.* Priapism associated with antipsychotics: Role of α_1-adrenergic affinity. *J Clin Psychopharmacol* 2010;30:68–71.

Andreasen NC, Pressler M, Nopoulos P, *et al.* Antipsychotic dose equivalents and dose-years: A standardized method for comparing exposure to different drugs. *Biol Psychiatry* 2010;67:255–262.

Baggaley M. Sexual dysfunction in schizophrenia: Focus on recent evidence. *Hum Psychopharmacol* 2008;23(3):201–209.

Baker RA, Pikalov A, Tran Q-V, *et al.* Atypical antipsychotic drugs and diabetes mellitus in the US Food and Drug Administration Adverse Event Database: A systematic Bayesian signal detection analysis. *Psychopharmacol Bull* 2009;42(1):1–21.

Ballard C, Hanney ML, Theodoulou M, *et al.* The dementia antipsychotic withdrawal trial (DART-AD): Long-term follow-up of a randomized placebo-controlled trial. *Lancet* 2009; 8:151–157.

Bay YM, Lin C-C, Chen JY, *et al.* Association of weight gain and metabolic syndrome in patients taking clozapine: An 8-year cohort study. *J Clin Psychiatry* 2010, doi:10.4088/JCP09m05402yel

Birkenaes AB, Birkeland KI, Engh JA, *et al.* Dyslipidemia independent of body mass in antipsychotic-treated patients under real-life conditions. *J Clin Psychopharmacol* 2008;28(2):132–137.

Bobes J, Arango C, Aranda P, *et al.* Cardiovascular and metabolic risks in outpatients with schizophrenia treated with antipsychotics: Results of the CLAMORS study. *Schizophr Res* 2007;90:162–173.

Buchholz S, Morrow AF, Coleman PL. Atypical antipsychotic-induced diabetes mellitus: An update on epidemiology and postulated mechanisms. *Int Med J* 2008, doi:10.1111/j.1445–5994.2008.01712.x

Bucur M, Mahmood T. Olanzapine-induced clitoral priapism. *J Clin Psychopharmacol* 2004;24(5):572–573.

Caroff SN, Hurford I, Lybrand J, *et al.* Movement disorders induced by antipsychotic drugs: Implications of the CATIE schizophrenia trial. *Neurol Clin* 2011;29:127–148.

Chew ML, Mulsant BH, Pollock BG, *et al.* Anticholinergic activity of 107 medications commonly used by older adults. *J Am Geriatr Soc* 2008;56:1333–1341.

Ciranni MA, Kearney TE, Olson KR. Comparing acute toxicity of first- and second-generation antipsychotic drugs: A 10-year, retrospective cohort study. *J Clin Psychiatry* 2009;70(1):122–129.

Correll CU, Frederickson AM, Kane JM, Manu P. Equally increased risk for metabolic syndrome in patients with bipolar disorder and schizophrenia treated with second-generation antipsychotics. *Bipolar Disord* 2008;10:788–797.

Correll CU, Manu P, Olshanskiy V, *et al.* Cardiometabolic risk of second-generation antipsychotic medications during first-time use in children and adolescents. *JAMA* 2009;302(16):1765–1773.

Correll CU. From receptor pharmacology to improved outcomes: Individualising the selection, dosing, and switching of antipsychotics. *Eur Psychiatry* 2010;25:S12–S21.

Croarkin PE, Emslie GJ, Mayes TL. Neuroleptic malignant syndrome associated with atypical antipsychotics in pediatric patients: A review of published cases. *J Clin Psychiatry* 2008;69(7):1157–1165.

Crossley NA, Constante M, McGuire P, *et al.* Efficacy of atypical *v.* typical antipsychotics in the treatment of early psychosis: meta-analysis. *Br J Psychiatry* 2010;196:424–439.

Davidson M, Galderisi S, Weiser M, *et al.* Cognitive effects of antipsychotic drugs in first-episode schizophrenia and schizophreniform disorder: A randomized, open-label clinical trial (EUFEST). *Am J Psychiatry* 2009;166(6):675–682.

De Hert M, Schreurs V, Sweers V, *et al.* Typical and atypical antipsychotics differentially affect long-term incidence rates of the metabolic syndrome in patients with schizophrenia: A retrospective chart review. *Schizophr Res* 2008;101:295–303.

De Hert M, Dockx L, Bernagie C, *et al.* Prevalence and severity of antipsychotic related constipation in patients with schizophrenia: A retrospective descriptive study. *BMC Gastroenterol* 2011;11(1):17.

Douglas IJ, Smeeth L. Exposure to antipsychotics and risk of stroke: Self controlled case series study. *BMJ* 2008, doi: 10.1136/bmj.a1227

Edwards SJ, Smith CJ. Tolerability of atypical antipsychotics in the treatment of adults with schizophrenia or bipolar disorder: A mixed treatment comparison of randomized controlled trials. *Clin Ther* 2009;31:1345–1359.

FDA Psychopharmacology Drugs Advisory Committee. Briefing document of Zeldox Capsules (Zyprasidone HCl), 19 July 2000. Retrieved on 18 October 2010 from www.fda.gov/ohrms/dockets/ac/00/transcripts/3619t1.rtf

Foley DL, Morley KI. Systematic review of early cardiometabolic outcomes of the first treated episode of psychosis. *Arch Gen Psychiatry* 2011, doi:10.1001/archgenpsychiatry.2011.2

Gaebel W, Riesbeck M, Wolwer W, *et al.* Maintenance treatment with risperidone or low-dose haloperidol in first-episode schizophrenia: 1-year results of a randomized controlled trial within the German Research Network on Schizophrenia. *J Clin Psychiatry* 2007;68:1763–1774.

Gao K, Kemp DE, Ganocy SJ, *et al.* Antipsychotic-induced extrapyramidal side effects in bipolar disorder and schizophrenia — a systematic review. *J Clin Psychopharmacol* 2008;28:203–209.

Gardner DM, Murphy AL, O'Donnell H, *et al.* International consensus study of antipsychotic dosing. *Am J Psychiatry* 2010;167(6):686–693.

Gebhardt S, Haberhausen M, Heinzel-Gutenbrunner M, *et al.* Antipsychotic-induced body weight gain: Predictors and a systematic categorization of the long-term weight course. *J Psychiatr Res* 2009;43:620–626.

Gentile S. Second-generation antipsychotics in dementia: Beyond safety concerns. A clinical, systematic review of efficacy data from randomized controlled trials. *Psychopharmacology* 2010;212:119–129.

Gillman PK. Neuroleptic malignant syndrome: Mechanisms, interactions, and causality. *Mov Disord* 2010;25(12):1780–1790.

Glassman AH, Bigger JT. Antipsychotic drugs: Prolonged QTc interval, torsade de pointes, and sudden death. *Am J Psychiatry* 2001;158:1774–1782.

Graham KA, Cho H, Brownley KA, *et al.* Early treatment-related changes in diabetes and cardiovascular disease risk markers in first episode psychosis subjects. *Schizophr Res* 2008;101:287–294.

Guanci N, Aggarwal R, Schleifer S. Atypical neuroleptic malignant syndrome associated with iloperidone administration. *Psychosomatics* 2012;53(6):603–605.

Guo X, Fang M, Zhai J, *et al.* Effectiveness of maintenance treatment with atypical and typical antipsychotics in stable schizophrenia with early stage: 1-year naturalistic study. *Psychopharmacology* 2011, doi: 10.1007/s00213–011–2242–3

Haukka J, Tiihonen J, Harkanen T, *et al.* Association between medication and risk of suicide, attempted suicide and death in a nationwide cohort of suicidal patients with schizophrenia. *Pharmacoepidemiol Drug Saf* 2008;17:686–696.

Hedges D, Jeppson K, Whitehead P. Antipsychotic medication and seizures: A review. *Drugs Today* 2003;39(7):551–557.

Hugenholtz GWK, Heerdink ER, Stolker JJ, *et al.* Haloperidol dose when used as active comparator in randomized controlled trials with atypical antipsychotics in schizophrenia: Comparison with officially recommended doses. *J Clin Psychiatry* 2006;67(6): 897–903.

Jolly K, Gammage MD, Cheng KK, *et al.* Sudden death in patients receiving drugs tending to prolong the QT interval. *Br J Clin Pharmacol* 2009;68(5):743–751.

Jones PB, Barnes TRE, Davies L, *et al.* Randomized controlled trial of the effect on quality of life of second- *vs.* first-generation antipsychotic drugs in schizophrenia. *Arch Gen Psychiatry* 2006;1079–1097.

Kales HC, Valenstein M, Kim HM, *et al.* Mortality risk in patients with dementia treated with antipsychotics versus other psychiatric medications. *Am J Psychiatry* 2007;164:1568–1575.

Kales HC, Kim HM, Zivin K, *et al.* Risk of mortality among individual antipsychotics in patients with dementia. *Am J Psychiatry* 2012;169:71–49.

Kane JM, Honigfeld G, Singer J, *et al.* Clozapine for the treatment-resistant schizophrenic: A double-blind comparison with chlorpromazine. *Arch Gen Psychiatry* 1988;45(9):789–796.

Kane JM, Fleishhacker WW, Hansen L, *et al.* Akathisia: An updated review focusing on second-generation antipsychotics. *J Clin Psychiatry* 2009;70(5):627–643.

Keefe RS, Bilder RM, Davis SM, *et al.* Neurocognitive effects of antipsychotic medications in patients with chronic schizophrenia in the CATIE trial. *Arch Gen Psychiatry* 2007;64:633–647.

Kelly HG, Fay JE, Lavery SG. Thioridazine hydrochloride (Mellaril): Its effects on the electrocardiogram and a report of two fatalities with electrocardiographic abnormalities. *Can Med Assoc J* 1963;89:546–554.

Krane-Gartiser K, Breum L, Glumrr C, *et al.* Prevalence of the metabolic syndrome in Danish psychiatric outpatients treated with antipsychotics. *Nord J Psychiatry* 2011;65(5):345–352.

Kumar R, Sachdev PS. Akathisia and second-generation antipsychotic drugs. *Curr Opin Psychiatry* 2009;22:293–299.

Landi F, Russo A, Liperoti R, *et al.* Anticholinergic drugs and physical function among frail elderly population. *Clin Pharmacol Ther* 2007;81(2):235–241.

Leucht S, Corves C, Arbter D, *et al.* Second-generation versus first-generation antipsychotic drugs for schizophrenia: A meta-analysis. *Lancet* 2009;373:31–41.

Leucht S, Wahlbeck K, Hamann J, *et al.* New generation antipsychotics versus low-potency conventional antipsychotics: A systematic review and meta-analysis. *Lancet* 2003;361: 1581–1589.

Lieberman JA, Scott Stroup T, McEvoy JP, *et al.* Effectiveness of antipsychotic drugs in patients with chronic schizophrenia. *N Engl J Med* 2005;353(12):1209–1223.

Lieberman JA, Merrill D, Parameswaran S. APA Guidance on the Use of Antipsychotic Drugs and Cardiac Sudden Death, 17 February 2009, Retrieved from www.omh.ny.gov/omhweb/advisories/asult_antipsychotic_use_attachement.html

Mackin P, Bishop D, Watkinson H, *et al.* Metabolic disease and cardiovascular risk in people treated with antipsychotics in the community. *Br J Psychiatry* 2007;191:23–29.

Madhusoodanan S, Parida S, Jimenez C. Hyperprolactinemia associated with psychotropics — a review. *Hum Psychopharmacol* 2010;25:281–297.

Margetic B, Margetic BA. Neuroleptic malignant syndrome and its controversies. *Pharmacoepidemiol Drug Saf* 2010;19:429–435.

Marras C, Gruneir A, Wang X, *et al.* Antipsychotics and mortality in Parkinsonism. *Am J Geriatr Psychiatry* 2012;20:149–158.

McEvoy JP, Meyer JM, Goff DC, *et al.* Prevalence of the metabolic syndrome in patients with schizophrenia: Baseline results from the Clinical Antipsychotic Trials of Intervention Effectiveness (CATIE) schizophrenia trial and comparison with national estimates from NHANES III. *Schizophr Res* 2005;80:19–32.

Meltzer HY, Alphs L, Green AI, *et al.* Clozapine treatment for suicidality in schizophrenia: International Suicide Prevention Trial (InterSePT). *Arch Gen Psychiatry* 2003;60(1):82–91.

Miyamoto S, Stroup TS, Duncan GE, *et al.* Acute pharmacological treatment of schizophrenia. In: Hirsch SR, Weinberger D, eds. *Schizophrenia*. 2nd ed., Blackwell Science, Hoboken, 2003, pp. 442–473.

Neuhut R, Lindenmayer J-P, Silva R. Neuroleptic malignant syndrome in children and adolescents on atypical antipsychotic medication: A review. *J Child Adolesc Psychopharmacol* 2009;19(4):415–422.

Nielsen J, Skadhede S, Currell CU. Antipsychotics associated with the development of type II diabetes in antipsychotic-naïve schizophrenia patients. *Neuropsychopharmacology* 2010;35:1997–2004.

Okuno S, Hamada H, Fujiki Y, *et al.* Transplacental exposure to antipsychotic drugs during pregnancy and megacystis in the fetus. *Prenat Diagn* 1999;19(10):980–982.

Padmavati R, McCreadie RG, Tirupati S. Low prevalence of obesity and metabolic syndrome in never-treated chronic schizophrenia. *Schizophr Res* 2010;121:199–202.

Penn DL, Keefe RSE, Davis SM, *et al.* The effects of antipsychotic medications on emotion perception in patients with chronic schizophrenia in the CATIE trial. *Schizophr Res* 2009;115:17–23.

Perlick DA, Rosenheck RA, Kaczynski R, *et al.* Impact of antipsychotic medication on family burden in schizophrenia: Longitudinal results of CATIE trial. *Schizophr Res* 2010;116:118–125.

Ray WA, Chung CP, Murray KT, *et al.* Atypical antipsychotic drugs and the risk of sudden cardiac death. *N Engl J Med* 2009;360:225–235.

Reist C, Mintz J, Albers LJ, *et al.* Second-generation antipsychotic exposure and metabolic-related disorders in patients with schizophrenia. *J Clin Psychopharmacol* 2007;27:46–51.

Rochon PA, Normand SL, Gomes T, *et al.* Antipsychotic therapy and short-term serious events in older adults with dementia. *Arch Intern Med* 2008;168(10):1090–1096.

Rondla S, Crane S. A case of clozapine-induced paralytic ileus. *Emerg Med* 2007;24:e12.

Rosebush PI, Mazurek MF. Catatonia and its treatment. *Schizophr Bull* 2010;36:239–242.

Rosenheck RA. Evaluating the cost-effectiveness of reduced tardive dyskinesia with second-generation antipsychotics. *Br J Psychiatry* 2007;191:238–245.

Rummel-Kluge C, Komossa K, Schwarz S, *et al.* Second-generation antipsychotic drugs and extrapyramidal side effects: A systematic review and meta-analysis of head-to-head comparisons. *Schizophr Bull* 2010, doi:10.1093/schbul/sbq042

Sacchetti E, Turrina C, Parrinello G, *et al.* Incidence of diabetes in a general practice population: A database cohort study on the relationship with haloperidol, olanzapine, risperidone or quetiapine exposure. *Int Clin Psychopharmacol* 2005;20:33–37.

Saha S, Chant D, McGrath J. A systematic review of mortality in schizophrenia: Is the differential mortality gap worsening over time? *Arch Gen Psychiatry* 2007;64(10): 1123–1131.

Schneider LS, Dagerman KS, Insel P. Risk of death with atypical antipsychotic drug treatment for dementia: Meta-analysis of randomized placebo-controlled trials. *JAMA* 2005;294(15):1934–1943.

Sierra Pena M, Yaltho TC, Jankovic J. Tardive dyskinesia and other movement disorders secondary to aripiprazole. *Mov Disord* 2011;26(1):147–152.

Sikich L, Fraziere JA, McClellan J, *et al.* Double-blind comparison of first- and second-generation antipsychotics in early-onset schizophrenia and schizoaffective disorder:

Findings from the Treatment of Early-Onset Schizophrenia Spectrum Disorders (TEOSS) study. *Am J Psychiatry* 2008;165:1420–1431.

Simpson G, Glick ID, Weiden PJ, *et al.* Randomized, controlled, double-blind multicenter comparison of the efficacy and tolerability of ziprasidone and olanzapine in acutely ill inpatients with schizophrenia or schizoaffective disorder. *Am J Psychiatry* 2004;161: 1837–1847.

Singh N, Wise TN. Neuroleptic malignant syndrome after exposure to asenapine: A case report. *Prim Care Companion J Clin Psychiatry* 2010;12(5), doi: PCC.10100966

Smith E, Rothschild AJ, Moonseong H, *et al.* Weight gain during olanzapine treatment for psychotic depression: Effects of dose and age. *Int Clin Psychopharmacol* 2008;23:130–137.

Strawn JR, Keck PE Jr., Caroff SN. Neuroleptic malignant syndrome. *Am J Psychiatry* 2007;164(6):870–876.

Sun SH, Nikolics L, Abbasi F, *et al.* Relationship between body mass index and insulin resistance in patients treated with second generation antipsychotic agents. *J Psychiatr Res* 2010;44:493–498.

Swartz MS, Perkins DO, Stroup TS, *et al.* Effects of antipsychotic medications on psychosocial functioning in patients with chronic schizophrenia: Findings from the NIMH CATIE trial. *Am J Psychiatry* 2007;164:428–436.

Szarfman A, Tonning JM, Levine JG, *et al.* Atypical antipsychotics and pituitary tumors: A pharmacovigilance study. *Pharmacotherapy* 2006;26(6):748–758.

Tarricone I, Serretti A, Ferrari Gozzi B, *et al.* Metabolic side effects of second generation antipsychotic agents in antipsychotic naïve patients: One month prospective evaluation. *Psychiatry Res* 2008;157:269–271.

Tenback DE, van Harten PN, Slooff CJ, *et al.* Evidence that early extrapyramidal symptoms predict later tardive dyskinesia: A prospective analysis of 10,000 patients in the European Schizophrenia Outpatient Health Outcomes Initiative (SOHO) study. *Am J Psychiatry* 2006;163:1438–1440.

Tran E, Rouillon F, Loze J-Y, *et al.* Cancer mortality in patients with schizophrenia. *Cancer* 2009;115:3555–3562.

Verma SK, Subramanian M, Liew A, Poon LY. Metabolic risk factors in drug-naïve patients with first-episode psychosis. *J Clin Psychiatry* 2009;70(7):997–1000.

Vinogradov S, Fisher M, Warm H, *et al.* The cognitive cost of anticholinergic burden: Decreased response to cognitive training in schizophrenia. *Am J Psychiatry* 2009;166:1055–1062.

Volavka J, Citrome L. Oral antipsychotics for the treatment of schizophrenia: Heterogeneity in efficacy and tolerability should drive decision-making. *Expert Opin Pharmacother* 2009;10(12):1917–1928.

Waddington JL, Kapur S, Remington GJ. The neuroscience and clinical psychopharmacology of first- and second-generation antipsychotic drugs. In Hirsch SR, Weinberger D, eds. *Schizophrenia.* 2nd ed. Blackwell Science, Hoboken, 2003, pp. 421–441.

Wang PS, Schneeweiss S, Avorn J, *et al.* Risk of death in elderly users of conventional *vs.* atypical conventional antipsychotics. *N Engl J Med* 2005;353(22):2335–2341.

Woods SW, Morgenstern H, Saksa JR, *et al.* Incidence of tardive dyskinesias with atypical versus conventional antipsychotic medications: A prospective cohort study. *J Clin Psychiatry* 2010;71(4):463–474.

Chapter 4

Description of Individual Antipsychotics

In the previous chapter, we provided a general overview and examined common aspects of antipsychotic medications. Here, we will discuss the distinctive characteristics of individual antipsychotic drugs currently in the U.S. market. For each drug and group of drugs, we will review issues related to pharmacokinetics/metabolism, dosing, and, in some cases, relevant clinical information on efficacy or adverse effects. As previously presented, we do not consider that the separation of antipsychotics into "old," "typical," "conventional," "traditional," or "first-generation," and "atypical" or "second-generation," is supported by existent pharmacological and clinical knowledge. We discuss the two groups separately simply because that is the current use.

4.1 Typical Antipsychotics

Despite the intense promotion and broad use of "atypical" antipsychotics, nearly a dozen "typical" or "conventional" antipsychotics remain in use in the USA, and a larger number of them are still used in Europe and the rest of the world. According to chemical structure, typical antipsychotics are usually divided into:

(1) Phenotiazines
- Aliphatic phenotiazines, such as chlorpromazine (Thorazine)
- Piperidine side-chain phenotiazines, such as thioridazine (Mellaril)
- Piperazine side-chain phenothiazines, such as fluphenazine (Prolixin), perphenazine (Trilafon), prochlorperazine, and trifluoperazine (Stelazine)

(2) Butyrophenones
- Haloperidol (Haldol) or droperidol (Inapsin)

(3) Miscellaneous
- Loxapine (Loxitane)
- Metoclopramide (Reglan)
- Molindone (Moban)
- Pimozide (Orap)
- Thiothixene (Navane)

Below, we review individually the "old" ("typical") antipsychotics currently available in the U.S. market.

4.1.1 *Chlorpromazine*

The first antipsychotic ever introduced, chlorpromazine (Thorazine, Largactil), is a middle-potency dopamine D_2 blocker with lower liability for EPS (extrapyramidal symptoms) than higher-potency agents, either typical or atypical. These characteristics as well as its propensity to induce weight gain, sedation, hypotension/tachycardia, and anticholinergic side effects, resemble middle-potency "atypical" antipsychotics (quetiapine, olanzapine). In the past, jaundice, retinitis pigmentosa, and skin pigmentation were described with chlorpromazine use, but these days they are rarely reported, possibly due to the limited use of the drug. These adverse effects were likely related to the huge doses of "typical" neuroleptics used in past decades, as discussed in the previous chapter on general characteristics of antipsychotics. The absorption of chlorpromazine after oral administration has been reported in the range of 4%–38% and it is dose-dependent, with a significant first-pass effect. Chlorpromazine is metabolized by CYP2D6 and has an elimination half-life of about 11 h.

A recent Chinese 12-month open-label trial compared chlorpromazine with several "atypical" antipsychotics in 1,133 subjects with schizophrenia or schizophreniform disorder, with treatment discontinuation as the primary outcome. Discontinuation rates within 12 months were 41.4% for chlorpromazine, 39.5% for sulpiride, 36.7% for clozapine, 40.2% for risperidone, 39.6% for olanzapine, 46.9% for quetiapine, and 40.2% for aripiprazole, with no significant statistical difference on discontinuation due to relapse, lack of tolerability, patient decision, or non-adherence. EPS were more common with chlorpromazine and sulpiride; anticholinergic side effects were more common with clozapine and chlorpromazine; and weight gain was more common with clozapine and olanzapine (Guo *et al.*, 2011).

The mean dose of chlorpromazine in the above-mentioned study was 334.7 mg/day. The dose recommendation for chlorpromazine in the International Consensus is 100–600 mg/day, with a maximum of 800 mg/day (see Table 3.1). Chlorpromazine is usually administered in two doses, with the larger one taken at night.

4.1.2 *Haloperidol*

Haloperidol (Haldol), at present, has been in use for over half a century. It is a relatively pure dopamine antagonist, with a potent D_2-blocking action and little or no affinity for adrenergic, cholinergic, or histamine receptors. Other than EPS, haloperidol has little potential for side effects/adverse reactions such as sedation, cognitive impairment, or cardiovascular adverse effects. This safety profile includes one of the lowest risks among currently marketed antipsychotics for QT prolongation and malignant arrhythmia (Glassman *et al.*, 2001). For these reasons, haloperidol is still the preferred antipsychotic in delirium and other medical and toxic conditions that affect the mental state and require antipsychotics.

Other positive aspects of haloperidol treatment are:

(1) It is very inexpensive; the cost ratio of daily treatment with haloperidol compared to "atypical" antipsychotics, in both oral and injectable preparations, can be higher than 1:100.
(2) It has a long record of large patient exposure, including pregnant women, with apparently no significant teratogenic effects.
(3) It is available in oral, injectable, and long-acting preparations.

Haloperidol is well absorbed after oral administration. It is metabolized by CYP2D6 with minor contribution by CYP3A4, 5, and 7. The elimination half-life seems to increase with prolonged use, from 1.2 to over 30 days, making it suitable for once-a-day dosing.

Like any other high-potency D_2 blocker, typical or atypical, haloperidol exhibits higher risk for EPS than low- to middle-potency agents. However, in the past, some factors have distorted the estimation of the risk for EPS with haloperidol; (1) until recent years, doses of haloperidol over 20 mg/day were routine (the Prescribing Information for haloperidol in the USA still mentions doses of 100 mg/day); and (2) the usual comparator in the initial studies with atypical antipsychotics was haloperidol used at doses over the current upper limit of the dosage range (Hugenholtz *et al.*, 2006).

Recent independent studies with haloperidol show no significant differences with high-potency "atypical" antipsychotics. In a controlled double-blind study of the German Research Network on Schizophrenia sponsored by the German government, 159 remitted patients were enrolled after treatment of an acute first episode of schizophrenia according to ICD criteria. Antipsychotic treatment with risperidone or haloperidol was maintained in a targeted dose of 2–4 mg/day for one year. One hundred and fifty one patients were eligible for analysis. The authors conclude that both antipsychotics were equally effective regarding significant symptom reduction and improvement in quality of life. EPS were slightly higher with haloperidol, but the overall dropout rate of 68% was not significantly different between the two drug groups (Gaebel *et al.*, 2007).

Regarding cognition, the European First Episode Schizophrenia and Schizophreniform Disorder Clinical Trial (EUFEST) compared the cognitive effects of antipsychotics in patients randomized to open-label haloperidol (1–4 mg/day, $N = 103$), amisulpride (200–800 mg/day, $N = 104$), olanzapine (5–20 mg/day, $N = 105$), quetiapine (200–750 mg/day, $N = 104$), or ziprasidone (40–160 mg/day, $N = 82$). The authors conclude: "Compared with scores at baseline, composite cognitive test scores improved for all five treatment groups at the 6-month follow-up evaluation. However, there were no overall differences among the treatment groups." (Davidson *et al.*, 2009)

The recommended dose of haloperidol in the International Consensus is 3–10 mg/day, with a maximum dose of 20 mg/day (see Table 3.1). The authors routinely start haloperidol at 2 mg daily, or even lower. The dosing recommendation for long-acting injectable haloperidol in the U.S. Prescribing Information is to give a monthly amount equivalent to 10–15 days of oral treatment.

4.1.3 *Loxapine*

Loxapine (Loxitane) has the curious distinction of being the first antipsychotic approved in the USA for inhalation in the treatment of agitation associated with schizophrenia and bipolar disorder.

Loxapine seems to have a lower liability for EPS than high-potency D_2 blockers, as well as moderate risk for sedation and autonomic side effects, and some risk for metabolic and cardiovascular side effects. All of this suggests a middle-potency agent not very different from chlorpromazine, olanzapine, or quetiapine. Oral loxapine is well absorbed in the gastrointestinal tract, but undergoes significant first-pass metabolism, resulting in a bioavailability of only 33%. The time to maximum concentration (T_{max}) after oral and IM (intramuscular) administration is 1–3 h. However, the effect of inhaled loxapine in the control of agitation appears within 10 min (see below). Loxapine seems to have several oxidative metabolic pathways involving

CYP1A2, 2D6, 2C19, and 3A4. These routes result in multiple metabolites, including 7-OH loxapine, which has 4–5 times the affinity of loxapine for the D_2 receptor, and amoxapine. The recommended dose for oral loxapine in the International Consensus is 17.5–100 mg/day with a maximum of 200 mg/day (see Table 3.1).

On 14 December 2012, the FDA approved inhaled loxapine (Adasuve) for use as a single 5 or 10 mg dose in 24 h for the treatment of agitation in patients with schizophrenia and bipolar disorder. The medication should be used with a Risk Evaluation and Mitigation Strategy (REMS). According to the Prescribing Information, Adasuve is very well tolerated. The reported incidence of EPS is very low, with only 1.7% of patients experiencing any EPS (versus 0.4% for placebo). The main risk for Adasuve seems to be bronchospasm in patients with active airway disease. Thus, it is contraindicated in patients with acute respiratory signs/symptoms (e.g., wheezing) or who are taking medications to treat asthma or COPD. The treatment of adverse airway reactions to loxapine is inhalation of a short-acting beta-agonist bronchodilator such as albuterol.

4.1.4 *Molindone*

Molindone (Moban), a high-potency conventional antipsychotic, seems to have the lowest potential for weight gain among all available antipsychotics, typical or atypical (Bagnall *et al.*, 2007). Molindone is a clean dopamine D_2 blocker, with little effect on histamine, cholinergic, or adrenergic receptors. Thus, clinically, the side effects of molindone are mainly EPS. Its elimination half-life is 1.5–2 h; however, it is generally effective in once-a-day dosing.

As discussed in the previous chapter on the general characteristics of antipsychotics, recently, in the USA, the publicly funded Treatment of Early-Onset Schizophrenia Spectrum Disorders (TEOSS) study compared the efficacy and safety of molindone with those of two second-generation antipsychotics, olanzapine and risperidone, in the treatment of early-onset schizophrenia and schizoaffective disorder. The atypicals showed no advantage in efficacy over molindone and, considering the metabolic risks of atypical antipsychotics in the youth, the authors questioned the tendency to use only atypical antipsychotics in the treatment of these disorders (Sikich *et al.*, 2008).

The dose of molindone in the TEOSS study was 10–140 mg/day (versus 2.5–20 mg/day for olanzapine and 0.5–6 mg/day for risperidone). The dosing recommendation for molindone in the International Consensus is 22.5–188 mg/day, with a maximum of 225 mg/day (see Table 3.1).

4.1.5 *Perphenazine*

Perphenazine (Trilafon) is a high-potency "typical" antipsychotic whose clinical side effects are mainly EPS. It was recently in the spotlight as the conventional comparator for the "atypicals" olanzapine, quetiapine, risperidone, and ziprasidone in the treatment of chronic schizophrenia in the publicy funded CATIE study. As discussed in the previous chapter, this study did not show any differences in effectiveness or cognitive effects between perphenazine and the four atypical antipsychotics in the treatment of schizophrenia. Regarding side effects, one of the greatest surprises from CATIE was the lack of statistically significant differences between perphenazine and olanzapine, quetiapine, risperidone, and ziprasidone in any of the scales used to measure EPS (AIMS, Barnes Akathisia Rating Scale, and Simpson Angus EPS). However, perphenazine had a higher rate of discontinuation due to EPS and a lower rate of discontinuation due to weight gain or metabolic effect (Lieberman *et al.*, 2005).

Perphenazine has an elimination half-life of 11–12 h, and is metabolized mainly by CYP2D6. The mean modal dose of perphenazine in the CATIE study was 20.8 mg/day in once-a-day dosing. The dose recommendation for perphenazine in the International Consensus is 8–24 mg/day, with a maximum of 42 mg/day (see Table 3.1).

A combination of perphenazine and amitriptyline (Etrafon) is still available in the USA. The authors see no justification for its use, especially because of toxicity issues. Let us remember that tricyclic antidepressants have significant cardiac toxicity that adds to that of antipsychotic agents, such as perphenazine.

4.1.6 *Pimozide*

Pimozide (Orap) has historical importance as it has traditionally been the preferred antipsychotic in Tourette's syndrome and in delusions involving the skin, such as delusions of parasitosis. However, it has a high potential for QT prolongation and malignant arrhythmia, a problem compounded by the fact that it is metabolized by CYP3A4, a cytochrome subject to inhibition by multiple substances. There are several reports of deaths in patients taking pimozide and cytochrome inhibitors. Considering that several high-potency antipsychotics, especially haloperidol and risperidone, have shown comparable efficacy in the treatment of Tourette's syndrome, the use of pimozide does not seem justified any longer in patients who are not clearly treatment-resistant. The recommended dose of pimozide in the International Consensus is 2–6 mg/day with a maximum of 10 mg/day (see Table 3.1).

4.1.7 *Other high-potency D_2 blockers: Fluphenazine, thiothixene, and trifluoperazine*

Fluphenazine (Prolixin), thiotixene (Navane), and trifluoperazine (Stelazine) are high-potency D_2 antagonists, which have low liability for anticholinergic, histaminergic, or adrenergic side effects, and whose main adverse effects are EPS. An important clinical advantage of fluphenazine is the existence of a long-acting injectable form (fluphenazine decanoate, Prolixin depot), in use in the USA for several decades.

The half-life of oral fluphenazine has been reported as 16.4 ± 13.3 h, and that of oral trifluoperazine as 12.5 ± 1.4 h. The dose recommendation for oral fluphenazine in the International Consensus is 3–15 mg/day, with a maximum of 20 mg/day; for trifluoperazine, it is 5–20 mg/day, with a maximum of 35 mg/day; and for thiothixene, 6–30 mg/day, with a maximum of 40 mg/day (see Table 3.1).

4.1.8 *Antipsychotics to avoid: Mesoridazine and thioridazine*

We mention here thioridazine (Mellaril) and mesoridazine (Serentil) only because these agents are still available in the USA. We see no justification to start new patients on either one of these medications that carry the highest risk for QT prolongation and fatal arrhythmias among all available antipsychotic agents, as well as high potential for seizures, sedation, hypotension, anticholinergic side effects, and degenerative retinopathy.

4.1.9 *"Hidden" antipsychotics: Metoclopramide and prochlorperazine*

Metoclopramide (Reglan, Metozolv) and prochlorperazine (Compazine) are used in gastrointestinal disorders such as nausea, vomiting, gastroparesis, and GERD, very often on a long-term basis. We mention them to remind prescribers that, despite the exclusive use in gastrointestinal conditions, they are antipsychotic drugs. All adverse reactions described for antipsychotics may occur with these two medications, including acute EPS, TD (tardive dyskinesia), and NMS (neuroleptic malignant syndrome). We must warn our patients about taking them simultaneously with antipsychotic treatment, as the combination is likely to trigger toxicity and adverse reactions. Though not approved for sale in the USA, domperidone, another dopamine blocker, is sold in a few other countries. It has an exceedingly high risk for QTc prolongation and malignant arrhythmia that makes its use, for any indication, unjustified.

4.2 Atypical Antipsychotics

As mentioned in the previous chapter, the unique characteristics of clozapine (higher efficacy, low liability for EPS) fueled the belief that a new generation of antipsychotics, safer and more efficacious, was coming to the market. Unfortunately, the "atypical" antipsychotics that followed clozapine have not replicated its superior effect. Besides this, low- to middle-potency "atypicals" (clozapine, quetiapine, and olanzapine) have a lower liability for EPS than pre-existing antipsychotics, yet they carry a high liability for metabolic side effects such as weight gain and the full metabolic syndrome. High-potency "atypical" antipsychotics, on the other hand, tend to show a similar profile to high-potency conventional antipsychotics, with low risk for metabolic side effects and high liability for acute and chronic EPS.

Here, we are describing the "atypical" antipsychotics in the approximate order they were introduced to the U.S. market. This way we are also listing them in descending order regarding the clinical experience and post-introduction information gained for each medication.

4.2.1 *Clozapine*

Clozapine (Clozaril, FazaClo) was introduced to the market in Northern Europe in the early 1970s, and promptly withdrawn, due to the observed high incidence of agranulocytosis among treated patients. After the initial withdrawal, the impression of a better response persisted and led to a U.S. multicenter trial, comparing clozapine with chlorpromazine in treatment-resistant patients. DSM-III schizophrenics who had failed to respond to at least three different antipsychotics were given treatment with haloperidol for six weeks. Those who did not respond entered a double-blind randomized comparison of clozapine (up to 900 mg/day) or chlorpromazine (up to 1,800 mg/day) for six weeks. In the final analysis, 30% of the clozapine-treated patients were categorized as responders compared with 4% of chlorpromazine-treated patients (Kane *et al.*, 1988). Clozapine was then approved for reintroduction in the USA with stringent guidelines.

More recently, the CATIE study confirmed the superiority of clozapine over other "atypical" antipsychotics in treatment-resistant schizophrenic patients. Ninety-nine patients who discontinued treatment with olanzapine, quetiapine, risperidone, or ziprasidone in phase 1 or 1B of CATIE, primarily because of lack of efficacy, were randomized to open-label treatment with clozapine or blinded treatment with another atypical that had not been received during the trial. Time to treatment discontinuation because of inadequate therapeutic effects was significantly longer for clozapine than for olanzapine, quetiapine, or risperidone (McEvoy *et al.*, 2006).

Another interesting positive aspect of clozapine is the possibility that it decreases the risk of suicide and hostility/aggressiveness. Several reports suggest that clozapine decreases suicidality in schizophrenia spectrum disorders. A recent prospective study involved an 18-month comparison of clozapine and olanzapine in 980 patients, a quarter of which were unresponsive to previous treatment and at high risk for suicide. Clozapine proved superior to olanzapine in preventing suicide attempts (Meltzer *et al.*, 2003).

Clozapine is metabolized by CYP1A2, and has an elimination half-life of about 12 h. Care needs to be exercised to avoid the combination with CYP1A2 inhibitors such as fluvoxamine, and with the sudden effect of smoking cessation, as smoking induces the activity of CYP1A2, decreasing the levels of clozapine. Thus, the increase in clozapine levels with smoking cessation may trigger toxicity. Because of its short half-life, but also to minimize its side effects, clozapine is always given in divided doses, at least twice daily, with the larger dose in the evening.

4.2.1.1 *Side effects of clozapine*

Though the risk of agranulocytosis is the most feared feature of clozapine, the drug has the potential for other disturbing side effects and adverse reactions, including seizures, syncope, and myocarditis. Because of the risk of agranulocytosis, the use of clozapine in the USA and industrialized countries is strictly regulated. In the USA, both patient and provider must be entered in a national registry, and the patient must have blood cell counts weekly for the first six months of treatment, biweekly for the next six months, and monthly afterwards. The pharmacy will not dispense the dose for the next period of treatment without a copy of the lab result. The U.S. guidelines for monitoring the white blood cell (WBC) count and absolute neutrophil count (ANC) are complex, but the core principle is stopping therapy when WBC count falls below 3,000/mm^3 and/or ANC falls below 1,500/mm^3.

The best estimate of clozapine-induced agranulocytosis in the first year of treatment seems to be around 0.8% of treated patients (Alvir *et al.*, 1993; Atkin *et al.*, 1998). Most cases of agranulocytosis seem to occur in the first weeks of treatment, with the incidence going down fast with continued treatment. However, the risk seems to persist for decades. A recent Finnish study reports that 10% of cases of agranulocytosis occurred after the second year of treatment, and mentions cases occurring after 13, 14, and 22 years of treatment (Lahdelma *et al.*, 2012). Factors that have been mentioned as increasing the risk for agranulocytosis are: older age at the beginning of treatment, female gender, and Asian ethnicity.

Clozapine has the potential to cause acute and chronic EPS and related syndromes, including TD and NMS. However, its risk for EPS seems to be the lowest among currently marketed antipsychotics. The reasons for this relatively low incidence of motor adverse effects are probably multiple. Clozapine seems to have the lowest affinity among available antipsychotics for the D_2 receptor. After occupation, it disassociates from the receptor faster than other antipsychotics. Thus, it is difficult to go beyond occupancy levels of 80%, the approximate threshold for EPS. Besides this, clozapine is the most anticholinergic among available antipsychotics. Actually, clozapine's affinity for M_1 receptors is higher than that for D_2 receptors. Thus, administering clozapine is equivalent to administering an antipsychotic plus an anticholinergic agent.

The low risk for EPS would make clozapine the preferred medication for the treatment of psychosis/impulsivity in dopamine-deficient patients, such as those with Parkinson's disease (PD) (usually induced by dopaminergic agents). However, because of the risk of agranulocytosis, quetiapine is considered the first-line agent, reserving clozapine for patients who do not tolerate or respond to quetiapine.

Some authorities recommend clozapine as a treatment for antipsychotic-induced TD. Considering that clozapine may cause all types of EPS, including TD, we do not support this practice, especially when taking into account the risks associated with clozapine therapy.

Regarding metabolic side effects, clozapine seems to have the highest potential, among all available antipsychotics, for weight gain, diabetes, and the full metabolic syndrome.

Cognitive side effects, especially, but not only, excessive sedation, are fairly common with clozapine for several reasons, including its anticholinergic and antihistamine effects. Peripheral anticholinergic side effects are also fairly common with clozapine and include difficult-to-treat constipation, dry mouth, urinary difficulty or retention, and ocular side effects such as blurry vision or exacerbation of narrow angle glaucoma. Vascular side effects, including orthostatic hypotension, tachycardia, and syncope, are also frequent with clozapine.

Myocarditis is an often-ignored risk with clozapine. It peaks at the beginning of treatment and goes down fast. The incidence has been estimated at 0.7%–1.2% or even 2% of treated patients, though it is likely that the risk is being underestimated for multiple reasons, including low rates of reporting to databases, variability in the clinical presentation which makes the diagnosis difficult, and low likelihood of psychiatric patients seeking medical attention. The mortality rate in cases of myocarditis has been estimated at about 10%. An Australian analysis including 10 fatal cases found that none of these had cardiac imaging done or was suspected of having myocarditis before death, and three of them had no symptoms of illness before death. Duration of treatment for the fatal cases was 14–33 days with an outlier case of 4.5 months. A significant factor for death in patients with myocarditis was obesity, present in 60% of the fatal, but only in 26% of the non-fatal cases (Ronaldson *et al.*, 2011).

Seizures have been reported to affect 5%–10% of patients taking clozapine. The risk seems to grow at high doses or serum levels or with rapid dose increases. The standard recommendation is to decrease the dose or switch medications. When this is not possible, patients must be given anticonvulsant treatment.

Drooling (sialorrhea) is a disturbing side effect of clozapine. It happens mainly at night but for some patients is a constant occurrence. A useful measure to minimize it is putting 1–2 drops of an ophthalmic preparation of atropine in the mouth before going to bed.

Because of its short half-life, clozapine should be given in several doses a day, with the largest dose in the evening to minimize the impact of adverse effects like sedation and hypotension. These adverse reactions are also a reason to start the medication at low daily doses, usually 50–100 mg/day in adults, going up by increments of 50–100 mg at regular intervals, until the target dose is reached, most frequently 500 mg/day. The maximum dose of clozapine, according to the U.S. Prescribing Information, is 900 mg/day. The recommended dose range of clozapine in the International Consensus is 25–500 mg/day, with a maximum of 800 mg/day (see Table 3.1). However, these limits apply when there is no drug monitoring with serum levels. When there is an unsatisfactory response at the high end of the dosage range, checking the serum levels can be useful. There is a consensus that effective levels start around 350–420 ng/mL. There is no unanimity about the existence of an upper therapeutic limit, with some authors suggesting that levels over 500 or, especially, 600 ng/mL are unlikely to add to the effectiveness but can increase the risk of side effects, especially seizures (Khan *et al.*, 2005).

The other critical indication of clozapine, psychosis or severe impulsivity in PD patients treated with dopamine agonists, usually requires lower doses. Besides this, these patients tend to be older and more vulnerable to adverse effects. Dosing in these patients usually start at 25–50 mg/day, and it is unlikely to go over 200 mg/day. In any case, use of clozapine in these patients has to follow the same rules as those of other indications.

4.2.2 *Risperidone and paliperidone*

Risperidone (Risperdal) is a high-potency D_2 antagonist with high liability for EPS and moderate propensity for vascular and metabolic side effects (it has comparable affinity for α_1-adrenergic and H_1 receptors than D_2 receptors). Paliperidone (Invega) is the main metabolite of risperidone. At bioequivalent doses, the two medications have a similar clinical profile, including effects and side effects.

The only significant difference between risperidone and paliperidone seems to be their metabolism. Risperidone is metabolized by CYP2D6, mainly to 9-hydroxyrisperidone (paliperidone). Paliperidone seems to be, for the most part, excreted unchanged, mainly in the urine. For this reason, it is recommended to decrease the dose of both paliperidone and risperidone in the elderly or in people with renal impairment. The half-lives of risperidone and paliperidone have been reported as 20 h and 23 h, respectively. These half-lives would make the immediate-release tablets suitable for once-a-day administration. Curiously, however, paliperidone (Invega) is marketed in the USA in sustained-release tablets only.

At high doses, the motor side effect profile of risperidone is very similar to that of the high-potency conventional antipsychotics, such as haloperidol. However, because of the affinity for H_1 receptors, risperidone has a higher risk for weight gain than other high-potency antipsychotics. And because of the affinity for adrenergic receptors, risperidone (and consequently paliperidone) have potential for vascular side effects, including priapism, and a large number of reports associate risperidone with this adverse effect. Besides this, risperidone, and possibly paliperidone, seem to have the highest risk for hyperprolactinemia among all available antipsychotics, both conventional and "atypical."

The recommended daily doses for risperidone and paliperidone in the International Consensus are 2–6 mg (with a maximum of 8.5 mg), and 3–9 mg (with a maximum of 12 mg), respectively (see Table 3.1). Both risperidone and paliperidone are available in long-acting injectable forms, Risperdal Consta and Invega Sustenna, respectively.

4.2.3 *Olanzapine*

Olanzapine (Zyprexa) is a middle-potency D_2 antagonist, which would imply less propensity for EPS, but higher risk for metabolic side effects than high-potency agents, both "typical" and "atypical." After clozapine, olanzapine seems to have the highest potential among all currently available antipsychotics for weight gain and diabetes/metabolic syndrome, which is partially due to its high affinity for H_1 receptors. Because of this high affinity for histamine receptors, olanzapine is also a sedative antipsychotic, which poses problems for long-acting preparations, as we will discuss further below. Because of its affinity for adrenergic vascular receptors, olanzapine may cause orthostatic hypotension and other cardiovascular adverse effects.

The mean half-life of olanzapine has been reported as 30 h. It is metabolized mainly by CYP1A2. Thus, similar to clozapine, both serum levels and risk of toxicity may go up when a patient taking olanzapine stops smoking.

The recommended dose for oral olanzapine in the International Consensus is 5–20 mg with a maximum of 30 mg (see Table 3.1). It is usually administered in once-a-day dosing in the evening, because of its sedative potential.

A combination of olanzapine and fluoxetine (Symbiax) has been introduced for the treatment of depressive bipolar I episodes and treatment-resistant depression in the USA. However, in the authors' opinion, the flexibility to titrate each medication individually is an important consideration that tilts the scale in favor of administering the medications separately instead of using a fixed-dose preparation.

Besides oral preparations, olanzapine is also available in short-term injectable and long-acting injectable forms. The long-acting injectable form, Zyprexa Relprevv, has been associated with a post-injection delirium/sedation syndrome. Because of this, in the USA, the use of Zyprexa Relprevv has been regulated this way:

(1) To receive Zyprexa Relprevv, patients need to be registered in a company program (Patient Care Program). The program requires prescriber, healthcare facility, patient, and pharmacy enrollment.
(2) After each injection, patients must be observed at the healthcare facility by a healthcare professional for at least 3 h.

Prolonged delirium/sedation after administration of Zyprexa Relprevv is not an idiosyncratic reaction, but something to be expected, considering the sedative and anticholinergic properties of olanzapine. This is the reason why all other depot antipsychotics available in the USA are high-potency agents with low risk for sedation and anticholinergic effects.

4.2.4 *Quetiapine*

Among antipsychotics currently marketed in the USA, quetiapine (Seroquel, Seroquel XR) has the second lowest risk, after clozapine, for causing EPS.

It has been postulated that this is due to a fast separation from the D_2 receptor, which means a higher dissociation constant. For this reason, quetiapine is the first-line antipsychotic in PD patients with psychosis/impulsivity induced by dopaminergic medications.

Quetiapine, though, has high affinity for H_1 and adrenergic receptors, and thus it has significant liability for sedation, weight gain/metabolic syndrome, and cardiovascular adverse effects such as orthostatic hypotension. There is debate regarding the anticholinergic properties of quetiapine, as some publications report no significant affinity of this antipsychotic for muscarinic receptors, while others find clear anticholinergic actions *in vitro* for quetiapine (Chew *et al.*, 2006). Clinically, however, patients treated with quetiapine show an appreciable incidence of anticholinergic side effects, such as constipation or dry mouth. Additionally, in reports of quetiapine intoxication, anticholinergic effects are prominent (Balit *et al.*, 2003; Rhyee *et al.*, 2010). Disregarding the anticholinergic properties of the parent compound, it is well established that norquetiapine, the most important active metabolite of quetiapine, is a potent anticholinergic drug (see the U.S. Prescribing Information for Seroquel XR).

The combination of cardiovascular and cognitive adverse effects seems to make overdose with quetiapine riskier than that with other commonly used antipsychotics. A case series report states: "In conclusion, acute quetiapine ingestion in adults was associated with coma, respiratory depression requiring intubation, hypotension, and a major outcome of death, and these complications were more likely to occur after quetiapine overdose compared with overdose by all other antipsychotic drugs as a group." (Ngo *et al.*, 2008)

Quetiapine is metabolized basically by CYP3A4, and is subject to interactions with grapefruit juice and other CYP3A4 inhibitors, which may significantly increase its levels and toxicity, and with CYP3A4 inducers, which may significantly decrease its effect. The mean terminal half-life has been reported as 7 h for quetiapine and 12 h for norquetiapine. Because of this short half-life, immediate-release quetiapine has to be given in bid dosing, and a sustained-release preparation (Seroquel XR) has been developed for once-a-day administration in the evening.

In the USA, besides the indications common to other antipsychotics, such as schizophrenia and mania, quetiapine is approved for the treatment of depression in bipolar patients. This last indication is discussed in detail in Chapter 14 on the treatment of bipolar depression. Quetiapine is also approved as "adjunctive treatment in major depressive disorder (MDD)." As discussed in the chapter on treatment of depression, the authors disagree with this use of quetiapine, except in cases of well-documented treatment resistance, for multiple reasons: (1) the efficacy is relatively small; (2) the risk and adverse reactions associated with the addition of antipsychotics are clearly higher than those of adding another antidepressant or a symptom-specific medication, such as a hypnotic; and (3) the cost of "atypical" antipsychotics, such as quetiapine, is exceedingly high. The recommended dose of quetiapine in the International Consensus is 100–800 mg/day, with a maximum of 1,000 mg (see Table 3.1).

4.2.5 *Ziprasidone*

Ziprasidone (Geodon) is a high-potency D_2 blocker with moderate affinity for α-adrenergic receptors, and little affinity for other receptors. Thus, it has high liability for EPS, moderate liability for vascular side effects, and very low liability for metabolic side effects, sedation, and other cognitive adverse effects. In the CATIE study, ziprasidone showed a significantly lower liability for weight gain and other metabolic adverse effects than the other "atypicals" in the study (olanzapine, quetiapine, and risperidone) and the "conventional" comparator, perphenazine. However, ziprasidone has significant liability for EPS, including restlessness/akathisia, and moderate liability for cardiovascular side effects such as hypotension and tachycardia (Tan *et al.*, 2009).

The actions of ziprasidone are due to the parent compound, and its reported half-life is short (about 7 h). Thus, the medication should be administered twice a day. Ziprasidone is metabolized mainly by aldehydeoxidase, with less than one-third oxidized by CYP450 enzymes, especially CYP3A4. Thus, CYP inhibitors such as grapefruit juice and ketoconazole may moderately increase, and CYP inducers such as carbamazepine may moderately decrease, the levels and effect of ziprasidone. The presence of food significantly improves the absorption of ziprasidone, and the medication should always be administered with meals.

The recommended total daily dose of ziprasidone in the International Consensus is 40–160 mg, with a maximum of 200 mg (see Table 3.1). Ziprasidone is given in two equal doses, preferably with food.

4.2.6 *Aripiprazole*

Aripiprazole (Abilify) is a high-potency D_2 blocker with negligible affinity for adrenergic, histamine, or muscarinic receptors. Thus, it should have high risk for EPS and very low risk for sedation, metabolic side effects, and cognitive impairment. The introduction of aripiprazole generated significant interest as it was the first antipsychotic with partial agonism at D_2 receptors. Reportedly, aripiprazole exerts an activity at D_2 receptors that is grossly 25% that of natural dopamine. This created the expectation that aripiprazole could have a risk for EPS significantly lower than other high-potency antipsychotics, and be better tolerated by dopamine-deficient patients, such as those with PD. None of these expectations was fulfilled in clinical practice. Patients on aripiprazole, even at low doses, show a significantly high rate of acute EPS, especially akathisia. In the relatively recent trials of aripiprazole in major depression, the rate of akathisia was 25% (versus 4% for placebo) plus a rate of 12% for "restlessness" (versus 2% for placebo) (see current U.S. Prescribing Information for Abilify). This higher-than-expected incidence of motor side effects with the use of aripiprazole also applies to late EPS such as TD (Sierra Pena *et al.*, 2011).

Contrary to expectations, aripiprazole was also found to significantly worsen the motor problems in patients with PD. Thus, the most recent publications on the treatment of psychosis/impulsivity in PD patients continue to recommend clozapine and quetiapine as the only safe antipsychotics in PD (Fernandez, 2012).

Aripiprazole is metabolized by CYP2D6 and 3A4. Thus, inhibitors for these enzymes may increase, and inducers may decrease, the levels and toxicity of the medication. For example, co-administration of quinidine, a CYP2D6 inhibitor, may grossly duplicate the levels of aripiprazole. On the other hand, co-administration of carbamazepine, a known CYP3A4 inducer, may decrease the levels of aripiprazole by two-thirds (see U.S. Prescribing Information). Aripiprazole has a very long half-life. Reported mean elimination half-lives for aripiprazole are 75 h for extensive CYP2D6 metabolizers, and 146 h for poor CYP2D6 metabolizers. This long half-life has the advantage that levels of aripiprazole fluctuate less than other antipsychotics with missed doses, but also the disadvantage that adverse reactions are longer lived and levels continue to increase for a longer period after the medication is started or the dose increased, with higher risk for late toxicity. Aripiprazole is also available in the USA in a long-acting injectable form (Abilify Maintena).

In the USA, besides the indications common to other antipsychotics (such as schizophrenia and mania), aripiprazole is approved for "adjunctive treatment of major depressive disorder (MDD)." As discussed in Chapter 10 on the treatment of depression, the authors disagree with this use of aripiprazole, except in cases of proven resistance to antidepressant treatment, for several reasons:

(1) The efficacy of adding aripiprazole in depression, as stated in one of the largest and most recent studies, is "marginal" (Fava *et al.*, 2012).

(2) In depression, the risks and adverse effects of adding antipsychotics are clearly bigger than those of adding another antidepressant or a symptom-specific medication (for example, sleeping aids).
(3) The cost ratio among brand antipsychotics, such as Abilify, and first-line generic antidepressants can be higher than 100:1.

The recommended dose for aripiprazole in the International Consensus is 10–30 mg/day (see Table 3.1). In schizophrenic or bipolar patients, the authors not infrequently start at a dose of 5 mg/day.

4.2.7 *Iloperidone*

Iloperidone (Fanapt) is a medication with high potency to block D_2 receptors, the main determinant of EPS with antipsychotics. This means that iloperidone should have a risk for EPS in line with other high-potency antipsychotics such as haloperidol, risperidone, ziprasidone, aripiprazole, asenapine, and lurasidone.

A significant problem with iloperidone is its high affinity for α-adrenergic receptors, especially α_2, which makes it a high-risk medication for adverse vascular reactions, including hypotension and syncope. To minimize this risk, iloperidone should be started at a very low dose of 1 mg bid, and increased gradually to the target dose of 6–12 mg bid (in the USA, the manufacturer offers a starting package). As is the case with other recently introduced antipsychotics, the therapeutic dose range initially recommended for iloperidone seems too narrow, and very likely will change as providers gain experience with the medication.

Iloperidone is metabolized sequentially by CYP2D6 and then CYP3A4. Of these two steps, the initial hydroxylation by CYP2D6 seems to be the most important. The elimination half-life has been reported as 18 h in extensive CYP2D6 metabolizers and 33 h in poor CYP2D6 metabolizers. Despite this relatively long half-life, the medication should be given twice a day, probably to minimize the risk of cardiovascular adverse events. Extreme care should be exercised when combining iloperidone with CYP2D6 inhibitors, such as fluoxetine, paroxetine, duloxetine, or bupropion.

4.2.8 *Asenapine*

Asenapine (Saphris) is a high-potency D_2 blocker that also shows high affinity for histamine H_1 and α_1- and α_2-adrenergic receptors. According to this receptor affinity profile, besides a high risk for EPS, asenapine should exhibit high risk for sedation and metabolic and vascular side effects (including weight gain/metabolic syndrome, and hypotension). However, the U.S. Prescribing Information reports a low risk for weight gain. The medication was introduced to the USA in a relatively recent date, and it is too early to estimate the actual risk for weight gain and other metabolic side effects. Regarding the very narrow range of therapeutic doses recommended, 5–10 mg bid, it will surely change, going up, as providers gain clinical experience with the medication.

Administration of asenapine is cumbersome. Intestinal absorption yields very poor serum levels and, when administered orally, the bioavailability is less than 2%. Because of this, asenapine is marketed in the USA in the form of sublingual tablets. This type of administration reportedly results in a bioavailability of 35%. Thus, unsupervised administration of asenapine requires a very cooperative patient. The tablets are to be put under the tongue only, and the patient has to avoid eating and drinking for 10 min afterwards.

Asenapine seems to be the only marketed antipsychotic eliminated through conjugation (glucuronidation). *In vitro* studies show that asenapine is metabolized mainly via glucuronidation by UGT1A4, with minor contributions by CYP enzymes, especially 1A2. However, the fact that smoking does not change the pharmacokinetics of asenapine *in vivo*, probably means that the contribution by CYP1A2 is insignificant.

4.2.9 *Lurasidone*

Lurasidone (Latuda) is a potent D_2 blocker with very low affinity for adrenergic receptors, and negligible affinity for histamine or muscarinic receptors. Thus, it has high liability for EPS but very low risk for sedation, metabolic, or cardiovascular adverse effects.

Lurasidone is metabolized mainly by oxidation by CYP3A4. The reported mean half-life is 18 h, and it has active metabolites. Thus, the medication is administered once a day.

Lurasidone has not been in the U.S. market long enough to allow clinicians to estimate a reliable range of therapeutic doses. The recommended initial dose in the U.S. Prescribing Information is 40 mg/day, with a maximum recommended dose of 160 mg/day. Considering the experience with other antipsychotics, this range seems too narrow, and very likely it will widen over time, by using a lower starting dose, or a higher maximum dose, or both.

References

Alvir JM, Lieberman JA, Safferman AZ, *et al.* Clozapine-induced agranulocytosis. Incidence and risk factors in the US. *N Engl J Med* 1993;329(3):162–167.

Atkin K, Kendall F, Gould D, *et al.* Neutropenia and agranulocytosis in patients receiving clozapine in the UK and Ireland. *Br J Psychiatry* 1996;169(4):483–488.

Bagnall A, Fenton M, Kleijnen J, *et al.* Molindone for schizophrenia and severe mental illness. *Cochrane Database Syst Rev* 2000;(2):CD002083.

Balit CR, Isbister GK, Hackett LP, *et al.* Quetiapine poisoning: A case series. *Ann Emerg Med* 2003;42:751–758.

Chew ML, Mulsant BH, Pollock BG, *et al.* A model of anticholinergic activity of atypical antipsychotic medications. *Schizophr Res* 2006;88:63–72.

Davidson M, Galderisi S, Weiser M, *et al.* Cognitive effects of antipsychotic drugs in first episode schizophrenia and schizophreniform disorder: A randomized open-label clinical trial (EUFEST). *Am J Psychiatry* 2009;166(6):675–682.

Fava M, Mischoulon D, Iosifescu D, *et al.* A double-blind, placebo-controlled study of aripiprazole adjunctive to antidepressant therapy among depressed outpatients with inadequate response to antidepressant therapy (ADAPT-A Study). *Psychother Psychosom* 2012;81(2):87–97.

Fernandez HH. Updates in the medical management of Parkinson's disease. *Cleve Clin J Med* 2012;79(1):28–53.

Gaebel W, Riesbeck M, Wolwer W, *et al.* Maintenance treatment with risperidone or low-dose haloperidol in first-episode schizophrenia: 1-year results of a randomized controlled trial within the German Network Research on Schizophrenia. *J Clin Psychiatry* 2007;68(11):1763–1774.

Glassman AH, Bigger JT. Antipsychotic drugs: Prolonged QTc interval, torsade de pointes, and sudden death. *Am J Psychiatry* 2001;158:1774–1782.

Guo X, Fang M, Zhai J, *et al.* Effectiveness of maintenance treatment with atypical and typical antipsychotics in stable schizophrenia with early stage: 1-year naturalistic study. *Psychopharmacology* 2011, doi: 10.1007/s002130-11-2242-3

Hugenholtz GW, Heerdink ER, Stolker JJ, *et al.* Haloperidol dose when used as active comparator in randomized controlled trials with atypical antipsychotics in schizophrenia: Comparison with officially recommended doses. *J Clin Psychiatry* 2006; 67(6):897–903.

Kane JM, Honigfeld G, Singer J, *et al.* Clozapine for the treatment-resistant schizophrenic: A double-blind comparison with chlorpromazine. *Arch Gen Psychiatry* 1988; 45(9):789–796.

Khan AY, Preskorn SH. Examining concentration-dependent toxicity of clozapine: Role of therapeutic drug monitoring. *J Psychiatr Pract* 2005;11:289–301.

Lahdelma L, Appelberg B. Clozapine-induced agranulocytosis in Finland, 1982–2007: Long-term monitoring of patients still warranted. *J Clin Psychiatry* 2012;73(6):837–842.

McEvoy JP, Lieberman JA, Stroup TS, *et al.* Effectiveness of clozapine versus olanzapine, quetiapine, and risperidone in patients with chronic schizophrenia who did not respond to prior atypical antipsychotic treatment. *Am J Psychiatry* 2006;163:600–610.

Meltzer HY, Alphs L, Green AL, *et al.* Clozapine for treatment of suicidality in schizophrenia: International Suicide Prevention Trial (InterSePT). *Arch Gen Psychiatry* 2003; 60(1):82–91.

Ngo A, Ciranni M, Olson KR. Acute quetiapine overdose in adults: A 5-year retrospective case series. *Ann Emerg Med* 2008;52:541–547.

Rhyee SH, Pedapati EV, Thompson J. Prolonged delirium after quetiapine overdose. *Pediatr Emerg Care* 2010;26(10):754–756.

Ronaldson KJ, Fitzgerald PB, Taylor AJ, *et al.* Clinical course and analysis of ten fatal cases of clozapine-induced myocarditis and comparison with 66 surviving cases. *Schizophr Res* 2011;128(1–3):161–165.

Sierra Pena M, Yaltho TC, Jankovic J. Tardive dyskinesia and other movement disorders secondary to aripiprazole. *Mov Disord* 2011;26(1):147–152.

Sikich L, Fraziere JA, McClellan J, *et al.* Double-blind comparison of first- and second-generation antipsychotics in early-onset schizophrenia and schizoaffective disorder: Findings from the Treatment of Early-Onset Schizophrenia Spectrum Disorders (TEOSS) study. *Am J Psychiatry* 2008;165:1420–1431.

Tan HH, Hoppe J, Heard K. A systematic review of cardiovascular effects after atypical antipsychotic medication overdose. *Am J Emerg Med* 2009;27:607–616.

Chapter 5

Treatment of Schizophrenia with Antipsychotic Medications

5.1 Choice of an Antipsychotic for the Initial Treatment of Schizophrenia

The authors feel that rather than simply making a choice between "typical" and "atypical" antipsychotics, the selection of an antipsychotic for the initial treatment of schizophrenia is essentially a trade-off between the risk for metabolic side effects (higher with low-to-moderate D_2-blocking potency agents such as chlorpromazine, clozapine, olanzapine, and quetiapine) and the risk for motor adverse effects (greater with high D_2-blocking potency agents such as haloperidol, fluphenazine, perphenazine, risperidone/paliperidone, ziprasidone, aripiprazole, lurasidone, asenapine, and iloperidone). For both large antipsychotic classes, "typical" and "atypical," there are agents with different degrees of dopaminergic-blocking potency. Therefore, we do not consider the distinction of "typical" versus "atypical" an essential factor when choosing an antipsychotic drug for the treatment of schizophrenia.

It must be kept in mind also, that besides the above-mentioned general risks, some individual antipsychotics bring drug-specific risks, such as the increased risk of hyperprolactinemia with risperidone/paliperidone, the higher risk of QT prolongation with thioridazine and ziprasidone, or the higher risk of orthostatic hypotension, syncope, and tachycardia with clozapine, iloperidone, chlorpromazine, and, to a lesser extent, quetiapine. Other factors that need to be considered when selecting an antipsychotic include access (e.g., cost and coverage by health insurers), dosing requirements that may impair compliance (e.g., more than one dose a day, medications that need to be given sublingually instead of orally such as asenapine, and medications that need to be titrated up carefully to avoid adverse effects such as iloperidone), and personal factors of the patient (e.g., illnesses such as obesity or diabetes, EPS [extrapyramidal symptoms] from previous antipsychotic treatment and, obviously, history of response). For a detailed discussion of the adverse effects and risks of antipsychotic drugs, please see Chapter 3 on general description of antipsychotics.

5.2 Dosing in the Initial Antipsychotic Treatment of Schizophrenia

The recommendations on the proper dosing for the initial antipsychotic treatment of schizophrenia have changed significantly in recent years. As mentioned in Chapter 3, high initial doses were recommended since the introduction of antipsychotics in the 1950s until the end of the 20th century, on the assumption that the higher the dopamine blockade, the better the therapeutic response. However, it is now recognized that initial high doses do not improve the chances of, or lessen the time to, response and significantly increase treatment risks and impair compliance with treatment. Regarding recommendations on initial, "target," and maximum doses of antipsychotics in schizophrenic patients, we refer the reader to Table 3.1, in the chapter on general description of antipsychotics. The authors, however, not infrequently, start patients at lower doses than those recommended by the consensus in that publication, especially when using high-potency "typical" antipsychotics. For example, an initial daily dose of 1 or 2 mg of haloperidol could be effective in many patients while minimizing the risk for adverse reactions, especially EPS (Emsley *et al.*, 2006).

5.3 How Long Does It Take to Respond to an Antipsychotic?

An aspect of antipsychotic treatment still highly debated is for how long we should administer an antipsychotic before deciding that a patient is unresponsive. In this regard, relatively recent evidence tells us that the time to response in schizophrenic patients treated with antipsychotics varies widely, with some patients responding in the first few days and others requiring several weeks or even months of treatment to respond.

Among recent studies of the time course for antipsychotic treatment response, we want to highlight a large multinational, randomized, double-blind comparison of risperidone and haloperidol, in 522 patients with first-episode schizophrenia, in which response was determined at weekly intervals for a median treatment length of 206 days. Both medications were started at a low dose of 1 mg/day that was increased, if necessary, by 1 mg/day after three days and then at weekly intervals to a maximum dose of 4 mg/day. In some cases of insufficient response with good tolerability, the weekly increases continued up to a maximum daily dose of 8 mg. Of the 522 patients, approximately three-quarters responded to treatment (defined as a ≥20% reduction in the PANSS total score). Of these responders, close to a quarter responded during the first week and another quarter during the second week, meaning that approximately half of the responders have done so in the first two weeks of treatment. The number of responders continued increasing after that, but at a lower rate; grossly 80% of responders have responded by the fourth week, grossly 90% by the eighth week, and the response rate seemed to plateau after approximately six months (Emsley *et al.*, 2006).

Another study of the time to response to antipsychotic treatment was designed by the German Research Network on Schizophrenia. It included 280 inpatients with both first- and multiple-episode schizophrenia, treated under naturalistic conditions with both typical and atypical antipsychotics combined with psychoeducation, social skills training, and family education. It showed a total response rate of 78.6%, similar to that in the study of the previous reference, though the progression of response was slower. Of the responders, almost half of them responded by the fourth week, and about 80% responded by the eighth week (Jager *et al.*, 2010).

An analysis of 112 patients with first-episode psychosis treated with low initial doses of olanzapine (2.5 mg/day) and risperidone (1mg/day) showed a more gradual response curve, with only 2.8% of subjects responding after one week, 21.8% responding after four weeks, 39.6% responding after eight weeks, 54.4% responding after 12 weeks, and 65.4% responding after 16 weeks (Gallego *et al.*, 2010).

Because of the above-mentioned evidence, the authors support an active but parsimonius approach for the initial treatment of schizophrenia, with initial monotherapy at low doses and regular increases (e.g., weekly or biweekly) according to response, for at least 8–16 weeks, unless exceptional circumstances are present, such as worsening symptoms, complete lack of response after several weeks, significant adverse reactions, suicidality, etc.

As mentioned in the discussion of abnormal movements in Chapter 3, the authors do not recommend starting prophylactic anticholinergic agents simultaneously with antipsychotic drugs to prevent EPS. The reason for this is our belief that early EPS are not a benign symptom because they predict late serious EPS such as tardive dyskinesia. For the same reason, when a patient experiences EPS, we prefer, whenever possible, to decrease the antipsychotic dose or switch to an agent with lower risk for motor adverse effects rather than adding anticholinergic agents.

5.4 Monitoring Antipsychotic Treatment

Around the time of antipsychotic treatment initiation, it is important to perform a baseline examination of abnormal movements; record vital signs such as height, weight/BMI, abdominal circumference, blood pressure, and cardiac frequency; ask for basic laboratory work including glucose, lipids, and electrolytes; and, in patients over 50 years old or with a history of cardiac illness or family history of prolonged QT interval, obtain an ECG. Follow-up determinations of all these parameters should be done at regular intervals. Prolactin should be measured in patients who report symptoms commonly associated with hyperprolactinemia such as sexual dysfunction, menstrual irregularities, or breast engorgement.

At every visit, patients on antipsychotics should be asked/screened for the most common adverse clinical effects of antipsychotic drugs, such as weight gain, motor adverse effects (EPS), sexual dysfunction, menstrual irregularities, and breast engorgement.

5.5 Maintenance of Antipsychotic Treatment of Schizophrenia

Schizophrenia is considered a chronic, progressive illness and the standard recommendation has been to continue treatment after the symptoms have improved or disappeared, to prevent relapses or exacerbations. The validity of this approach seems to be confirmed in a recent analysis of 116 randomized placebo-controlled studies of antipsychotic treatment after stabilization, in patients with a diagnosis of schizophrenia. The primary outcome was relapse between seven and 12 months. Antipsychotic drugs significantly reduced relapse rates at one year (27% *vs.* 64% for placebo; RR: 0.40, 95% CI: 0.33–0.49; NNT to benefit 3, 95% CI: 2–3). Depot preparations reduced relapse more than oral drugs (Leucht *et al.*, 2012).

However, prolonged treatment with antipsychotic medications carries significant risks, especially, but not exclusively, for abnormal movements and metabolic adverse effects. Thus, as concluded in the above study, "the advantages of these drugs must be weighed against their side effects." Considering that the risk for the most important adverse reactions to antipsychotics, including motor and metabolic, is dose-dependent, periodic attempts should be made in all patients, but particularly in those who require high doses for stabilization, to find the minimum necessary dose to keep the patient stable.

Besides this, as mentioned before, regular clinical and laboratory monitoring of adverse reactions is mandatory, including periodic examinations for abnormal movements; measurement of vital signs including height, weight/BMI, abdominal circumference, blood pressure, and pulse; and laboratory determinations of glucose, lipids, electrolytes, and, if indicated, prolactin (for a detailed discussion of the adverse reactions and risks associated with antipsychotic drug treatment, see Chapter 3).

5.6 Combination of Antipsychotic Drugs in Schizophrenia ("Polypharmacy")

The combined administration of two or more antipsychotic drugs seems to be on the rise worldwide, despite the lack of evidence to support its therapeutic benefits. The authors disallow the concomitant administration of antipsychotic medications for multiple reasons, including:

(1) Lack of evidence about any therapeutic benefit. Other than combinations with clozapine, *where the data is weak anyway*, there is no evidence to support the practice.
(2) Increased risk for adverse effects. Because of the common underlying mechanisms of action, the risk for adverse reactions with antipsychotic "polypharmacy" is additive.
(3) Increased risk for drug–drug interactions (DDIs). Combinations of medications increase the stress on common metabolic pathways and the number of potential DDIs.
(4) Decreased medication adherence. It has been demonstrated that the higher the number of medications and doses, the lower the medication compliance with all of the drugs.
(5) Substantially increased cost, especially when the newer "atypical" medications are used.
(6) Difficult dose adjustments, both in case of symptom exacerbation or adverse reactions.

A common medication addition these days is that of a sedative antipsychotic as a sleeping aid. This practice creates liability for the prescriber and unjustified risks for the patient, as significantly safer and cheaper hypnotic medications are available. Another frequent justification for keeping patients on several antipsychotics is the observation of symptomatic improvement when a new drug is added. Considering that the improvement is likely due to the most recent medication, the sound approach is completing the switch as planned instead of keeping the patient on both medications indefinitely.

5.7 Pharmacological Management of Treatment-Resistant Schizophrenia

Another critical subject in the treatment of schizophrenia is the number of antipsychotic trials a patient must have before concluding that he/she is "treatment-resistant" so that clozapine treatment may be considered. Clozapine is a useful and, very often, necessary medication, but its use entails significant practical difficulties and medical risks. Besides this, the total number of available antipsychotics, including "typical" and "atypical," keeps growing. Because of these facts, unless exceptional circumstances are present, the authors consider that the threshold of two failed antipsychotic trials before recurring to clozapine, which is supported by many experts, is too low. We favor multiple trials, that are long enough and that use doses up to the high range, unless there is poor tolerability. Even though there is no well-documented evidence to support this recommendation, the authors believe that the various antipsychotics tried should be as heterogeneous as possible. For example, this process should include both high- and low-to-moderate-potency agents, both typical and atypical antipsychotics, drugs with different metabolic pathways, and so on.

We must point out that there are several non-pharmacological interventions that should be considered, as they have been proven to be very helpful as a complement for pharmacological treatment. However, these are beyond the scope of this handbook.

Regarding medications, the only helpful approach to treatment-resistant schizophrenia appears to be the use of clozapine. The authors consider that currently, the only valid reasons for the clinical use of clozapine are treatment-resistant psychoses, either schizophreniform or affective, or in special circumstances, when clozapine's little potential for EPS brings a particular advantage (e.g., psychosis in patients with Parkinson's disease). For a description of the use of clozapine, we refer the reader to Chapter 4.

5.8 Use of Long-Acting Injectable Antipsychotics in Schizophrenia

The usefulness of long-acting injectable (LAI) antipsychotics to solve the problem with medication adherence, so prevalent with oral antipsychotics, has been a matter of debate for decades, and recent evidence still provides contradictory information. On the negative side, we have a prospective randomized comparison of oral antipsychotics and LAI risperidone in patients with schizophrenia or schizoaffective disorder who had been hospitalized within the previous two years or were at imminent risk of hospitalization, at the U.S. Veterans Administration. Of 369 participants, 40% were hospitalized at randomization, 55% were hospitalized within the previous two years, and 5% were at risk of hospitalization. The rate of hospitalization after randomization was not different among patients on LAI risperidone and patients on oral antipsychotics (39% after 10.8 months *vs.* 45% after 11.3 months; hazard ratio: 0.87; 95% CI: 0.63–1.20). There were no differences either in psychiatric symptoms, quality of life, scales of personal and social performance, and neuropsychological side effects. Patients on LAI risperidone reported more EPS (Rosenheck *et al.*, 2011).

On the positive side, we wish to mention a Finnish nationwide study of oral and depot antipsychotics examining the risk of rehospitalization and drug discontinuation in a cohort of 2,588 consecutive patients hospitalized for the first time with a diagnosis of schizophrenia. In a pairwise comparison between LAIs and the equivalent oral formulations, the risk of rehospitalization for patients receiving LAIs was about one-third of that for patients receiving oral medications (adjusted hazard ratio: 0.36; 95% CI: 0.17–0.75). An important limitation of this study, however, is that a minority of patients adhered to the initial antipsychotic in the first 60 days after discharge (only 58.2% of patients collected a prescription for an antipsychotic during the first 30 days post-discharge and only 45% continued treatment for 30 days or longer) (Tiihonen *et al.*, 2011).

A possible explanation for these contrasting results can be found in a systematic review of LAI antipsychotics in the treatment of schizophrenia and special populations at risk for treatment non-adherence of both randomized and naturalistic studies that included among its conclusions the following statement: "They [the results] also suggest that LAIs reduce risk of relapse versus oral antipsychotics in schizophrenia outpatients when combined with quality psychosocial interventions." (Zhornitsky *et al.*, 2012) Thus, it is likely that starting patients on LAIs and sending them back to treatment as usual makes little difference with oral antipsychotics, while using enriched approaches to improve compliance can show additional benefits for LAI antipsychotics.

References

Emsley R, Rabinowitz J, Medori R. Time course for antipsychotic treatment response in first-episode schizophrenia. *Am J Psychiatry* 2006;163:743–745.

Gallego JA, Robinson DG, Sevy SM, *et al.* Time to treatment response in first-episode schizophrenia: Should acute treatment trials last several months? *J Clin Psychiatry* 2011; 72(12):1691–1696.

Jager M, Riedel M, Obermeier M, *et al.* Time course of antipsychotic treatment response in schizophrenia: Results from a naturalistic study in 280 patients. *Schizophr Res* 2010;118:183–188.

Leucht S, Tardy M, Komossa K, *et al.* Antipsychotic drugs versus placebo for relapse prevention in schizophrenia: A systematic review and meta-analysis. *Lancet* 2012;379: 2063–2071.

Rosenheck RA, Krystal JH, Lew R, *et al.* Long-acting injectable risperidone and oral antipsychotics in unstable schizophrenia. *N Engl J Med* 2011;364:824–851.

Tiihonen J, Haukka J, Taylor M, *et al.* A nationwide cohort study of oral and depot antipsychotics after first hospitalization for schizophrenia. *Am J Psychiatry* 2011;168: 603–609.

Zhornistky S, Stip E. Oral versus long-acting injectable antipsychotics in the treatment of schizophrenia and special populations at risk for treatment non-adherence: A systematic review. *Schizophr Res Treat* 2012;2012:407171.

Chapter 6

Antidepressants: Selective Serotonin Reuptake Inhibitors and Serotonin–Norepinephrine Reuptake Inhibitors

6.1 Introduction

Since the almost simultaneous introduction of the first antidepressants, antipsychotics, and tranquillizers in the 1950s, the most dramatic single event in clinical psychopharmacology has been perhaps the introduction of the first selective serotonin reuptake inhibitor (SSRI), fluoxetine (Prozac), in 1988. Its vastly superior safety and tolerability profile radically changed the public's view of antidepressant treatment and even depression itself. Today, SSRIs are the most widely used psychotropic medications, with a range of indications going from depression and anxiety to aggression and menstrual mood disturbances. Seven SSRIs are currently available in the USA: fluoxetine (Prozac), fluvoxamine (Luvox), paroxetine (Paxil), sertraline (Zoloft), citalopram (Celexa), citalopram's isomer S-citalopram (Lexapro), and vilazodone (Viibryd).

Serotonin–norepinephrine reuptake inhibitors (SNRIs) have been around for almost as long as SSRIs. Immediate-release venlafaxine (Effexor) was introduced in 1994 and extended-release preparations (Effexor XR) were introduced three years later. Duloxetine (Cymbalta) was introduced in 2004, desvenlafaxine (Pristiq) in 2008, and milnacipram (Savella) in 2009. Different from SSRIs, which only inhibit serotonin reuptake, SNRIs inhibit both the serotonin and norepinephrine reuptake pumps, working in a way similar to a group of old antidepressants, the tricyclic antidepressants (TCAs). However, as with SSRIs, the main advantage of SNRIs over the first-generation antidepressants is not increased efficacy, but an improved safety and tolerability profile. SNRIs are relatively safe and tolerable medications, though less so than SSRIs, for reasons we will discuss in detail later in this chapter.

6.2 Pharmacodynamics of SSRIs and SNRIs (Receptor Affinity)

SSRIs. As the name indicates, SSRIs are highly selective blockers of the serotonin reuptake pump (5-HT transporter) compared to other monoamine transporters, especially the norepinephrine (NE) and dopamine (DA) transporters. Different studies give variable figures regarding the affinity of the various SSRIs for each of the three main monoamine transporters, and some authors emphasize that paroxetine has the highest affinity among SSRIs for the NE transporter, and sertraline the highest for the DA transporter. However, regardless of the method used to measure it, for all SSRIs, receptor affinity for the 5-HT transporter is >100 times higher than those for the NE and DA transporters. Regarding other receptors, among SSRIs, paroxetine shows the highest affinity for the M_1 receptor and sertraline the highest for the α_1 receptor. Nevertheless, the scarcity of anticholinergic effects such as constipation or urinary retention with paroxetine, and vascular side effects such as hypotension with sertraline, probably indicate that this affinity does not have major clinical significance.

Regarding their effect on the serotonin transporter, citalopram and escitalopram are very similar medications. Citalopram is the racemic mixture of two enantiomers, R- and S-citalopram. However, only the S-isomer is biologically active at the transporter. This was the rationale to offer purified S-citalopram, which needs only half of the citalopram dose in weight. At bioequivalent doses (citalopram 2 mg = escitalopram 1 mg), the clinical effect of the two preparations is probably similar. However, they may differ in other aspects, such as the risk for QT prolongation, as we discuss later in this same chapter.

Apparently, the SSRI vilazodone is also a partial agonist at serotonin 5-HT_{1A} receptors. This agonism is unlikely to bring about a significant difference between vilazodone and other SSRIs or SNRIs, as all of them, by increasing the amount of extracellular serotonin, increase agonism at serotonin receptors, including $5HT_{1A}$. In any case, the side effect and adverse reaction profile of vilazodone seems identical to that of other SSRIs.

SNRIs. The distinctive characteristic of SNRIs is their ability to inhibit the reuptake of both serotonin and NE. Pharmacologically, SNRIs are more heterogeneous than SSRIs. All SNRIs exert a potent action at the serotonin transporter, but they differ in their potency at the NE transporter. Venlafaxine and desvenlafaxine have a significantly higher affinity for the 5-HT than the NE transporter. It has been argued that these two medications are basically serotonergic at low doses and that the noradrenergic effect appears gradually as the dose increases. Duloxetine has a moderately higher affinity for the 5-HT than the NE transporter, and milnacipram seems to show an affinity in the same order of magnitude for both transporters.

Regarding possible differences in the effects of venlafaxine and desvenlafaxine, let us remember that desvenlafaxine is the main metabolite of venlafaxine, and it has a longer half-life (10 h) than that of venlafaxine (4 h). Because of this, patients who take venlafaxine have a longer exposition to desvenlafaxine than to the parent compound. This poses the question of what is the contribution of desvenlafaxine to the therapeutic effect of venlafaxine. In line with this, some publications suggest that CYP2D6 poor metabolizers, which have a low venlafaxine to desvenlafaxine conversion rate, tend to respond poorly to venlafaxine.

Some authorities, when comparing SNRIs with SSRIs, argue that medications having two potential antidepressant or anti-anxiety mechanisms at work should be better than those having just one. As of yet, no individual second-generation antidepressant agent has been proved conclusively better either in its own group or compared to others for the treatment of depression or anxiety disorders. Besides this, though very safe and tolerable, because of their additional adrenergic action, SNRIs have a wider range of potential side effects and are more toxic than SSRIs.

6.3 Pharmacokinetics of SSRIs and SNRIs

All SSRIs are well absorbed after oral administration. The absorption of vilazodone seems to increase by approximately 150% when administered with food. SSRIs are eliminated basically through oxidation by the CYP450 system: fluvoxamine by CYP1A2, paroxetine and fluoxetine by CYP2D6, sertraline and vilazodone mainly by CYP3A4 (though reportedly vilazodone is also a substrate for non-CYP enzymes such as carboxylesterase), and citalopram/escitalopram by CYP3A4, CYP2C19, and other cytochromes. The SSRI with the shortest elimination half-life is fluvoxamine (15 h); citalopram/escitalopram, paroxetine, sertraline, and vilazodone have half-lives close to one day (20–30 h); and fluoxetine has a significantly longer half-life (3–4 days for the parent compound, up to two weeks counting active metabolites). Another pharmacokinetic difference among SSRIs is that while fluvoxamine, paroxetine, and vilazodone do not have active metabolites, citalopram/escitalopram, fluoxetine, and sertraline do. Thus, the last four drugs have a pharmacological effect longer than the half-life of the parent compounds would suggest. This lack of active metabolites is another possible explanation, for example, for the high incidence of discontinuation syndrome observed with paroxetine, as will be discussed later.

All SNRIs — venlafaxine, desvenlafaxine, duloxetine, and milnacipram — are well absorbed after oral administration. Venlafaxine is transformed by CYP2D6 into desvenlafaxine (O-desmethylvenlafaxine). Desvenlafaxine is then eliminated mainly through conjugation and, to a minor extent, through oxidation by CYP3A4. Duloxetine is metabolized by CYP1A2 and 2D6. Milnacipram is eliminated mostly unchanged in urine, and, a minor part, through conjugation. All available SNRIs have short half-lives. The elimination half-lives for venlafaxine, desvenlafaxine, duloxetine and milnacipram are 4 h, 10 h, 12 h, and 8 h, respectively. Immediate-release SNRIs need to be administered in several doses a day. Regular venlafaxine (Effexor) must be given in two or three doses a day, and milnacipram (Savella) is given twice a day. Effexor XR capsules, venlafaxine ER tablets, Cymbalta capsules, and Pristiq tablets, scheduled for once-a-day dosing, are all extended-release preparations.

6.4 Use of SSRIs in Mental Disorders

Below are the U.S. FDA approved indications for SSRIs:

(1) Major Depressive Disorder (MDD)
(2) Generalized Anxiety Disorder (GAD)
(3) Obsessive–Compulsive Disorder (OCD)
(4) Panic Disorder
(5) Post-Traumatic Stress Disorder (PTSD)
(6) Social Anxiety Disorder (SAD)
(7) Bulimia Nervosa
(8) Premenstrual Dysphoric Disorder
(9) Bipolar Depression (fluoxetine plus olanzapine)

We must notice that no SSRI carries all the indications. Fluvoxamine, for example, is approved for OCD only. However, the therapeutic effect of SSRIs seems to be a class effect. Thus far, there is no clear proof that any one SSRI is more effective than others for a given condition.

Besides depression and anxiety, SSRIs seem to be helpful in a wide range of mental disorders, reflecting the importance of serotonin systems in the brain. Though serotonin-producing neurons are not as widely disseminated in the brain as glutamate or GABA neurons or even DA and NE, they modulate or control several other neurotransmitter systems.

6.4.1 *SSRIs in the treatment of depression*

As discussed in Chapter 10 on the individualized treatment of depression, the antidepressant efficacy of all currently available antidepressants is roughly the same. Thus, the choice of an antidepressant can be based on patient-specific information, such as comorbid psychiatric conditions, comorbid medical conditions and their medications, physical condition (for example, being over- or underweight), history of response to psychiatric medications, etc. Cases of depression where an SSRI could be the best choice include patients with significant comorbid anxiety or OCD symptoms (including repetitive self-injurious behaviors), significant impulsivity/aggressiveness (excluding bipolar patients), and patients with serious physical illness, especially cardiovascular ones. An important consideration in favor of SSRIs, at least in the USA, is the fact that most of them are now available in generic form, with resulting cost benefits.

6.4.2 *SSRIs in the treatment of anxiety disorders*

As discussed in detail in Chapter 12 on anti-anxiety medications, we generally recommend SSRIs as the first-line treatment for anxiety both on the basis of safety (regarding lethality and potential for dependence/addiction), and efficacy in treating these disorders. Here, also, the relatively low cost of SSRIs is a significant positive factor. Among anxiety disorders for which SSRIs should be the best option, we include health anxiety, the unwarranted fear of having a disease, a disorder formerly called hypochondriasis and classified with the somatoform disorders. Concerning the use of individual SSRIs in specific anxiety disorders, we try to avoid fluvoxamine which some psychiatrists still consider the first-line medication in OCD patients. First, fluvoxamine has the shortest half-life among SSRIs, and is the only drug in their class needing twice-daily dosing, or administration in a sustained-release preparation. Additionally, fluvoxamine significantly inhibits several CYP450 enzymes, with high risk of DDIs, and this risk goes up with the high doses needed for OCD. Thus, when treating OCD, unless the patient is already stable on fluvoxamine, we prefer trying other SSRIs first, knowing that we will need to use a robust dose for the anti-OCD effect.

6.4.3 *Use of SSRIs in other disorders or conditions*

SSRIs have also been used to manage symptoms and conditions such as impulsivity, anger, aggression, self-injurious behaviors, repetitive behaviors, and behavioral addictions. The rationale for this use is that diminished serotonergic function may be one of the biological substrates for these behaviors. In sexual disorders, such as pedophilia, exhibitionism, voyeurism, and frotteurism (paraphilias), characterized by poor impulse control, SSRIs may be helpful because of their potential to decrease both impulsive behaviors and sex drive. Because of their potential to delay orgasm, SSRIs are also tried in premature ejaculation. In pain syndromes, all SSRIs as well as other types of antidepressants may help alleviate chronic pain, including neuropathies, though this action seems to be particularly salient for dual-action agents, such as the SNRIs. Paralleling the treatment of OCD, SSRIs may be useful in conditions characterized mainly by compulsions, such as trichotillomania, or skin picking.

6.5 Use of SNRIs in Mental Disorders

The FDA-approved indications of the four SNRIs available in the USA are:

(1) venlafaxine (Effexor, Effexor XR, venlafaxine ER tablets): MDD, GAD, SAD, and panic disorder;
(2) desvenlafaxine (Pristiq): MDD.
(3) duloxetine (Cymbalta): MDD, GAD, diabetic neuropathic pain, and fibromyalgia; and
(4) milnacipram (Savella): fibromyalgia.

In general, the clinical use of SNRIs parallels that of SSRIs, with the most significant difference being that of OCD and other repetitive and compulsive behaviors. In these disorders, serotonergic actions such as those of SSRIs seem to be the critical factor, and it makes no sense to expose our patients to the additional noradrenergic effects of SNRIs or other types of antidepressants. Moreover, these additional adrenergic side effects limit our ability to reach the high doses that are usually needed in OCD and behavioral disorders.

Regarding the analgesic effect of SNRIs and other antidepressants, we must keep in mind these observations:

(1) Practically all antidepressants, including SSRIs, seem to have some effect in neuropathic pain. However, the effect seems to be more marked with dual-action agents, such as SNRIs or TCAs.

(2) The analgesic effect of antidepressants, even dual-action agents, is limited to neuropathic pain. In neuropathic pain, it is not comparable to specific analgesics.
(3) To work on neuropathic pain, SNRIs may require relatively large doses. In a review on neuropathic pain, daily doses of 60 and 90 mg of duloxetine had an effect, but 30 mg did not.
(4) Antidepressants have no significant effect on other types of pain. The makers of duloxetine, approved for fibromyalgia and neuropathic pain, applied for the indication as an analgesic, but the FDA denied it.

6.6 Dosing of SSRIs and SNRIs

Regarding recommended doses for SSRIs and SNRIs, to avoid duplication, we refer the reader to Table 10.3, in the chapter on the individualized treatment of depression. The only caveat is remembering that, in anxious patients, serotonergic medications may initially exacerbate the anxiety, including panic-like symptoms. To improve treatment compliance, anxious patients should be informed about this risk and, if necessary, the medication should be started at a dose below the usual initial antidepressant dose.

6.7 Adverse Effects of SSRIs and SNRIs

Despite their low toxicity, SSRIs and SNRIs show many bothersome serotonergic side effects. Reasons for this include the fact that they increase activity in practically all the types of 5-HT receptors identified so far, which are involved in myriad functions and, in some cases, even have opposite actions. Additionally, because serotonergic neurons modulate the activity of other neurotransmitter circuits, for example dopaminergic ones, SSRIs and SNRIs may also induce non-serotonergic side effects, such as EPS (extrapyramidal symptoms). As with any other type of medication, side effects with SSRIs and SNRIs threaten treatment adherence. Thus, even if they are not risky, the frequency of side effects is the main clinical problem in therapy with SSRIs and SNRIs and, as a rule, we can assume that the frequency is higher than reported. For multiple reasons, patients are not good at reporting side effects. For example, they are unlikely to establish an association between a medication and decreased sexual desire, teeth-grinding, headaches, or excessive yawning. Thus, to locate side effects, clinicians or researchers must actively and specifically look for them systematically.

6.7.1 *Antidepressants and the risk of suicide*

We discuss this subject in the present chapter because SSRIs and SNRIs are by far the most widely used antidepressants. However, the reader must keep in mind that the warning about suicide risk, as discussed below, applies to all antidepressants and even to some non-antidepressant medications approved for use in depressed patients.

In 2004, the FDA issued a black box warning, expanded in 2007, stating that antidepressants increase "suicidality" in young people. Today, this warning affects all medications known to have an antidepressant mechanism, including the SNRI milnacipram (Savella, approved in the USA only for the treatment of fibromyalgia), or approved for the treatment of any type of depressive disorder, including the atypical antipsychotics quetiapine and aripiprazole (Seroquel and Abilify, respectively, approved for bipolar depression or as adjunctive treatment in unipolar depression), or the combination of the antipsychotic olanzapine and the antidepressant fluoxetine (Symbyax, approved for the treatment of bipolar depression). This is the current version of the warning:

> WARNING: SUICIDALITY AND ANTIDEPRESSANT DRUGS
> Antidepressants increased the risk compared to placebo of suicidal thinking and behavior (suicidality) in children, adolescents, and young adults in short-term studies of Major Depressive Disorder (MDD) and other psychiatric disorders. Anyone considering the use of [Insert established name] or any other antidepressant in a child, adolescent, or young adult must balance this risk with the clinical need. Short-term studies did not show an increase in the risk of suicidality with antidepressants compared to placebo in adults beyond age 24; there was a reduction in risk with antidepressants compared to placebo in adults aged 65 and older. Depression and certain other psychiatric disorders are themselves associated with increases in the risk of suicide. Patients of all ages who are started on antidepressant therapy should be monitored appropriately and observed closely for clinical worsening, suicidality, or unusual changes in behavior. Families and caregivers should be advised of the need for close observation and communication with the prescriber.

The warning, when carefully read, is sort of tepid. As some critics have noted, it states that "depression and certain other psychiatric disorders are themselves associated with increases in the risk of suicide," which makes it the first black box warning to note that a disease itself carries risk — and implies that there is risk in not using the very medication being warned about (Friedman *et al.*, 2007).

Whatever the actual wording of the warning, the simplified and distorted view offered in the mass media — that antidepressants induce suicide — led to a steep reduction in the number of antidepressant prescriptions for both children and adults, and a heated public health debate ensued. On the one hand, opponents of medication treatment for psychiatric disorders, especially in children, saw in this a confirmation of their misgivings. On the other, mental health researchers and practitioners argued that the harm caused by the reduction in the number of treated depressed patients clearly outweighed the risk of an unproven or, at the most, a very modest increase in suicides, due to antidepressant treatment.

Problems here start with the use of the newly coined term 'suicidality' (suicidal thinking and behavior), instead of the more categorical 'suicide' or 'completed suicide.' Actually, in the original pediatric study that led to the initial warning, there were no completed suicides. It is true that other studies have also reported an increase in suicidal ideation or non-lethal self-injurious behaviors in the young treated with antidepressants, but, again, these ideas and behaviors have many gradations, and are liable to multiple interpretations. Maybe more importantly, suicides in these studies, including large ones, were exceedingly rare. A recently published large German pharmacovigilance study, which was carried out from 1993 until 2008 in 85 hospitals and included 142,090 adult patients on antidepressants, documents only three completed suicides (Stübner *et al.*, 2010). A large meta-analysis of 27 randomized placebo-controlled trials of antidepressants for pediatric depression, OCD, and anxiety, with over 5,000 subjects, concludes: "While there was increased risk difference of suicidal ideation/suicide attempt across all trials and indications for drug vs. placebo... There were no completed suicides." (Bridge *et al.*, 2007) Besides this, the correlation between suicidal thinking or behavior and completed suicide is not unequivocal, and may even be opposite. This conundrum is well exemplified by the conclusions of a nationwide study in Finland, with 15,390 patients with a mean follow-up of 3.4 years: "Among suicidal subjects who had ever used antidepressants, the current use of any antidepressant was associated with a markedly increased risk of attempted suicide and, at the same time, with a markedly decreased risk of completed suicide and death." (Tiihonen *et al.*, 2006)

Meanwhile, epidemiological studies in several industrialized countries, including the USA, Denmark, and Japan, have shown a temporal association between an increase in prescriptions for second-generation antidepressants and a decrease in suicide rates.

Thus, the association between antidepressant treatment and completed suicide in people up to the age of 24, in our opinion, is still possible but not clearly proven, and it does not seem to exist for older groups. An analysis of FDA data with almost 100,000 patients, two-thirds on antidepressants and one-third on placebo, concludes that: "Risk of suicidality associated with use of antidepressants is strongly age dependent. Compared with placebo, the increased risk for suicidality and suicidal behavior among adults under 25 approaches that seen in children and adolescents. The net effect seems to be neutral on suicidal behavior but possibly protective for suicidal ideation in adults aged 25–64 and to reduce the risk of both suicidality and suicidal behavior in those aged ≥65." (Stone *et al.*, 2009) A serious shortcoming of this report is that although it mentions eight completed suicides, these are not analyzed separately (they are not even assigned to medication or placebo groups), but are lumped together, with other less significantly but more frequent "suicidality" events.

Because of the above, we generally agree with the conclusions in the consensus statement of the section on pharmacopsychiatry of the World Psychiatric Association:

> In surveying this important problem, three problems were posed. First, should we expect further restrictions for the use of SSRIs in adults? This is basically a political question. The cautions in children seem based less on high risk than an over-interpretation of what suicidality actually means. Many drugs carrying a real risk of serious harm are marketed without black boxes, but with accepted risks balanced against known benefits. We need to be alert to the possibility that such an unusual emphasis on this aspect of drug safety for antidepressants is driven by a broader anti-psychiatric agenda. Of course, on the other hand, we can only examine the published data. There may well be unpublished data which we are not aware of but which convinced the regulatory agencies that a black box warning was necessary. Second, is there solid evidence that SSRIs carry a higher risk of inducing/aggravating suicidality compared to other ADs, especially TCAs? The simple answer appears to be 'no.' Finally, is the risk of SSRI use or the use of other ADs acceptable when balanced against the beneficial consequences of treatment with ADs accordingly to the principles of good clinical practice? In the opinion of this expert group the answer is a clear 'yes.' (Möller *et al.*, 2008)

6.7.2 *Serotonergic side effects of SSRIs and SNRIs*

6.7.2.1 *Mental (cognitive)*

The adverse cognitive effects of serotonergic antidepressants are usually overlooked. They include apathy (or "indifference syndrome"), tiredness/fatigue, inattentiveness/difficulty concentrating, memory problems, and mental slowing (Fava *et al.*, 2006). Apathy or indifference, characterized by excessive emotional detachment (as one of our patients put it, "I am not depressed any longer, but I don't care"), is often disturbing to the patients, and usually responds to reductions in the dose or, if necessary, medication change (Padal *et al.*, 2012). Fatigue is usually part of the depressive or anxiety symptoms; however, fatigue that gets worse after starting antidepressant treatment or persists long after other symptoms have remitted is probably medication-induced (increased serotonin in the brain seems to produce a feeling of fatigue, and serotonin antagonists have been tried to reduce fatigability in sportspeople). Significant insomnia, whether part of the disorder or medication-induced, warrants treatment with hypnotics. Other mental adverse effects, such as memory loss, difficulty thinking, confusion, and mental slowing, are likely early signs of toxicity. The antidepressant dose should be reduced or, if they are severe, the medication stopped.

It is important to keep in mind that both SSRIs and SNRIs, as well as practically all antidepressants, are considered to be the main cause of the acute form of REM sleep behavior disorder (RBD).

6.7.2.2 *Neuromuscular*

These are relatively common with SSRIs and SNRIs (let us remember that serotonin neurons modulate dopaminergic motor pathways in the basal ganglia). They include typical EPS, such as those observed with antipsychotics, and unusual ones, such as restless legs syndrome, bruxism, yawning, or myoclonus (sudden, isolated muscle jerks, usually in the head, neck, or limbs). Uncontrollable yawning is very disturbing for patients. Bruxism (grinding of the teeth) may cause dental fractures and wear. Often, the association between SSRI/SNRI treatment and restless legs, bruxism, and other movement disorders goes unnoticed, and the abnormal movements are treated as separate disorders.

6.7.2.3 *Gastrointestinal*

Serotonin plays a huge role in the digestive tract, including gastric production of acid and intestinal movement. Thus, the high frequency of gastrointestinal side effects with SSRIs/SNRIs is not surprising. These effects usually appear in the very first days of treatment and include heartburn, nausea, vomiting, and diarrhea. Gastrointestinal adverse reactions with SSRIs/SNRIs are practically the only type that tends to disappear in a matter of days or weeks, despite continuation of treatment at the same or even higher doses. As mentioned before, besides these serotonergic gastrointestinal side effects, SNRIs also show adrenergic gastrointestinal effects, especially constipation.

6.7.2.4 *Sexual*

Sexual side effects are common and disturbing, and to elicit them we have to ask specific questions because patients are often embarrassed to discuss them. These include decreased sexual interest or delayed orgasm (anorgasmia) in males and females, and erectile dysfunction in men. A prospective open-label study including 1,022 patients (610 women and 412 men) with previously normal sexual function, found these incidences of sexual dysfunction for diverse antidepressants: fluoxetine 57.7%, sertraline 62.9%, fluvoxamine 62.3%, paroxetine 70.7%, citalopram 72.7%, the SNRI venlafaxine 67.3%, and the non-SSRI/SNRI mirtazapine 24.4% (Montejo *et al.*, 2001). A more recent international study, comparing SSRIs and the SNRI duloxetine in sexually active MDD patients without sexual dysfunction at entry found lower incidences of antidepressant-associated sexual dysfunction but the figures are still significant: SSRI monotherapy 23.4% and duloxetine 28.7% (Duenas *et al.*, 2011). Phosphodiesterase inhibitors may be useful in antidepressant-associated erectile dysfunction, and addition of bupropion may be tried for decreased sex drive, both in males and females. However, sexual side effects often require dose reduction or medication change.

6.7.2.5 *Syndrome of inappropriate antidiuretic hormone secretion*

Together with antipsychotics and antiepileptic drugs, serotonergic antidepressants have been associated with syndrome of inappropriate antidiuretic hormone secretion (SIADH), a condition characterized by the release of excessive amounts of antidiuretic hormone, which increases the retention of water by the kidneys, lowering serum sodium levels (hyponatremia). Sodium levels below 135 mOsm/kg are considered abnormal, but symptoms appear usually under 130 mOsm/kg. The clinical symptoms include malaise and myalgia, but the most dramatic are neurological and mental, from nausea, headache, lethargy, and confusion/disorientation to loss of consciousness and convulsions. The reported incidence varies wildly, from 0.5% to 32% (Jacob *et al.*, 2006). In any case, it seems to be more frequent in the elderly and in females. Another important risk factor is the concomitant use of serotonergic antidepressants and medications that lower serum sodium by a different mechanism, such as thiazide diuretics (Rosner, 2004).

6.7.2.6 *Headaches*

Headaches are a complex issue. Some depressed and particularly, anxious patients report frequent headaches that are clearly associated with the mood episode. These very often improve with any type of antidepressant/anti-anxiety treatment, including SSRIs/SNRIs. Besides this, some studies have shown benefits with SSRI treatment of tension headaches and migraines, though TCAs clearly have a better effect on these pain symptoms (Jackson *et al.*, 2010). However, some patients will report increased frequency and/or severity of headaches, especially migraines, with SSRI/SNRI use. Thus, establishing a pre-treatment baseline and examining trends in severity/frequency of headaches are critical to decide if continuation of treatment with SSRIs/SNRIs is likely to reduce or worsen this worrisome symptom.

6.7.2.7 *Weight changes*

In general, SSRIs and SNRIs are weight-neutral. However, occasionally, some patients report increased or decreased appetite/weight while on these medications.

6.7.2.8 *Risk of bleeding*

Serotonin receptors are involved in platelet adhesion, especially 5-HT_{2A}, and platelets release serotonin at sites of bleeding and vascular damage. However, platelets do not synthesize serotonin but obtain it from the bloodstream. Thus, inhibition of the serotonin reuptake transporter by medications may decrease platelet stores of serotonin. Because of this, potential bleeding problems with SSRIs have received a lot of attention. A comparison of 1,321 patients with upper gastrointestinal bleeding and 10,000 matched controls showed an increase in the risk for patients taking SSRIs (paroxetine) or SNRIs (venlafaxine). An interaction with nonsteroidal anti-inflammatory drugs (NSAIDs) was observed, in particular among those not using acid-suppressing agents (de Abajo *et al.*, 2008). Regarding risk of bleeding during surgical procedures, a retrospective study of orthopedic patients undergoing surgery found that the risk of blood transfusion almost quadrupled for patients on serotonergic antidepressants, while patients using non-serotonergic antidepressants had no increase in risk (Movig *et al.*, 2003). A recent retrospective cohort study followed 27,058 patients discharged from the hospital with antiplatelet therapy after acute myocardial infarction. Compared to both ASA alone and ASA–clopidogrel combination, the addition of an SSRI significantly increased the risk of bleeding (Labos *et al.*, 2011). The consensus seems to be that, though systemic anticoagulation effects of SSRIs are not relevant in healthy subjects, SSRIs (as well as TCAs and SNRIs) may increase the general risk of bleeding in surgical patients or patients on anticoagulation, or upper gastrointestinal bleeding in patients taking NSAIDs or aspirin. Thus, though there is no absolute contraindication, care should be exerted in these cases. As this adverse effect on coagulation seems specific of SSRIs, SNRIs, and TCAs, switching to a different type of antidepressant could be considered in these patients.

6.7.2.9 *QT prolongation and risk of malignant arrhythmia*

On 24 August 2011 and 28 March 2012, the U.S. FDA issued communications regarding the risk of QT prolongation and malignant arrhythmia with citalopram. They included a table comparing the change in QT induced by bioequivalent doses of citalopram and its purified active S-isomer, escitalopram. According to these data, the QT change induced by a citalopram dose is roughly twice as high as that induced by the equivalent dose of the purified S-isomer. This likely means that both isomers contribute to this risk, and by giving the purified isomer, S-citalopram, we cut the risk in half.

These are the Revised Recommendations from the most recent communication regarding use of citalopram:

(1) Citalopram is not recommended for use at doses greater than 40 mg/day because such doses cause too large an effect on the QT interval and confer no additional benefit.
(2) Citalopram is not recommended for use in patients with congenital long QT syndrome, bradycardia, hypokalemia or hypomagnesemia, recent acute myocardial infarction, or uncompensated heart failure.
(3) Citalopram use is also not recommended in patients who are taking other drugs that prolong the QT interval.
(4) The maximum recommended dose of citalopram is 20 mg/day for patients with hepatic impairment, patients who are older than 60 years of age, patients who are CYP2C19 poor metabolizers, or patients who are taking concomitant cimetidine (Tagamet) or another CYP2C19 inhibitor, because these factors lead to increased blood levels of citalopram, increasing the risk of QT interval prolongation and torsades de pointes.

Actually, reviews mentioning the risk of QT prolongation with citalopram have been in the public domain since at least 2004 (Isbister *et al.*, 2004; Kelly *et al.*, 2004). Thus, if there is something to be criticized in the FDA warning, it is its lateness. More importantly, this warning raises significant questions regarding other antidepressants. Other SSRIs seem to be safer than citalopram regarding QT prolongation, but we need good studies (note that the Prescribing Information for vilazodone reports that treatment with doses up to 80 mg/day did not prolong the QT interval). Other types of antidepressants need to be examined, especially SNRIs, as mortality after overdose is higher with SNRIs than SSRIs. Additionally, we need to be concerned about antipsychotics, as the QT prolongation reported with high doses of citalopram seems to be in the same range as that reported for some currently marketed antipsychotics, including "atypicals."

6.7.2.10 *Osteoporosis and risk of fractures*

Serotonin receptors play an important role in the activity of all bone cell types. For this reason, the possibility that serotonergic antidepressants affect the risk for osteoporosis and fractures has been periodically discussed. The issue is a complex one, as depression itself seems to increase the risk by decreasing bone mineral density (BMD) and increasing the occurrence of falls. However, recent reviews and meta-analyses coincide in the conclusion that SSRIs and TCAs enhance fracture risk. Use of these types of medications could increase the risk of fractures by as much as twofold versus nonusers. The increase in risk would be greater in the early stages of treatment, and the risk would decrease toward baseline in the year following discontinuation (Rizzoli *et al.*, 2012; Rabenda *et al.*, 2011; Tsapakis *et al.*, 2010). These publications do not consider SNRIs, but we need to apply their conclusions to this antidepressant group.

6.7.2.11 *Diabetes*

Several reports have suggested that SSRIs may complicate the management of diabetes. This subject needs to be approached with extreme care, as there is great intra- and inter-individual variability in the condition of diabetic patients, including insulin needs. A recent retrospective study with careful subject selection, comparing pre- and during antidepressant treatment, actually showed a decrease in the amount of insulin administered during SSRI use, and no change in the amount administered during TCA use (Knol *et al.*, 2008). Thus far, our opinion is that there is no reasonable evidence that SSRIs induce or worsen diabetes, but this needs further study.

6.7.2.12 *Cataracts*

A large retrospective study reported an increase in the risk for cataracts in patients taking SSRIs. However, the probable increase in risk was very modest, with an OR for cataracts among current SSRIs users versus controls of 1.15 (95% CI: 1.08–1.23). Besides this, some confounding factors, such as smoking, were not ruled out (Etminam *et al.*, 2009). Therefore, our opinion is that there is no clear evidence regarding the association of cataracts with SSRIs.

6.7.3 *Noradrenergic side effects of SNRIs*

Besides the serotonergic adverse effects discussed above, SNRIs may also induce adrenergic side effects. Because of this, the authors think that SSRIs should be generally preferred to SNRIs in clinical practice.

Regarding adrenergic side effects of SNRIs, the most common, risky, or bothersome are:

(1) Increases in pulse and blood pressure, both systolic and diastolic, which are more likely to occur at high doses.
(2) Ocular side effects. The most troublesome of these is increased intraocular pressure, which can result in acute glaucoma symptoms. Others are blurred vision, likely due to impaired accommodation, and mydriasis.
(3) Dry mouth.
(4) Insomnia.
(5) Constipation.
(6) Urinary hesitancy and retention. Some clinicians report urinary incontinence with SNRIs; the mechanism is likely urinary retention with overflowing of a full bladder.

6.8 Discontinuation Syndrome with SSRIs and SNRIs

The appearance of multiple general symptoms shortly after stopping an SSRI/SNRI indicate discontinuation syndrome. The most common discontinuation symptoms are malaise, fatigue, chills, arthralgias, myalgias, tremors, paresthesias, electric-like shocks, sleep disturbances, headaches, lightheadedness, flu-like symptoms, decreased appetite, nausea, and vomiting. Risk for discontinuation syndrome seems to increase with duration of therapy and short half-life of the antidepressant involved. Paroxetine is associated with discontinuation syndrome more often than other SSRIs with comparable half-life, probably due to the lack of active metabolites. Venlafaxine, even in extended-release form, is known for its protracted discontinuation syndrome, which often requires a very gradual tapering (in the order of 37.5 or even 25 mg reductions per week). Treatment for discontinuation syndrome consists of simply restarting the antidepressant at the last dose taken and tapering it gradually over several days. This means, for example, cutting the dose by 25% to 50% at weekly intervals, though some very sensitive patients may require an even more gradual process. Other authorities recommend substituting fluoxetine at an equivalent dose, and then tapering or even just stopping, as fluoxetine, due to its long half-life, is unlikely to induce discontinuation syndrome. Sensitive patients may report some discontinuation symptoms when they miss doses of any SSRI/SNRI other than fluoxetine. Strategies to improve medication adherence must be developed with such patients, or they may be switched to fluoxetine.

6.9 Toxicity of SSRIs and SNRIs and Serotonin Syndrome

SSRIs have very low toxicity in general. The lethal dose for all SSRIs is estimated to be in the order of several grams. Reported SSRI-associated deaths are usually not due to intrinsic drug toxicity, but to drug interactions in the CYP450 oxidation system. Though clearly safer than monoamine oxidase inhibitors (MAOIs) or TCAs, SNRIs seem to be less safe than SSRIs. For example, significantly more deaths per million prescriptions are reported with SNRIs than SSRIs. A likely factor for this is the adrenergic cardiovascular effects of SNRIs. In non-fatal overdose with SNRIs, findings have included QT prolongation, bundle branch block, QRS prolongation, arrhythmias, hypotension, and seizures.

The most severe toxicity with SSRIs/SNRIs is serotonin syndrome, caused by excessive serotonin input in the brain. It may be due to the combination of, or overdose with, serotonergic drugs, or to DDIs inhibiting the metabolism of serotonergic drugs. Serotonin syndrome is characterized by the triad of *changes in mental status* (disorientation/confusion and agitation), *neuromuscular abnormalities* (hyperreflexia, tremor, clonus, myoclonus, and finally, rigidity), and, in approximately 50% of cases, *autonomic hyperactivity* (diaphoresis, fever, tachycardia, and tachypnea). Results of autopsy show that serotonin syndrome shares neuropathological features (loss of cerebellar Purkinje cells) with heat stroke and neuroleptic malignant syndrome, two conditions characterized by hyperthermia, suggesting that hyperthermia is a major factor for damage in serotonin syndrome.

A risk factor for antidepressant-induced serotonin syndrome these days is the promotion of serotonergic antidepressants for non-psychiatric indications. Thus, patients may be simultaneously prescribed one of these medications for a mental disorder, and another one, usually duloxetine or milnacipram, for fibromyalgia or pain. The case of milnacipram in the USA is particularly troubling, as it is being promoted only for fibromyalgia, and providers may be unaware of the fact that it is actually an SNRI.

Medications and substances reported as contributing to serotonin syndrome include MAOIs, TCAs, SSRIs, SNRIs, other serotonergic antidepressants, buspirone, sibutramine, stimulants, and ecstasy (especially in combination with amphetamines or cocaine). We must also remember that the herbal preparation St. John's wort, has serotonin reuptake inhibition properties and should not be combined with antidepressants.

Regarding other potential contributors to serotonin syndrome, note that:

(1) Some, but not all opiates, may contribute to serotonin syndrome: meperidine, tramadol, methadone, dextromethorphan, and propoxyphene appear to be weak SRIs and have been reported as contributing to serotonin toxicity (including deaths). Morphine, codeine, oxycodone, and buprenorphine are not considered SRIs, and do not seem to cause serotonin toxicity.
(2) Despite an alert from the FDA, some authorities have concluded that there is not enough evidence to limit the use of tryptans combined with SSRIs and other serotonergic antidepressants, with adequate patient information and monitoring. In support of this position, some argue that tryptans are agonists of 5-HT_{1B}, 5-HT_{1D}, and 5-HT_{1F} receptors, whereas serotonin syndrome is believed to be due to activation of 5-HT_{1A} and 5-HT_{2A} receptors.

Some 5-HT_2 blockers such as cyproheptadine or chlorpromazine, have been recommended for the management of serotonin syndrome. However, treatment is mainly supportive, including IV (intravenous) fluids, cooling measures, management of delirium, and, if necessary, ventilation. Serotonin syndrome has a shorter course than neuroleptic malignant syndrome, as, in most cases it subsides in one day, though some patients (40%) may have a longer course.

6.10 Precautions with SSRIs and SNRIs

All SSRIs and SNRIs except milnacipram must be used with care in significant hepatic disease, decreasing dosages, as they are mainly metabolized by the CYP450 system. Milnacipram must be used with care in renal insufficiency.

SSRIs and SNRIs have potential for DDIs by interfering with the CYP450 cytochromes. Fluvoxamine inhibits, moderately or strongly, CYP1A2, 2C9, 2C19, and 3A4. Fluoxetine and paroxetine may cause strong inhibition, and duloxetine moderate inhibition, of CYP2D6. Sertraline and citalopram/escitalopram exhibit some potential to inhibit CYP2D6. Vilazodone has shown potential to inhibit CYP2C8, a cytochrome involved in the oxidation of some medications such as amodiaquin, amiodarone, cerivastatin, montelukast, paclitaxel, and several oral antidiabetic drugs. In Chapter 19, the reader may review the main substrates for the above-mentioned cytochromes. Regarding the important DDIs between antidepressants and the anticancer drug tamoxifen, converted by CYP2D6 to the active form endoxifen, we remind the reader that safe antidepressant options seem to be venlafaxine, desvenlafaxine, vilazodone, mirtazapine, trazodone, and milnacipram (for this subject, see also Chapter 10).

SNRIs are contraindicated in narrow angle glaucoma. SNRIs should be used with care in patients with history of dysuria (lower urinary tract obstruction, prostate hypertrophy, prostatitis, etc.), and also those with conditions that might be compromised by hemodynamic changes (e.g., hyperthyroidism, heart failure, or recent myocardial infarction). We must also keep in mind that liver toxicity has been reported with duloxetine, and elevation of liver enzymes has been reported with milnacipram.

SSRIs and SNRIs should not be combined with MAOIs. A wash-out period of 14 days is recommended between the discontinuation of one of these groups of medications and the start of the other (one month when discontinuing fluoxetine).

6.11 Use of SSRIs and SNRIs During Pregnancy and Lactation

For the treatment of depression and anxiety during pregnancy and lactation, SSRIs are probably the best choice, because they have both the lowest toxicity among all antidepressant groups and the larger exposure among second-generation antidepressants without showing clear deleterious effects on pregnancy. We do not recommend SNRIs for use during pregnancy because of some evidence suggesting they may pose a higher risk for preeclampsia than SSRIs (see below). However, there are some caveats about the use of SSRIs during pregnancy that we are going to synthesize here. The main question about the use of SSRIs and other serotonergic antidepressants during pregnancy is their possible association with persistent pulmonary hypertension of the newborn (PPHN) (Chambers *et al.*, 2006). This issue is considered unsettled, as some studies suggest that depression in pregnant women *per se* could contribute to PPHN. However, we need to take into account the results of a recent large cohort study from the five Nordic countries, considering all singletons born after 33 weeks of pregnancy, between 1996 and 2007. It included the children of around 30,000 women using SSRIs during pregnancy, with 11,014 using them after gestational week 20. This study found that exposure to SSRIs late in pregnancy increased the risk for PPHN, with an adjusted OR of 2.1 of (95% CI: 1.5 to 3.0), and the increase in risk was of similar magnitude for all SSRIs (sertraline, citalopram, paroxetine, and fluoxetine) (Kieler *et al.*, 2011). The risk, if it indeed exists, may be mainly related to the use of serotonergic medications in the last weeks of pregnancy. Thus, the safest course regarding PPHN is, whenever possible, discontinuing or decreasing the dose of the antidepressant in the last trimester of pregnancy.

There are also reports of heterogeneous mental and behavioral symptoms in children born to mothers on SSRIs, that range from increased flaccidity to irritability. As some of these symptoms may correspond to discontinuation syndrome, it seems to be advisable, for patients taking serotonergic antidepressants in late pregnancy, to try to discontinue or decrease the dose of the antidepressant before delivery, restarting, if necessary, immediately afterwards.

Regarding the choice of antidepressant for use during pregnancy, we generally avoid citalopram because of the controversy about QT prolongation; paroxetine because of reports of cardiac malformations; fluoxetine because of its very long half-life; and fluvoxamine because of the significantly elevated risk for DDIs. This leaves sertraline as the preferred choice. Sertraline, reportedly, has also one of the lowest concentrations in milk, making it the preferred option during lactation.

6.11.1 *SSRIs and SNRIs and risk for preeclampsia*

Regarding this issue, a retrospective analysis of data from 5,731 women with non-malformed infants and no underlying hypertension, including 199 treated with SSRIs, found an adjusted relative risk for preeclampsia of 1.4 for women who received SSRI treatment only during the first trimester, and 4.9 for women who continued treatment beyond that point (Toh *et al.*, 2009). However, it was difficult to draw conclusions from this study regarding causality as some studies suggest that mood disorders *per se* may cause preeclampsia. This gives more importance to the results of a recent and larger study of 69,448 pregnancies in women with depression, comparing the risk of preeclampsia in women treated with SSRIs, SNRIs, or TCAs between gestational weeks 10 and 20 with the risk in depressed women not using antidepressants. Compared to women with untreated depression, the relative risk for preeclampsia in women treated with SSRIs was 1.22 (95% CI: 0.97–1.54), with SNRIs 1.95 (95% CI: 1.25–3.03), and with TCAs 3.23 (95% CI: 1.87–5.59) (Palmsten *et al.*, 2012). Even if we accept that causality is still not proven, the difference in risk among SSRIs and SNRIs/TCAs is striking, and a likely explanation for this is the fact that while SSRIs increase only serotonergic activity, SNRIs and TCAs increase both serotonergic and noradrenergic activity. This is another reason for us to recommend SSRIs and try to avoid SNRIs and TCAs, in the treatment of mood disorders during pregnancy.

References

Belmaker RH, Agam G. Major depressive disorder. *N Engl J Med* 2008;358:55–68.

Bridge JA, Iyengar S, Salary CB, *et al.* Clinical response and risk for reported suicidal ideation and suicide attempts in pediatric antidepressant treatment: A meta-analysis of randomized controlled trials. *JAMA* 2007;297:1683–1696.

Chambers CD, Hernandez-Diaz S, Van Marter LJ, *et al.* Selective serotonin-reuptake inhibitors and risk of persistent pulmonary hypertension of the newborn. *N Engl J Med* 2006;354(6):579–587.

De Abajo FJ, Garcia-Rodriguez LA. Risk of upper gastrointestinal track bleeding associated with selective serotonin reuptake inhibitors and venlafaxine therapy. *Arch Gen Psychiatry* 2008;65(7):795–803.

Duenas H, Brnabic AJ, Lee A, *et al.* Treatment-emergent sexual dysfunction with SSRIs and duloxetine: Effectiveness and functional outcomes over a 6-month observational period. *Int J Psychiatry Clin Pract* 2011;15(4):242–254.

Etminam M, Mikelberg FS, Brophy JM. Selective serotonin reuptake inhibitors and the risk of cataracts — a nested case control study. *Ophtalmology* 2010;117(6):1251–1255.

Evans CE, Sebastian J. Serotonin syndrome. *Emerg Med J* 2007;24:e20.

Evans RW, Tepper SJ, Shapiro RE, *et al.* The FDA alert on serotonin syndrome with use of tryptans combined with selective serotonin reuptake inhibitors or selective serotonin-norepinephrine reuptake inhibitors: American Headache Society position paper. *Headache* 2010;50:1089–1099.

Fava M. A cross-sectional study of the prevalence of cognitive and physical symptoms during long-term antidepressant treatment. *J Clin Psychiatry* 2006;67:1754–1759.

——. Prospective studies of adverse events related to antidepressant discontinuation. *J Clin Psychiatry* 2006;67(Suppl. 4):1421.

Filip M, Bader M. Overview on 5-HT receptors and their role in physiology and pathology of the central nervous system. *Pharm Rep* 2009;61:761–777.

Isbister GK, Bowe SJ, Dawson A, *et al.* Relative toxicity of selective serotonin reuptake inhibitors (SSRIs) in overdose. *J Toxicol Clin Toxicol* 2004;42(3):277–285.

Kelly CA, Dhaun N, Laing WJ, *et al.* Comparative toxicity of citalopram and the newer antidepressants after overdose. *J Toxicol Clin Toxicol* 2004;42(1):67–71.

Koolschinj PC, van Haren NE, Lensvelt-Mulders GJ, *et al.* Brain volume abnormalities in major depressive disorder: A meta-analysis of magnetic resonance imaging studies. *Hum Brain Mapp* 2009;30(11):3719–3735.

Jackson JL, Shimeall W, Sessums L, *et al.* Tricyclic antidepressants and headaches: Systematic review and meta-analysis. *BMJ* 2010;341:c5222, doi: 10.1136/bmj.c5222

Jacob S, Spinler SA. Hyponatremia associated with selective serotonin-reuptake inhibitors in older adults. *Ann Pharmacother* 2006;40:1618–1622.

Knol MJ, Derijks HJ, Geerlings MI, *et al.* Influence of antidepressants on glycaemic control in patients with diabetes mellitus. *Pharmacoepidemiol Drug Saf* 2008;17:577–586.

Looper KJ. Potential medical and surgical complications of serotonergic antidepressant medications. *Psychosomatics* 2007;48:1–9.

Möller H-J, Baldwin DS, Goodwin G, *et al.* Do SSRIs or antidepressant in general increase suicidality? WPA Section on Psychopharmacology: Consensus statement. *Eur Arch Psychiatry Clin Neurosci* 2008;258(Suppl. 3):3–23.

Montejo AL, Llorca G, Izquierdo JA, *et al.* Incidence of sexual dysfunction associated with antidepressant agents: A prospective multicenter study of 1022 outpatients. *J Clin Psychiatry* 2001;62(Suppl. 3):10–21.

Movig KL, Janssen MW, de Waal Malefijt J, *et al.* Relationship of serotonergic antidepressants and need for blood transfusion in orthopedic surgical patients. *Arch Intern Med* 2003;163(19):2354–2358.

Padala PR, Padala KP, Monga V, *et al.* Reversal of SSRI-associated apathy syndrome by discontinuation of therapy. *Ann Pharmacother* 2012;46(3):e8, doi: 10.1345/aph.1Q656

Palmsten K, Setoguchi S, Margulis AV, *et al.* Elevated risk of preeclampsia in pregnant women with depression: Depression or antidepressants? *Am J Epidemiol* 2012;175(10): 988–997.

Qiu C, Williams MA, Calderon-Margalit R, *et al.* Preeclampsia risk in relation to maternal mood and anxiety disorders before or during early pregnancy. *Am J Hypertens* 2009;22(4):397–402.

Rabenda V, Nicolet D, Beaudart C, *et al.* Relationship between use of antidepressants and risk of fractures: A meta-analysis. *Osteoporos Int* 2013;24(1):121–137.

Rizzoli R, Cooper C, Reginster J-Y, *et al.* Antidepressants medications and osteoporosis. *Bone* 2012, doi:10.1016/j.bone.2012.05.018

Rosner MH. Severe hyponatremia associated with the combined use of thiazide diuretics and selective serotonin reuptake inhibitors. *Am J Med Sci* 2004;327(2):109–111.

Safarinejad MR. The effects of adjunctive bupropion on male sexual dysfunction induced by a selective serotonin reuptake inhibitor: A double-blind placebo-controlled and randomized study. *BJU Int* 2010;106:840–847.

——. Reversal of SSRI-induced female sexual dysfunction by adjunctive bupropion in menstruating women: A double-blind, placebo controlled and randomized study. *J Psychopharmacol* 2011;25(3):370–378.

Sen S, Duman R, Sanacora G. Serum BDNF, depression and antidepressant medications: Meta-analyses and implications. *Biol Psychiatry* 2008;64(6):527–532.

Stübner S, Grohmann R, von Stralendorf I, *et al.* Suicidality as rare adverse event of antidepressant medication: Report from the AMSP multicenter drug safety surveillance project. *J Clin Psychiatry* 2010;71(10):1293–1307.

Targownik LE, Bolton JM, Metge CJ, *et al.* Selective serotonin reuptake inhibitors are associated with a modest increase in the risk of upper gastrointestinal bleeding. *Am J Gastroenterol* 2009;104:1475–1482.

Tiihonen J, Lonnqvist J, Wahlbeck K, *et al.* Antidepressants and the risk of suicide, attempted suicide, and overall mortality in a nationwide cohort. *Arch Gen Psychiatry* 2006;63: 1358–1367.

Toh S, Mitchell AA, Louik C, *et al.* Selective serotonin reuptake inhibitor use and risk of gestational hypertension. *Am J Psychiatry* 2009;166:320–328.

Tsapakis EM, Gamie Z, Tran GT, *et al.* The adverse skeletal effects of selective serotonin reuptake inhibitors. *Eur Psychiatry* 2012;27(3):156–159.

Wongpakaran N, van Reekum R, Wongpakaran T, *et al.* Selective serotonin reuptake inhibitor use associates with apathy among depressed elderly: A case-control study. *Ann Gen Psychiatry* 2007;6:7.

Xiong GI, Jiang W, Clare RM, *et al.* Safety of selective serotonin reuptake inhibitor use prior to coronary artery bypass grafting. *Clin Cardiol* 2009;33(6):E94–E98.

Chapter 7

Bupropion

7.1 Introduction

In 2005, the *Journal of Clinical Psychiatry* published an article entitled "Why isn't bupropion the most frequently prescribed antidepressant?" (Zimmerman *et al.*, 2005) In our view, it remains a pertinent question. Besides showing an efficacy comparable to that of other antidepressant drugs without having serotonergic side effects, bupropion also improves concentration and energy, decreases appetite, reduces craving for nicotine and, likely, cocaine and stimulant drugs, and enhances sexual function. Additionally, due to its unique mechanism of action, bupropion can be combined with practically any other antidepressant medication. Thus, the answer to the initial question is found in the early history of this, the only dopaminergic antidepressant. Bupropion, a compound structurally related to stimulants, was developed by Burroughs Wellcome researchers in the 1960s. A patent for the substance, initially named amferobutamone, was granted in 1974. It was approved by the FDA for depression in December 1985, in the form of an immediate-release formulation (Wellbutrin) with a suggested dose of 400–600 mg/day. While the launch of the new drug was being prepared, reports of seizures in patients taking the medication were reported, including a study of bupropion in bulimia nervosa patients, in which four of 55 subjects taking bupropion had grand mal seizures (Hornet *et al.*, 1988). The manufacturer voluntarily withdrew the medication in 1986. It was subsequently learned that the incidence of seizures rises five- or sixfold when dosages between 450 and 600 mg/day are used. Immediate-release bupropion was reintroduced in 1989, this time dosed three times a day, with a maximum recommended daily dose of 450 mg (150 mg tid), and even safer twice-a-day and once-a-day sustained-release preparations were introduced a few years later. However, bupropion remains associated with seizures in the minds of clinicians, and, despite its extended use in obesity, it has remained contraindicated in bulimia or anorexia nervosa patients.

7.2 Pharmacology

Bupropion and several of its metabolites work as weak inhibitors of norepinephrine (NE) and dopamine (DA) reuptake. The affinity of bupropion for the NE transporter is grossly four times that for the DA transporter. However, the inhibition of norepinephrine reuptake by bupropion is significantly less potent than that of TCAs or SNRIs. Bupropion does not affect serotonin reuptake, and does not bind post-synaptic receptors (including histamine, α- or β-adrenergic, serotonin, dopamine, or muscarinic receptors). Bupropion is a noncompetitive inhibitor of nicotinic cholinergic receptors. This action may contribute to the antidepressant and smoking cessation effects of the drug (see Table 7.1). In contrast to stimulant medications, bupropion does not seem to increase the release of DA.

Table 7.1 Pharmacological properties of bupropion (modified from Dhillon *et al.,* 2008).

Mechanism of action
Weak inhibitor of DA reuptake
Weak inhibitor of NE reuptake
Noncompetitive inhibitor of nicotinic receptors
No significant effect on serotonin neurotransmission
No binding of postsynaptic receptors (histamine, α- or β-adrenergic, serotonin, dopamine, or muscarinic)
Effects related to dopaminergic and adrenergic function
Antidepressant activity
Resolution of sleepiness and fatigue
Improved attention (ADHD)
Enhanced sexual functioning, anti-craving, and anti-withdrawal effects
Maybe associated with weight loss
Improvement in extrapyramidal symptoms (EPS)
No serotonergic effects
No significant effect on anxiety
No memory loss or apathy
Devoid of adverse effects on sexual function

The importance of dopaminergic actions in the effects of bupropion has been confirmed by different tests *in vivo* and *in vitro*. In humans, for example, PET studies have confirmed a decreased occupancy of the DA transporter by other ligands when bupropion is administered. Studies in rats have shown that D_1 and, especially, D_2 receptors are central to the effects of bupropion. A related observation which could have clinical implications is the reduction of the pharmacological effects of bupropion in mice by the antipsychotic pimozide, which, like all other available antipsychotics, is a D_2 blocker (Martin *et al.*, 1990).

7.2.1 *Pharmacokinetics*

Absorption of bupropion in the digestive track is fast and close to 100%, though it suffers a significant first-pass metabolism in the gut and liver. Bupropion is metabolized mainly by CYP2B6, to hydroxybupropion, an active metabolite. Other metabolic pathways, most likely CYP2C19 and non-CYP enzymes, produce two other active metabolites, erythrohydrobupropion and threohydrobupropion. These three active metabolites have longer half-lives than the parent compound, leading to greater C_{max} and AUC values, as well as steady-state concentrations, for them than those of bupropion. Though the metabolites are less potent than bupropion, the fact that they have higher systemic exposure than bupropion may enhance their activity. Bupropion is an inhibitor for CYP2D6.

All currently marketed forms of bupropion (immediate-release, twice-a-day sustained-release, and once-a-day sustained-release) are considered bioequivalent, meaning that the percentage of medication absorbed is grossly the same for all of them (bioavailability). However, there are pharmacokinetic differences between them which likely have implications in the safety of the medication. The slower the absorption, the longer the time to maximum plasma levels and the lower these maximum plasma levels. This difference is important as risk of seizures is surely related to plasma levels. With the immediate-release preparation, maximum plasma levels (C_{max}) are reached 2 h after administration. Absorption is slower for Wellbutrin SR (3 h to C_{max}), and even more so for Wellbutrin XL (5 h to C_{max}).

7.3 Approved Indications and Other Possible Uses

In Table 7.2, we list the approved indications and other potential uses of bupropion. Below, we provide some observations in this regard.

Table 7.2 Approved indications and other possible uses of bupropion.

Approved indications
Major depressive disorder (MDD)
Seasonal affective disorder
Aid in smoking cessation
Other current possible uses
Adjunctive treatment in partial response to other antidepressants
Attention deficit hyperactivity disorder (ADHD)
Sexual dysfunction
— Treatment of sexual side effects of serotonergic medications
— Treatment of hypoactive sexual desire
Weight loss (in combination with naltrexone)
Decreasing the cravings in addictions (cocaine, amphetamine)
Restless legs syndrome (RLS)
Generalized anxiety disorder (GAD) (?)

7.3.1 *Major depressive disorder*

Bupropion is approved for the treatment of MDD, and it has shown comparable efficacy to other antidepressants in the treatment of this disorder. However, some characteristics of bupropion, for example, decreasing appetite and enhancing/preserving energy, concentration, and alertness more effectively than other types of antidepressants, make it a good choice for depression presenting with prominent lack of energy (anergia), sleepiness, apathy, poor concentration, overeating, and anhedonia. Another practical advantage of bupropion over all other antidepressants is the lack of significant sexual side effects. On the other hand, its main disadvantage is the lack of a significant clinical effect on anxiety. Because of its multiple positive aspects, in our opinion, bupropion should be among the first-line medications for depressive disorder not accompanied by significant anxiety symptoms.

7.3.2 *Bupropion as an add-on in depression*

Due to its unique mechanism of action, bupropion can be combined with practically any other second-generation antidepressant (we would recommend caution only in the case of SNRIs, because of the theoretical possibility of added noradrenergic effects). Adding bupropion is safer, and likely more effective, than adding non-antidepressant medications, such as antipsychotics.

Another advantage of bupropion is its ability to address directly residual symptoms such as low energy, poor concentration, increased appetite, or daytime sleepiness.

7.3.3 *Anxiety disorders*

A meta-analysis of 10 double-blind placebo-controlled studies of bupropion and SSRIs in patients with major depression and associated anxiety, found that bupropion and SSRIs led to a similar degree of improvement in anxiety symptoms with no differences in the time to anxiolysis (Papakostas *et al.*, 2008). Even though we do not have good-quality studies of bupropion in anxiety disorders (meaning prospective, placebo-controlled), considering the benefit/risk profile of bupropion compared to non-antidepressant medications, in cases of difficult-to-treat anxiety, the addition of bupropion must be considered, in our opinion, before resorting to riskier medications such as TCAs or anticonvulsants.

7.3.4 *Seasonal affective disorder*

Wellbutrin XL is the only antidepressant approved for seasonal affective disorder. Ideally, the administration of bupropion should start in fall, while the mood is still good, and continue through the winter until springtime.

7.3.5 *Smoking cessation*

Bupropion, under the brand name Zyban, is approved as an aid to smoking cessation treatment. According to the Prescribing Information, the dose of Zyban is 150 mg once daily for three days, and then 150 mg twice a day (Zyban is an "SR" form). This total daily dose of 300 mg should not be exceeded. In practice, however, the uses of bupropion in depression and smoking cessation have become commingled, and all forms of bupropion are used for the latter indication.

7.3.6 *Attention deficit hyperactivity disorder*

Double-blind placebo-controlled studies have shown bupropion to be useful in the treatment of ADHD. For the use of bupropion in ADHD, three observations are relevant:

(1) Meta-analyses and clinical experience show that bupropion is less effective than stimulants.

(2) However, some meta-analyses/reviews suggest that bupropion is in the same range of efficacy as non-stimulant medications approved for ADHD, such as the NRI atomoxetine (Strattera).
(3) Studies of bupropion in ADHD have mainly used sustained-release preparations. However, it has been suggested that efficacy could be improved by using immediate-release bupropion administered in several doses, timed to the intellectual tasks, as we do with stimulant medications.

7.3.7 *Sexual dysfunction*

As mentioned in Chapter 6, a few randomized placebo-controlled studies suggest that bupropion may be useful in the treatment of sexual side effects of SSRIs, SNRIs, and other serotonergic medications, in both genders. Other studies have shown bupropion useful in the treatment of primary sexual disorders, in males and females, including hypoactive sexual desire disorder.

7.3.8 *Weight loss*

Over the last decade, several studies of bupropion, alone or in combination, have shown some usefulness of bupropion for weight loss in obese patients. Recently, a large, multicenter, 56-week, randomized placebo-controlled study in 1,742 subjects, using 360 mg of bupropion combined with two doses of naltrexone (16 or 32 mg), showed a weight change of –6.1% for BN32 and –5.0% for BN16, versus –1.3% for placebo (Greenway *et al.*, 2010). A criticism of this study is that the benefit/risk balance, measured as the difference between number needed to treat and number needed to harm, seems to diminish quickly when the magnitude of weight loss goes up (Citrome, 2010).

7.3.9 *Addictions (cocaine and amphetamines)*

For over a decade, case reports, open studies, and randomized placebo-controlled studies of bupropion in combination with psychosocial interventions have suggested a role for bupropion in the treatment of cocaine and amphetamine addictions. However, because two recent studies showed no benefit of bupropion in the treatment of cocaine or amphetamine abuse/dependence, the issue remains unsettled.

7.3.10 *Restless legs syndrome*

A number of case reports suggest that bupropion is useful in restless legs syndrome, both primary and secondary to antidepressant serotonergic medications.

7.4 Dosing and Available Forms of Bupropion

In the USA, bupropion is available as:

(1) immediate-release form (Wellbutrin 75 and 100 mg tablets); high doses need to be given in three daily doses;
(2) sustained-release form (Wellbutrin SR 100, 150, and 200 mg tablets); high doses need to be administered in two daily doses;
(3) extended-release form (Wellbutrin XL 150, 300 mg, and 450 mg tablets); all doses for once-a-day administration; and
(4) sustained-release form (Zyban 150 mg tabs); with a target dose in smoking cessation of 150 mg twice a day.

In depression, the dose range is 150–450 mg/day. In our practice, we almost exclusively prescribe the once-a-day formulation of bupropion (XL). There are several reasons for this preference. First, for any medication, the number of doses is inversely proportional to medication adherence. Second, a medication that increases alertness and may delay sleep onset, such as bupropion, should be administered shortly after getting up in the morning. Third, due to lower plasma peak levels, the XL formulation is likely to pose a lower risk for seizures than other forms. In healthy adult patients, we usually start with one 150 mg tablet a day, in the morning, increasing the dose to 300 mg/day after two weeks. We generally make the decision about going up to the maximum dose, 450 mg/day, by carefully assessing the patient after at least a month on 300 mg/day.

7.5 Side Effects and Adverse Reactions

According to the Prescribing Information for Wellbutrin XL, the side effects with the highest difference in frequency (percentage) from placebo were:

(1) gastrointestinal: especially dry mouth, nausea, and constipation;
(2) nervous: especially headaches and tremor;
(3) mental: especially insomnia, anxiety, and agitation;
(4) decreased appetite;
(5) tinnitus; and

(6) hypertension: according to the Prescribing Information for Wellbutrin XL, the difference between medication and placebo for hypertension is 2%. The risk seems to be particularly high for the combination of bupropion with transdermal nicotine (3% difference with placebo).

7.5.1 *Risk of seizures*

Other than for high doses of the immediate-release form, the incidence of seizures with bupropion seems to be in the same range of other antidepressants. The Prescribing Information puts the risk of seizures for Wellbutrin SR up to 300 mg/day at 0.1% (1:1,000). For immediate-release Wellbutrin, 300–450 mg/day, the mentioned risk is 0.4%.

Patient factors associated with increased risk of seizures include history of seizures; CNS lesions; severe hepatic cirrhosis; diabetes treated with oral medications or insulin; abuse of opiates, cocaine, and stimulants; use of supplement or over-the-counter stimulants and appetite suppressants; abuse of sedatives or alcohol; and concomitant use of medications known to decrease the seizure threshold.

7.6 Contraindications, Warnings, and Precautions

Combination with antipsychotics. Considering the evidence from studies in animals that antipsychotics may block the effects of bupropion, the authors wonder if it is advisable to combine bupropion and antipsychotics in clinical practice. The safer course seems to be, for patients on antipsychotics, to use a serotonergic antidepressant instead.

Bulimia and anorexia nervosa. Bupropion is contraindicated in patients with a current or prior diagnosis of bulimia or anorexia nervosa. However, as mentioned above, this contraindication is related to the seizures observed with doses up to 600 mg of immediate-release bupropion. It is possible that, with the proper information and vigilance, bupropion can be used safely in these patients.

Combination with monoamine oxidase inhibitors (MAOIs). Like any other antidepressant, bupropion is contraindicated in patients taking MAOIs. A washout period of at least 14 days should elapse between discontinuation of an MAOI and initiation of treatment with bupropion.

Liver and renal disease. Bupropion should be used with care in patients with liver disease. Regarding precautions in renal disease, the issue is unclear, with some studies showing no effect while others showing changes in the elimination of bupropion or, especially, its metabolites.

Drug–drug interactions. Bupropion is an inhibitor for CYP2D6 and must be used with care in combination with drugs metabolized by this enzyme.

7.7 Use of Bupropion During Pregnancy

Reportedly, bupropion is used during 0.7% of pregnancies in the USA, second only to SSRIs (3.8% of pregnancies) (Reefhuis *et al.*, 2011). This high use is surely related, at least in part, to the increasingly interventionist approach to smoking during pregnancy (Clark *et al.*, 2011). However, although the incidence of malformations, including cardiac ones, with the use of bupropion during pregnancy seems to be in the same range of that seen with other types of antidepressants, we must keep in mind that the pharmacological mechanisms of bupropion are completely different from other antidepressants, especially SSRIs. DA and NE underlie different systems compared to serotonin in the body and, before concluding on the safety of bupropion, we need studies paying attention to the main body functions served by adrenergic and dopaminergic circuits, especially, but not only, cardiovascular function. Regarding epinephrine/NE, as discussed in the previous chapter, some studies suggest that use of adrenergic antidepressants during pregnancy may increase the risk of preeclampsia. Regarding the metabolic effects of bupropion, such as appetite suppression, there exists at least one worrisome report of hyperinsulinism in a baby whose mother was given bupropion for smoking cessation during pregnancy. The infant presented with profound hypoglycemia and seizures on its third day of life (Gisslen *et al.*, 2011).

References

Citrome L. Miracle pills for weight loss: What is the number needed to treat, number needed to harm and likelihood to be helped or harmed for naltrexone-bupropion combination? (Editorial). *Int J Clin Pract* 2010;64(11):1461–1465.

Clark SM, Nakad R. Pharmacotherapeutic management of nicotine dependence in pregnancy. *Obstet Gynecol Clin North Am* 2011;38(2):297–311.

Dhillon S, Yang PH, Curran MP. Bupropion: A review of its use in the management of major depressive disorder. *Drugs* 2008;(68)5:653–689.

Dopheide JA, Pliszka SR. Attention-deficit-hyperactivity disorder: An update. *Pharmacothrapy* 2009;29(6):656–679.

Faraone SV, Glatt SJ. A comparison of the efficacy of medications for adult attention-deficit-hyperactivity disorder using meta-analysis of effect sizes. *J Clin Psychiatry* 2010;71(6):754–763.

Gisslen T, Nathan B, Thompson T, *et al.* Hyperinsulinism associated with gestational exposure to bupropion in a newborn infant. *J Pediatr Endocrinol Metab* 2011;24(9–10): 819–822.

Greenway FL, Fujioka K, Plodkowski RA, *et al.* Effect of naltrexone plus bupropion on weight loss in overweight and obese adults (COR-I): A multicentre, randomised, double-blind, placebo-controlled, phase 3 trial. *Lancet* 2010;376:595–695.

Horne RL, Ferguson JM, Pope HG, *et al.* Treatment of bulimia with bupropion: A multicenter controlled trial. *J Clin Psychiatry* 1988;49(7):262–266.

Lee JJ, Erdos J, Wilkosz MF, *et al.* Bupropion as a possible treatment for restless legs syndrome. *Ann Pharmacother* 2009;43:370374.

Martin P, Massol J, Colin JN, *et al.* Antidepressant profile of bupropion and three metabolites in mice. *Pharmacopsychiatry* 1990;23(4):187–194.

Papakostas GI, Trivedi MH, Alpert JE, *et al.* Efficacy of bupropion and selective serotonin reuptake inhibitors in the treatment of anxiety symptoms in major depressive disorder: A meta-analysis of individual patient data from 10 double-blind, randomized clinical trials. *J Psychiatr Res* 2008;42:134–140.

Reefhuis AS, Rasmussen SA, Friedman JM, *et al.* Patterns of antidepressant medication use among pregnant women in a United States population. *J Clin Pharmacol* 2011;51(2):264–270.

Shoptaw S, Heinzerling KG, Rotheram-Fuller E, *et al.* Bupropion hydrochloride versus placebo, in combination with cognitive behavioral therapy, for the treatment of cocaine abuse/dependence. *J Addict Dis* 2008;27(1):13–23.

——. Randomized, placebo-controlled trial of bupropion for the treatment of metamphetamine dependence. *Drug Alcohol Depend* 2008;96(3):222–232.

Tripp AC. Bupropion, a brief history of seizure risk. *Gen Hosp Psychiatry* 2010;32:216–217.

Tsoi DT, Porwal M, Webster AC. Efficacy and safety of bupropion for smoking cessation and reduction in schizophrenia: Systematic review and meta-analysis. *Br J Psychiatry* 2010; 196(5):346–353.

Zimmerman M, Posternak MA, Attiullah N, *et al.* Why isn't bupropion the most frequently prescribed antidepressant? *J Clin Psychiatry* 2005;66(5):603–610.

Chapter 8

Mirtazapine, Trazodone, and Nefazodone

8.1 Mirtazapine

Mirtazapine (Remeron) was developed by Organon, in the Netherlands, and first used in Europe. It was approved for clinical use in depression in the USA in 1996. Mirtazapine is a serotonergic and adrenergic antidepressant with no monoamine reuptake inhibition properties. Mirtazapine is an antagonist for serotonin 5-$HT_{2(A, B, C)}$ and 5-HT_3, as well as norepinephrine $\alpha_{2(A,B,C)}$-adrenergic receptors. The end result of these various actions is an increase in the activity of 5-HT_{1A} receptors, and in the release of both serotonin and norepinephrine in the brain. Mirtazapine also blocks histamine H_1 receptors, with an affinity even higher than that for serotonin and norepinephrine receptors, and has low affinity for cholinergic muscarinic M_1 receptors.

There is an important consideration regarding the multiple effects of mirtazapine. Due to its high affinity for H_1 receptors, the antihistaminic effects of mirtazapine, such as sedation and increased appetite, are appreciable at low doses. However, the noradrenergic effects that may counter them, at least partially, appear with intermediate and high doses. This leads to the clinical paradox that sedation and increased appetite, both common side effects with starting doses of mirtazapine, may decrease as the dose goes up.

Mirtazapine's action at serotonin 5-HT_3 may have significant clinical effects. Serotonin 5-HT_3 antagonism has an antiemetic effect (this is the mechanism of action of the antiemetic ondansetron). 5-HT_3 antagonism also seems to decrease anxiety and improve cognition.

8.1.1 *Pharmacokinetics*

Mirtazapine is well absorbed after oral administration but undergoes significant first-pass elimination, all of which results in an absolute bioavailability of approximately 50%. Mirtazapine has an elimination half-life of 20–40 h. It is metabolized by several enzymes in the CYP450 system, mainly CYP1A2, 2D6, and 3A4. So far, no significantly active metabolites have been identified. The final conjugated metabolites are eliminated in urine. Mirtazapine is not a significant inhibitor for any metabolic enzyme.

8.1.2 *Indications and uses*

In Table 8.1, we list the indications, generally accepted uses, and possible uses of mirtazapine. Below, we offer some comments on these indications.

8.1.2.1 *Depression*

In the USA, depression is mirtazapine's only approved indication. Mirtazapine seems to be as effective as other antidepressants for treating depression. However, because of its therapeutic profile, it deserves special consideration in depressed patients with significant insomnia, anorexia, emesis, or intestinal irritability, and in depressed patients with anxiety who do not tolerate well SSRIs or SNRIs.

8.1.2.2 *Anxiety disorders*

Considering its serotonergic and adrenergic properties, it is not surprising that both randomized and open-label studies have shown mirtazapine to be effective in anxiety disorders, including generalized anxiety disorder, panic

Table 8.1 Approved indication, and accepted and suggested uses of mirtazapine.

Approved indication	Major depressive disorder (MDD)
Generally accepted uses	Generalized anxiety and other anxiety disorders (panic disorder, social anxiety disorder, PTSD, etc.)
Suggested uses	Antiemetic
	Coadjuvant to antipsychotics in schizophrenia
	Neuropathic pain
	Insomnia
	Treatment of antipsychotic-induced akathisia

disorder, and social phobia. More ambiguous results have been found in post-traumatic stress disorder and obsessive–compulsive disorder.

8.1.2.3 *Emesis*

As mentioned above, the mechanism of action of some widely used antiemetic drugs, such as ondansetron, is serotonin 5-HT_3 antagonism. Some authors have emphasized that mirtazapine could be a cheaper alternative to ondansetron in the treatment of hyperemesis, such as that induced by chemotherapy. In combined therapy, mirtazapine has the additional advantage of causing no significant drug–drug interactions. Thus, there are several reasons for mirtazapine to be considered early in the treatment of patients receiving other treatments, or suffering from illnesses, that may cause nausea, vomiting, diarrhea, and intestinal irritability.

8.1.2.4 *Antipsychotic-induced akathisia*

Several studies point to the usefulness of mirtazapine for neuroleptic-associated akathisia. However, as mentioned in Chapter 3, because acute EPS predict the emergence of serious late EPS (e.g., tardive dyskinesia) we prefer to decrease the dose of the antipsychotic drug or switch medications in patients with akathisia.

8.1.2.5 *Neuropathic pain*

Some publications suggest a benefit from mirtazapine in neuropathic pain. This fits the drug's profile in terms of its dual action on serotonergic and adrenergic systems. Thus, if depression and/or insomnia are important clinical considerations, mirtazapine could be considered in patients with neuropathic pain, such as depressed diabetics.

8.1.2.6 *Add-on to antipsychotics in schizophrenia*

Some placebo-controlled Nordic studies have reported improvement in both positive and negative symptoms after adding mirtazapine to typical antipsychotics in patients with schizophrenia. However, an Australian randomized, placebo-controlled study in schizophrenic patients on atypical antipsychotics showed no benefit when adding on mirtazapine.

8.1.2.7 *Insomnia*

Some studies report clinical benefits from using mirtazapine in patients with sleep disorders, such as the insomnia associated with obstructive sleep apnea. However, as with the treatment of movement disorders, because of the multiplicity of effects of mirtazapine, unless it is indicated also for a comorbid depressive or anxious disorder, we prefer to use more specific hypnotic drugs. An additional factor discouraging the use of mirtazapine as the primary medication for insomnia is its long half-life which increases the risk of next-day sedation/cognitive impairment.

8.1.3 *Dosing*

Mirtazapine is administered once a day, in the evening. The recommended initial dose is 15 mg, which can be increased, after several weeks, to 30 mg, and then 45 mg/day. However, in patients with partial response and no side effects at 45 mg/day, daily doses of 60 mg have been used successfully.

8.1.4 *Side effects, adverse reactions, warnings, and precautions*

The most common side effects with mirtazapine are those related to its antihistaminic and, less frequently, to its anticholinergic actions. These include somnolence, increased appetite and weight gain, dry mouth, and constipation.

Serotonergic side effects such as sexual dysfunction or EPS may occur with mirtazapine, but they are significantly less frequent than with SSRIs and SNRIs (for serotonergic side effects, we refer the reader to Chapter 6).

Abrupt suspension of mirtazapine may induce discontinuation symptoms. However, this syndrome is less likely to occur and less severe than those induced by SSRIs or SNRIs. As with other antidepressants, the treatment for discontinuation symptoms is restarting mirtazapine at the last dose, and then tapering it gradually (see Section 6.8 for details).

The Prescribing Information for mirtazapine (Remeron) includes a warning about reversible granulocytopenia, mentioning that in pre-marketing trials, three patients developed agranuloctytosis or severe neutropenia, all of whom recovered when mirtazapine was stopped. This emphasis on blood dyscrasias is probably related to the fact that mirtazapine's predecessor, mianserin, was taken off the market due to the occurrence of agranulocytosis. After 14 years of widespread use in the USA, however, we have found very scarce reports of neutropenia with mirtazapine.

Mirtazapine should be used with caution in patients with liver disease. Also, careful monitoring is recommended in renal disease.

Mirtazapine may also cause serotonin syndrome in overdose or when coadministered with other serotonergic medications (for serotonin syndrome, see Section 6.9).

Mirtazapine, as with every other antidepressant, should never be co-administered with MAOIs (monoamine oxidase inhibitors).

8.1.5 *Use of mirtazapine during pregnancy*

Although there are no large studies examining this issue, mirtazapine seems to be a relatively safe medication during pregnancy, with similar caveats to other serotonergic antidepressants (for example, risk for pulmonary hypertension of the newborn). However, there exist isolated reports of rare adverse effects, such as a case of neonatal prolonged hypothermia in twins born to a mirtazapine-treated mother. According to the authors of that report, mirtazapine has the potential to influence thermoregulation through serotonin and adrenergic receptors (Sokolover *et al.*, 2008). On the positive side, there are reports on the successful treatment of hyperemesis gravidarum with mirtazapine.

8.2 Trazodone

Trazodone was actually the first second-generation antidepressant introduced in the USA in 1982, under the brand name Desyrel. It was initially developed in Italy by investigators seeking common pathways for depression and pain and marketed in the USA by Mead Johnson Laboratories. At first, trazodone was broadly used as an antidepressant and took a good share of the market, but then declined after the appearance of the SSRIs and also due to the strong sedation induced by the therapeutic dosages needed to treat depression. However, these may not have been the only reasons for trazodone's decline. Immediate-release (IR) trazodone had to be given in several doses a day, and as it induced significant sleepiness with each dose, daytime sleepiness became a practical problem. In any case, use of trazodone gradually shifted from the treatment of depression to the treatment of insomnia, in single doses of 50–300 mg given before bedtime. However, recently, a sustained-release (SR) preparation of trazodone, under the name Oleptro, has been introduced for the indication of depression, and this can be administered in one daily dose at night.

The antidepressant mechanism of trazodone is not completely clear. Trazodone is a potent antagonist at 5-HT_{2A} (some consider this its predominant antidepressant mechanism). Trazodone also seems to be an agonist or partial agonist at 5-HT_{1A}, which may also contribute to its antidepressant and anti-anxiety action. Trazodone is a weak serotonin (5-HT) reuptake inhibitor and a weak antagonist at 5-HT_{2C} receptors (which would be a reason for its small effect on appetite). Trazodone blocks histamine H_1 receptors. It is a weak antagonist of α_2- but a potent blocker of α_1-adrenergic receptors (this last action may contribute to sedation and cardiovascular side effects). Besides this, it has been proposed that some metabolites of trazodone, especially m-chlorophenylpiperazine (m-CPP), which is a potent agonist at serotonin receptors, including 5-HT_{1A}, play a role in the clinical effects of the drug. m-CPP poses special problems, as it may cause side effects such as anxiety, anorexia, and depression; some argue that the potential presence of m-CPP should be considered as a negative factor when prescribing trazodone.

8.2.1 *Pharmacokinetics*

Trazodone is well absorbed after oral administration. Its half-life is 4–9 h. Peak concentration (C_{max}) occurs 1–2 h after oral administration of IR trazodone and 9 h after administration of Oleptro. However, the total amount of trazodone that is absorbed is grossly the same for three 100 mg individual doses of IR trazodone and one single 300 mg dose of Oleptro. Trazodone is metabolized mainly by CYP3A4, and the metabolites are eliminated in urine. Trazodone is not a significant inhibitor of metabolic enzymes.

8.2.2 *Indications and uses*

8.2.2.1 *Depression*

Trazodone is approved for the treatment of major depression. When discussing this use, we will focus on the SR preparation, Oleptro. The recommended dose of Oleptro is 150–375 mg/day, in one dose at night. Despite their SR formulation, the tablets (150 and 300 mg) may be split in half.

8.2.2.2 *Anxiety disorders*

Trazodone has been shown, in randomized placebo-controlled studies, to have anti-anxiety effects. Thus, even though we would not recommend it as a primary treatment for anxiety, trazodone may offer an additional benefit in depressed patients with coexistent anxiety and insomnia.

8.2.2.3 *Insomnia*

The broad use of trazodone for insomnia grew in the last decades thanks to its sedating, sleep-inducing properties, and to the fact that it is not addictive (unlike the benzodiazepines) and requires no special controls. A 14-day comparison of trazodone and zolpidem with placebo in primary insomnia showed at week 1 an advantage for both medications over placebo in shortening sleep latency and prolonging sleep time; at week 2, only zolpidem showed an advantage over placebo in sleep latency, and neither zolpidem nor trazodone had an advantage over placebo in sleep duration. However, this loss of the significant difference with placebo may have been related to continued improvement in the placebo group rather than loss of efficacy in the medication groups (Walsh *et al.*, 1998). Some experts question the use of trazodone as a primary hypnotic agent, mainly because of its side effect profile. In our opinion, trazodone should be considered especially in the case of depressed patients and patients at higher risk of dependence in which we want to avoid addictive medications.

8.2.2.4 *Other uses of trazodone*

Due to the lack of significant anticholinergic effects, trazodone has been suggested as an appropriate choice for managing depression in the elderly, and it is often used for the treatment of behavioral problems (agitation) in older patients, particularly those with dementia. The issue has not yet been settled. Furthermore, in the elderly, we have to keep in mind that trazodone has a relatively high incidence of antihistaminic and adrenergic (cardiovascular) side effects.

8.2.3 *Side effects and adverse reactions*

Trazodone may cause serotonergic side effects, such as sexual dysfunction (see Chapter 6 for details), antihistaminic side effects, and adrenergic side effects like hypotension/syncope.

Below, we list the most common side effects reported with Oleptro (in parenthesis the frequency with placebo):

(1) Somnolence/Sedation 8 (4.0%)
(2) Dizziness 7 (3.5%)
(3) Confusional state 2 (1.0%)
(4) Coordination abnormal 2 (1.0%)
(5) Headache 2 (1.0%)

(6) Nausea 2 (1.0%)
(7) Balance disorder/Gait disturbance 2 (1.0%)

Abrupt discontinuation of trazodone may induce discontinuation syndrome. As with other antidepressants, treatment is restarting at the last dose, and tapering gradually (see Section 6.8).

Serotonin syndrome (Section 6.9) may be an issue with trazodone in overdose or when co-administered with other serotonergic medications.

The Prescribing Information for Oleptro gives a warning regarding the potential of trazodone to prolong the QT/QTc interval, and cause malignant arrhythmia (torsades de pointes). Considering that a major factor for this dangerous reaction is the number of QT-prolonging medications taken concomitantly, co-administration of trazodone with other QT-prolonging medications requires careful consideration (see Chapters 6 and 19). Administration of trazodone is also not recommended in patients with cardiac disease.

A rare but serious side effect of trazodone in males is priapism, a prolonged painful erection that may cause penile lesion and impotence (see Section 3.11 for more details). It seems to occur more often in young males. In studies with Oleptro, no cases of priapism were found, possibly because concentration peaks, which are likely to trigger side effects, are lower with Oleptro than IR trazodone. However, all patients on any formulation of trazodone must receive a clear warning in lay language. Our standard advice is for patients to go to the Emergency Room if they have an erection that lasts longer than 3–4 h. A parallel side effect, persistent genital arousal, has been described in females.

Trazodone should be used with care in patients with significant hepatic or renal disease.

As with any other antidepressant, trazodone should never be co-administered with MAOIs.

8.3 Nefazodone

Nefazodone is an antidepressant with standard efficacy and good tolerability, introduced in the USA in 1996 under the brand name Serzone. Unfortunately, reports of irreversible hepatitis needing liver transplant have led to its withdrawal in Canada and restricted its use in the USA.

Nefazodone is a potent antagonist for all 5-HT_2 receptors, and a moderate antagonist at the α_1-adrenergic and 5-HT_{1A} receptors. Because of its lower affinity for α_1 receptors, nefazodone has less sedative and cardiovascular side effects than trazodone. Nefazodone is a weak inhibitor of 5-HT reuptake.

Its affinity for H_1 and M_1 receptors is negligible, and thus it has no clinical antihistaminic or anticholinergic effects.

8.3.1 *Pharmacokinetics*

Nefazodone has an almost complete absorption after oral administration, but has also a fast metabolism, resulting in a low bioavailability and short half-life (2–4 h). Similarly to the case of trazodone, active metabolites, including m-CPP, may play a role in the adverse effects of nefazodone.

Nefazodone is metabolized by the oxidative enzyme CYP3A4, and is a strong inhibitor for CYP3A4 and a weak inhibitor for CYP2D6.

8.3.2 *Indications and uses*

Nefazodone is approved for the treatment of depression. Several studies have shown the benefits of nefazodone in anxiety and other disorders. However, considering the liabilities derived from the risk of liver failure, probably the only judicious use of nefazodone these days is in depressed patients with documented poor tolerance of, or response to, other second-generation antidepressants.

8.3.3 *Dosing*

The recommended initial dose of nefazodone is 200 mg/day, in two divided doses of 100 mg. The maximum dose is 600 mg/day, in two 300 mg doses.

8.3.4 *Adverse reactions, side effects, and precautions*

The side effects of nefazodone with the highest difference in frequency regarding placebo were, in descending order: dry mouth, somnolence, dizziness, nausea, constipation, headache, lightheadedness, asthenia, confusion, and postural hypotension (but not syncope).

Regarding liver failure, this is the paragraph about its incidence, in the Prescribing Information for nefazodone:

> The reported rate in the United States is about 1 case of liver failure resulting in death or transplant per 250,000 to 300,000 patient-years of Nefazodone treatment. This represents a rate of about 3 to 4 times the estimated background rate of liver failure. This rate is an underestimate because of under reporting, and the true risk could be considerably greater than this. A large

> cohort study of antidepressant users found no cases of liver failure leading to death or transplant among Nefazodone users in about 30,000 patient-years of exposure. The spontaneous report data and the cohort study results provide estimates of the upper and lower limits of the risk of liver failure in Nefazodone-treated patients, but are not capable of providing a precise risk estimate.

When prescribing nefazodone, we urge the reader to review the section on 'Hepatotoxicity' in the Prescribing Information, regarding the monitoring of patients taking nefazodone.

Abrupt discontinuation of nefazodone may induce discontinuation syndrome. As with other antidepressants, treatment is restarting at last dose, and tapering gradually (see Section 6.8).

Nefazodone may also cause serotonin syndrome in overdose or when coadministered with other serotonergic medications (see Section 6.9).

Nefazodone is both a substrate and a strong inhibitor for CYP3A4; the combination of nefazodone with substrates or inhibitors of CYP3A4 can lead to toxicity.

Nefazodone use should be avoided in patients with liver disease.

As with every other antidepressant, nefazodone should not be combined with MAOIs.

References

Mirtazapine

Alderman CP, Condon JT, Gilbert AL. An open-label study of mirtazapine as a treatment for combat-related PTSD. *Ann Pharmacother* 2009;43(7):1220–1226.

Berk M, Gama CS, Sundram S, *et al.* Mirtazapine add-on therapy in the treatment of schizophrenia with atypical antipsychotics: A double-blind, randomised, placebo-controlled clinical trial. *Hum Psychopharmacol* 2009;24(3):233–238.

Gambi F, De Berardis D, Campanella D, *et al.* Mirtazapine treatment of generalized anxiety disorder: A fixed dose, open label study. *J Psychopharmacol* 2005;19(5):483–487.

Joffe G, Terevnikov V, Joffe M, *et al.* Add-on mirtazapine enhances antipsychotic effect of first generation antipsychotics in schizophrenia: A double-blind, randomized, placebo-controlled trial. *Schizophr Res* 2009;108:245–251.

Ostacher MJ, Eisner L, Nierenberg AA. Mirtazapine in the treatment of mood and anxiety disorders. *Expert Review Neurother* 2003;3(4):425–433.

Poyurovsky M, Pashinian A, Weizman R, *et al.* Low-dose mirtazapine: A new option in the treatment of antipsychotic-induced akathisia. A randomized, double-blind, placebo- and propranolol-controlled trial. *Biol Psychiatry* 2006;59(11):1071–1077.

Sokolover N, Merlob P, Klinger G. Neonatal recurrent prolonged hypothermia associated with maternal mirtazapine treatment during pregnancy. *Can J Clin Pharmacol* 2008; 15(2):e188–e190.

Trazodone

Ghanbari R, El Mansari M, Blier P. Sustained administration of trazodone enhances serotonergic neurotransmission: *In vivo* electrophysiological study in the rat. *J Pharmacol Exp Ther* 2010;335(1):197–206.

Kast RE. Trazodone generates m-CPP: In 2008 risks from m-CPP might outweight benefits of trazodone. *World J Biol Psychiatry* 2009;10(4):682–685.

Mendelson WB. A review of the evidence for the efficacy and safety of trazodone in insomnia. *J Clin Psychiatry* 2005;66(4):469–476.

Odagaki Y, Toyoshima R, Yamauchi T. Trazodone and its active metabolite m-chlorophenylpiperazine as partial agonists at 5-HT_{1A} receptors assessed by [35S]GTPgammaS binding. *J Psychopharmacol* 2005;19(3):235–241.

Rosenberg RP. Sleep maintenance insomnia: Strengths and weaknesses of current pharmacological therapies. *Ann Clin Psychiatry* 2006;18(1):49–56.

Nefazodone

Taylor DP, Carter RB, Eison AS, *et al.* Pharmacology and neurochemistry of nefazodone, a novel antidepressant drug. *J Clin Psychiatry* 1995;56(Suppl. 6):3–11.

Vieweg WV. Nefazodone and depression. *Drugs Today* 1998;34(10):845–853.

Chapter 9

Monoamine Oxidase Inhibitors and Tricyclic Antidepressants

In this chapter, we will examine the two antidepressant groups introduced 60 years ago, during the psychopharmacology explosion of the 1950s: tricyclic antidepressants (TCAs) and monoamine oxidase inhibitors (MAOIs). TCAs were the mainstay in the treatment of depression, and MAOIs the option in patients unresponsive to them, until the 1980s, when, mainly for safety and tolerability considerations, they were displaced by SSRIs and other second-generation antidepressants. Though the advantages of the new antidepressants regarding toxicity and side effects are large, the antidepressant efficacy has not improved, and the old antidepressants still have a role to play in patients who respond poorly to the new medications. However, in recent times, in the case of difficult-to-treat depressed patients, the old antidepressants are being gradually replaced by non-antidepressant medications such as "atypical" antipsychotics. This trend is not justified by the available evidence. It involves an overvaluation of the antidepressant effect of the new antipsychotics, and a false sense of security derived from the erroneous belief that these new "atypical" antipsychotics are significantly safer than the old ones. Thus, until the advent of more efficacious antidepressant and anti-anxiety medications, TCAs and MAOIs will have a role to play in patients with difficult-to-treat mood disorders.

9.1 Monoamine Oxidase Inhibitors

The first antidepressant ever introduced, during the psychopharmacology explosion of the 1950s, was iproniazide (Marsilid), an MAOI related to the anti-infective drug isoniazide, launched in 1954 and later withdrawn due to liver toxicity. Nonselective irreversible MAOIs still in use in the USA, such as tranylcypromine (Parnate) and phenelzine (Nardil), were introduced in the early 1960s, and isocarboxazid (Marplan), with a more checkered history, followed shortly afterwards. More recently, selegiline, a selective MAO-B inhibitor long used for the treatment of Parkinson's disease, was introduced in a new formulation — transdermal patch — for the treatment of depression (Emsam). Significantly safer selective MAO-A reversible inhibitors, such as brofaromine and moclobemide, have long been in use in Europe for the treatment of depression, but were never introduced in the USA.

Phenelzine, tranylcypromine, and isocarboxazid increase the amount of free serotonin, norepinephrine, and dopamine in the brain by inhibiting the MAOs that primarily metabolize them. Two MAO types, A and B, are recognized, with different affinity for the monoamines and other substrates. Serotonin, norepinephrine, and epinephrine are metabolized primarily by MAO-A, while dopamine is metabolized by both types. Because the inhibition of the enzymes by these drugs is irreversible and the body's production of MAOs is a slow process, when these medications are discontinued, it takes several weeks for MAO activity to go back to normal. An important factor for adverse reactions with these antidepressants is that, besides neurotransmitter monoamines, MAOs also metabolize a number of other amines with physiological effects, especially cardiovascular. Thus, MAO-A and B are abundant in the brain, but are also present in some compartment barriers, such as the blood–brain and blood–gut barriers, exerting a protective role.

The potential to inhibit the metabolism of monoamines with cardiovascular actions has been the main factor curtailing the therapeutic use of MAOIs. The best-known of these amines is tyramine, present in a number of foods and drinks, especially those that are aged. Tyramine is metabolized primarily by MAO-B. Ingestion of food or beverage rich in tyramine, in conditions of generalized MAO inhibition, produces a hypertensive crisis that can be fatal. Because of this, all nonselective MAOIs and selective MAO-B inhibitors are subject to severe dietary restrictions, mainly of liver and aged foods and beverages, including cheese and alcoholic drinks (see Table 9.1). MAOIs should not be combined either with any adrenergic, serotonergic, or dopaminergic medications/supplements/substances of abuse. This means all the antidepressants, the anti-anxiety medication buspirone, stimulant medications, cocaine, and many cardiovascular and respiratory drugs or combinations of drugs (see Table 9.2). A two-week washout period is recommended when switching from other antidepressants to MAOIs or vice versa (longer for medications with a long half-life, such as fluoxetine).

Table 9.1 Food groups to avoid or restrict while on MAOIs.

Avoid	Restrict
Liver	Coffee
Aged cheese	Tea
Aged and processed meats	Cola
Red wine and aged wine liqueurs	Bottled and canned beer
Overripe and dried fruit	White wine
Fermented and pickled products (incl. sauerkraut)	Soy milk
Tap beer	
Soup packages	
Fava beans	
Yeast extract (OK yeast in bakery or pasteurized beer)	
Processed soy products	
Monosodium glutamate (MSG)	

Table 9.2 Medications and supplements to avoid in combination with MAOIs.

Medications	Supplements and substances of abuse
Antidepressant medications	L-tryptophan
Stimulants (includes "ecstasy")	St. John's wort
Carbamazepine	Yeast extract
Cyclobenzaprine	Anorexigenic ("weight-reducing") and stimulant ("energy") supplements
Buspirone	Cocaine
Meperidine	
D-metorphan	
Fenfluramine, sibutramine, and other anorexiants	
Dopaminergic medications	
Serotonergic medications	
Adrenergic medications (remember cold medications and anti-asthma medications)	

9.1.1 *Pharmacokinetics of the nonselective irreversible MAOIs: Isocarboxazid, phenelzine, and tranylcypromine*

Oral MAOIs approved for psychiatric use in the USA include the hydrazine derivatives isocarboxazide and phenelzine, and the non-hydrazine tranylcipromine. Phenelzine has structural similarities to amphetamine, and some animal evidence suggests that it may have stimulant-like effects and affect the release and reuptake of dopamine, norepinephrine, and, to a lesser extent, serotonin. MAOIs have short biological half-lives, in the order of single digits in hours, and need to be given several times a day. The metabolic pathway of MAOIs is not completely clear. Phenelzine is likely a substrate for MAO, but the issue is not settled. Tranylcypromine seems to be eliminated by CYP450 oxidation, and is an inhibitor for CYP2C19.

9.1.2 *Partially selective irreversible transdermal MAOI: Selegiline*

Oral selegiline, also called L-deprenyl (Eldepryl), has long been used, concurrent with L-DOPA, for the treatment of the motor symptoms of Parkinson's disease. In Parkinson's disease, selegiline has also shown some benefit for depressive and demented symptoms. An irreversible MAOI, low-dose selegiline is selective for MAO-B, but as the dose goes up it gradually inhibits also MAO-A. Selegiline has both a very short half-life and a large first-pass elimination at the gut and liver. Selegiline is metabolized by several CYP450 enzymes to amphetamine and methamphetamine, and there is some indication that these metabolites could contribute to its therapeutic effects.

In 2006, a transdermal formulation (patch) of selegiline (Emsam) was approved in the USA for the treatment of depression. Administration through the skin has a dual benefit; it increases the bioavailability of selegiline, avoiding the first-pass elimination at the gut and liver, and reduces interactions with food and oral drugs due to the inhibition of MAO in these organs. At the lowest transdermal dose, one 6 mg patch every 24 h, Emsam does not require dietary limitations.

9.1.3 *Side effects and adverse reactions*

MAOIs may induce the side effects described for serotonergic, adrenergic, and dopaminergic antidepressants, and several others. An uncomfortable side effect is ankle edema, which may require the administration of diuretics. Orthostatic hypotension may require the addition of salt and mineralocorticoids such as fludrocortisone. Other side effects/adverse reactions include weight gain or loss, headaches, cognitive disturbances, dizziness, constipation, urinary difficulty, sexual dysfunction, dry mouth, blurry vision, muscle cramps, weakness, and extrapyramidal symptoms. Hepatotoxicity is seen infrequently, but liver function tests must be performed whenever there are symptoms pointing in this direction.

9.1.4 *Precautions*

MAOIs should not be used in patients with pheochromocytoma, their use is relatively contraindicated in patients with hypertension or significant cerebral or coronary artery disease.

9.1.5 *Hypertensive crisis*

Hypertensive crisis is usually due to the combination of MAOIs with certain foodstuffs, drugs, substances of abuse or supplements (see Tables 9.1 and 9.2). It is characterized by occipital headache, neck stiffness and soreness, hypertension, tachycardia, mydriasis, photophobia, nausea, vomiting, and sometimes chest pain. Traditionally, treatment has been parenteral administration (IM or IV) of 5 mg of the α-adrenergic receptor blocker phentolamine, with the option of repeating after 30 min; however, recently some authors recommend sublingual captopril (at 25mg doses) or nifedipine (at 10 mg doses). The patient could be kept in an erect position to additionally lower the blood pressure. Other medications, such as beta-blockers or diuretics may also be used for tachycardia or fluid retention.

9.1.6 *Use of MAOIs during pregnancy*

Because of the risk for serious adverse events, especially cardiovascular ones, the authors do not consider MAOIs be used during pregnancy. For severely depressed pregnant patients, when reasonably safe pharmacological options have been exhausted, other effective and safe somatic treatments, especially ECT, are available.

9.1.7 *What is the role of MAOIs in today's clinical practice?*

With the introduction of new drugs with an improved safety profile that are well tolerated and easy to use, MAOIs have continued to go further down the list of preferred agents. Today, MAOIs are "last-ditch" medications, to be tried in difficult-to-treat depressed patients, when all other pharmacological measures have failed. However, until the advent of antidepressants with higher efficacy, MAOIs will likely have a role to play in the management of depression. Regarding other disorders, considering their wide mechanism of action, it is not surprising that MAOIs seem to be useful in a range of mental illnesses that includes anxiety, panic, social phobia, obsessive–compulsive disorder, post-traumatic stress disorder, chronic pain, etc. However, as in the case of depression, the use of MAOIs in these disorders is warranted only when safer and better-tolerated options have been exhausted.

9.2 Tricyclic Antidepressants

The TCAs derive their group name from the fact that their molecule has three central rings. However, included in this group are some compounds such as maprotiline (Ludiomil) which, despite having a somewhat different molecular structure, are clinically similar to the true TCAs.

9.2.1 *General characteristics and classification*

When we think of the TCAs, we tend to forget how similar their mechanism of action is to that of newer drugs such as the SSRIs and SNRIs. The main differences between old antidepressants such as TCAs and the ones introduced more recently reside not as much in their mechanism of action or clinical efficacy as in their safety and tolerability profile. The TCAs inhibit the reuptake of serotonin and norepinephrine, in a similar way to SSRIs and SNRIs. However, different from SSRIs and SNRIs, which are rather selective for the serotonin (5-HT) and norepinephrine transporters, the TCAs, at clinical doses, affect a number of other receptors, causing disturbing side effects and creating risks not seen with newer antidepressants. These receptors include adrenergic (α_1), histaminic (H_1), and muscarinic/cholinergic (M_1).

TCAs are divided into **tertiary TCAs**, which have two terminal methyl groups, and **secondary TCAs,** which have only one terminal methyl group. *In vivo*, the first pass in the metabolism of tertiary tricyclics involves the loss of one of these methyl groups, to become secondary TCAs. Tertiary TCAs show a significantly higher affinity for the 5-HT reuptake pump, while secondary TCAs show higher affinity for the norepinephrine transporter. Thus, because of their *in vivo* transformation to a secondary TCA, administering a tertiary TCA is, in essence, very similar to administering an SNRI. In general, tertiary TCAs tend to bind more receptors, besides the 5-HT and norepinephrine transporters, than the secondary TCAs, and because of this they tend to have more side effects. For example, it is usually said that the tertiary TCA amitriptyline is the "dirtiest" psychotropic available, due to the high number of receptors it binds. In Table 9.3, we list the TCAs available in the USA.

9.2.1.1 *Receptor binding profile*

In Table 9.4, we present the relative affinity of TCAs for the main types of receptors. As we can see, clomipramine has the highest affinity for the 5-HT

Table 9.3 Tricyclic antidepressants available in the USA.

Both tertiary and secondary TCAs available	Amitriptyline (Elavil) → nortriptyline (Pamelor)
	Imipramine (Tofranil) → desipramine (Norpramin)
Only tertiary TCAs available	Clomipramine (Anafranil)
	Doxepin (Sinequan)
	Trimipramine (Surmontil)
Only secondary TCAs available	Protriptyline (Vivactil)
Tetracyclic	Maprotiline (Ludiomil)
Heterocyclic, related to antipsychotics	Amoxapine (Asendin)

Table 9.4 Relative affinity of TCAs for the receptors they tend to bind.

Drug	5-HT trans.	NE trans.	H_1	M_1	α_1	5-HT_2
Amitriptyline	+++	++	+++	++	++	++
Amoxapine	++	++	++	---	++	+++
Clomipramine	++++	++	++	++	++	++
Desipramine	++	++++	+	+	+	+
Doxepin	++	++	++++	++	+	++
Imipramine	+++	++	++	++	+	+
Maprotiline	---	++	+++	+	++	+
Nortriptyline	++	+++	+++	+	++	++
Protriptyline	++	+++	++	++	+	++
Trimipramine	+	---	++++	++	++	++

transporter, which explains the superior effect of this drug in obsessive–compulsive disorder, a disorder that responds mainly to serotonergic drugs. Amitriptyline and clomipramine have significant affinity (++ to ++++) for all the transporters and receptors listed, thus they are more likely to have a variety of side effects. However, as we can deduce from this table, all TCAs have the potential for disturbing side effects. Doxepin and trimipramine have significantly higher affinity for the histamine H_1 than any other receptor, and clinically they exhibit potent antihistaminic and sedative actions. In fact, doxepin has one of the highest affinities for the histamine H_1 receptor among available drugs in all of medicine; its affinity for H_1 receptors is two orders of magnitude (at least 100:1) higher than for the 5-HT or norepinephrine transporters. Because of this, doxepin is also offered as an antipruritic cream and was recently introduced as a sleeping aid. Following doxepin and trimipramine in the potency of antihistaminic effects are amitriptyline, maprotiline, and nortriptyline. Amoxapine is a pharmacological rarity. Besides its serotonergic and dopaminergic activity, amoxapine, directly and, especially through its metabolite 7-OH amoxapine, exerts dopaminergic-blocking properties. Thus, it also has antipsychotic properties.

9.2.2 *Pharmacokinetics*

TCAs undergo an almost complete intestinal absorption, but also a significant first-pass effect at the liver, which reduces the serum levels. Due to their anticholinergic effect, TCAs slow the intestinal transit, furthermore enhancing absorption, an important consideration in overdose, when signs of toxicity may continue or go up long after admission. The elimination half-life of TCAs, with the exception of amoxapine, is 24 h or longer. Thus, they can be administered once a day, preferably at night, because of their sedative effects.

TCAs are eliminated mainly through CYP450 oxidation (see CYP tables in Chapter 19). Several cytochromes have the ability to oxidize TCAs, with the main ones being CYP2C19 for tertiary TCAs, and CYP2D6 for secondary TCAs. In general, TCAs are not significant inhibitors or inducers for oxidative or other metabolic enzymes.

9.2.3 *Dosing*

In Table 9.5, we give the daily dose ranges for TCAs, including starting and target doses. Starting doses for insomnia or neuropathic pain are significantly lower, 10 or 25 mg qhs. TCAs can be given once a day, preferably at night. As with any other serotonergic medication, the initial dose should be reduced (usually cut in half) in patients with panic or severe anxiety, to minimize the

Table 9.5 Usual effective antidepressant dose and, between parenthesis, starting dose of TCAs in adults.

Drug	Starting dose (mg/day)	Usual final antidepressant dose (mg/day)
Amitriptyline	50–75	150–300
Amoxapine	50–75	150–300
Clomipramine	50–75	150–300
Desipramine	50–75	150–300
Doxepin	50–75	150–300
Imipramine	50–75	150–300
Maprotiline	50–75	75–225
Nortriptyline	25–50	50–150
Protriptyline	10–20	20–60
Trimipramine	50–75	150–300

risk of exacerbation of anxiety or panic attacks. When stopping treatment, the dose must be tapered gradually (for example, cut in half every 4–7 days) to minimize the risk of discontinuation symptoms.

9.2.3.1 *Therapeutic drug monitoring*

A therapeutic window in serum levels was reported for some TCAs decades ago, especially for nortriptyline. Interest in this concept has declined with the decrease in TCA use, but some authorities still recommend targeting a range of serum levels when using nortriptyline and other TCAs. The authors do not put too much stock in therapeutic drug monitoring (TDM) for TCAs. First, the evidence for its validity is weak, as the ranges were generally assessed long ago in small studies in inpatient populations, using definitions of depression different from the current ones. Second, for all TCAs, most patients show significant side effects at medium and maximum doses, so the possibility of increasing the dose further if the levels are low is generally limited.

9.2.4 *Side effects*

Besides serotonergic and adrenergic side effects derived from their ability to increase serotonin and norepinephrine levels, TCAs may cause a wide array of adrenergic, antihistaminic, anticholinergic, and cardiovascular adverse reactions, related to their ability to block histamine, cholinergic, and circulatory adrenergic receptors. They also have significant potential to block the fast sodium channels in the heart, inducing malignant arrhythmias, as we will discuss below. The possibility and severity of the side effects and adverse reactions of TCAs, including seizures and cardiac toxicity, increase directly with the doses and serum levels.

Potential side effects and adverse reactions of TCAs include:

Cognitive. Sedation, cognitive impairment, and delirium. TCAs have a significantly higher risk than new antidepressants for sedation and delirium because of their antihistaminic and anticholinergic effects. Risk is even higher in patients already showing cognitive impairment, the elderly, and those taking other anticholinergic or antihistaminic drugs.

Neurologic. Seizures, paresthesias, numbness, fine tremor, akathisia, ataxia, myoclonus, and other EPS.

Gastrointestinal. Dry mouth, which can be severe enough to produce cavities and other dental problems, and constipation.

Genitourinary. Urinary retention and sexual dysfunction.

Ocular. Blurred vision, dry eye, and exacerbation of narrow angle glaucoma.

Skin. Excessive sweating.

Cardiovascular. Hypertension, tachycardia, orthostatic hypotension and syncope, and cardiac arrhythmias (including malignant such as torsades de pointes). TCAs are contraindicated in children and adults with pre-existent cardiac disease, especially conduction delay, as cardiac deaths have been reported at all ages.

9.2.5 *Serotonin syndrome with TCAs*

TCAs are serotonergic reuptake inhibitors; hence, in overdose or in combination with other serotonergic medications, they may induce serotonin syndrome (see Section 6.9).

9.2.6 *Precautions with TCAs in liver disease*

Due to their significant toxicity and narrow therapeutic margin, TCAs should be used with extreme care, or not at all, in patients with significant liver disease.

9.2.7 *Contraindications*

TCAs should not be used in patients with cardiac disease, and should never be combined with MAOIs. A washout period of 14 days must elapse between uses of these two types of medications.

9.2.8 *Toxicity*

TCAs are significantly more toxic than newer antidepressants. TCAs have a relatively narrow therapeutic margin (distance between therapeutic and harmful doses). The general estimate for the relationship between maximum daily doses and lethal doses for TCAs is approximately 1:10. A standard recommendation in potentially suicidal patients, in the pre-SSRI days, when TCAs were the most widely used antidepressants, was for the pharmacy to dispense these medications at weekly or even shorter intervals to decrease the chances of overdose. In a recent British study, fatal toxicity, defined as the ratio of deaths to prescriptions, was almost 30 times higher for TCAs compared to SSRIs (Hawton *et al.*, 2010). The reported toxic levels for TCAs vary considerably, both between compounds and subjects. This, in general, is not attributable to the test used to measure them, but the huge pharmacokinetic variability in any population. TCA overdose is associated with seizures, respiratory depression, and cardiac toxicity. Additionally, TCAs, as is often the case with medications used for suicide, are frequently ingested with alcohol and other drugs, whose respiratory, neurotoxic, and cardiac effects add to those of TCAs.

Cardiac arrhythmias with TCAs deserve special consideration as this is the usual cause of death in overdose. Cardiac toxicity of TCAs is due mainly to blockade of cardiac fast sodium channels, delaying the conduction of the electric impulse in the heart, an action similar to that of type I antiarrhythmics such as quinidine. This is further compounded by the M_1, H_1, and α_1 antagonism of TCAs. Same as quinidine and other antiarrhythmics, TCAs may induce malignant arrhythmias, especially torsades de pointes, with high lethality. TCAs also affect, to a lesser extent, delayed potassium channels in the heart, which can add to the risk of medications with potential to block potassium channels, such as antipsychotics. The TCA risk for malignant arrhythmias is additive with that of other medications. Several risk factors for torsades de pointes and other malignant arrhythmias have been identified, including pre-existing prolonged QT, female sex, age, metabolic and cardiac disease, and electrolytic imbalance (especially hypokalemia). However, a critical risk factor is the co-administration of medications with the potential to block sodium channels. These medications are numerous, and they include cardiovascular drugs, some antihistamines, and some antibiotics. Particular care should be exercised not to prescribe TCAs to patients taking antipsychotics and non-psychiatric medications known to increase the risk for malignant arrhythmias.

9.2.9 *Use of TCAs during pregnancy*

For 30 years, TCAs were the first option for pharmacological treatment of depression/anxiety during pregnancy. Although those years of wide use did not expose significant teratogenic effects, the use of TCAs in pregnancy should take into account their toxicity and potential for serious adverse events. Neonatal complications seem to be more common with TCAs than with newer antidepressants (Reis *et al.*, 2010). However, in difficult-to-treat depressed or anxious pregnant patients already stable on them, TCAs likely have a more positive benefit/risk ratio than non-antidepressant drugs such as antipsychotics. There are at least two caveats to the use of TCAs during pregnancy. First, they likely increase the risk for persistent pulmomary hypertension of the newborn in the same range as SSRIs/SNRIs. Second, in a similar way to SNRIs, their noradrenergic effects probably make them a high risk for preeclampsia (Palmsten *et al.*, 2012).

9.2.10 *What is the role of TCAs in today's clinical practice?*

Some experts maintain that TCAs seem to show higher efficacy in some types of depression, such as melancholic depression. However, this is supported mainly by anecdotal or small clinical observations. The controlled studies are few, including very small samples, and they date back several years, which poses the question of the comparability with populations selected using our current definition of depression. Second, and most importantly, we consider that, with their significant toxicity and tolerability issues, TCAs cannot, reasonably, be considered first-line treatment for any mental disorder. They have a role, though, in the management of difficult-to-treat ("treatment-resistant") mood disorders, such as depression, anxiety, panic, or obsessive–compulsive disorder, when multiple second-generation antidepressants have failed. TCAs are never first-choice hypnotic medications. However, because of their high H_1 affinity (especially doxepin, trimipramine, amitriptyline, and nortriptyline), they are also useful for the treatment of insomnia, in patients who should avoid addictive drugs, or who have not responded to other hypnotics. Hypnotic doses of TCAs are usually significantly lower than antidepressant doses to avoid side effect and toxicity risks. TCAs also seem more effective than the new antidepressants in the treatment of migraines. Finally, as other dual-action antidepressants, TCAs could be helpful in the management of neuropathic pain.

It does not seem realistic to expect that recently trained psychiatrists will be as knowledgeable about TCAs or MAOIs as the older generation of practitioners was at a time when there were no better options. However, in our opinion, in the case of TCAs, practitioners need to be familiar with at least one or two tertiary and one or two secondary TCAs. The obvious candidate among the tertiary TCAs is clomipramine. Clomipramine has the highest affinity for the 5-HT transporter among TCAs. It also exerts significant norepinephrine reuptake inhibition, both directly and through metabolites. Finally, it is the TCA to switch to when SSRIs prove unsatisfactory in treating obsessive–compulsive disorder. Among secondary TCAs, the obvious choice is nortriptyline, as it is the most widely used secondary TCA, the one with the most information available, the one with a potential therapeutic "window," and also, the one with a reasonably good side effect profile compared to other TCAs.

Regarding amoxapine, because of its dual antidepressant–antipsychotic effect, it was of interest during pre-SSRI times. We do not consider it justifiable these days to start a patient on a medication that combines the potential toxicity and side effects of TCAs and antipsychotics.

References

Flanagan RJ. Fatal toxicity of drugs used in psychiatry. *Hum Psychopharmacol Clin Exp* 2008;23:43–51.

Gillman PK. Tricyclic antidepressant pharmacology and therapeutic drug interactions updated. *Br J Pharmacol* 2007;151:737–748.

Hawton K, Bergen H, Simkin S, *et al.* Toxicity of antidepressants: rates of suicide relative to prescribing and non-fatal overdose. *Br J Psychiatry* 2010;196(5):354–358.

Reis M, Kallen B. Delivery outcome after maternal use of antidepressant drugs in pregnancy: An update using Swedish data. *Psychol Med* 2010;40(10):1723–1733.

Palmsten K, Setoguchi S, Margulis AV, *et al.* Elevated risk of preeclampsia in pregnant women with depression: Depression or antidepressants? *Am J Epidemiol* 2012;175(10): 988–997.

Vieweg WVR, Wood MA. Tricyclic antidepressants, QT prolongation, and torsade de pointes. *Psychosomatics* 2004;45:371–377.

Chapter 10

Individualized Treatment of Depression

All clinically available antidepressants have shown similar efficacy in the treatment of depression, and all have a "latency period" of several weeks before a full clinical effect is attained (possibly, the "experimental" drug ketamine will be the exception in this instance). However, there are broad differences across antidepressants in terms of safety, side effects/adverse reactions, and their effect on certain symptoms (e.g., anxiety, insomnia or hypersomnia, anorexia or increased appetite, poor concentration, energy, etc.).

Available guidelines on treatment of depression give clinicians ample room to make choices among second-generation antidepressants (SGAs). For example, an International Consensus Algorithm recommends, as a first step, "to prescribe an SSRI, SNRI, or NDRI" (Nutt *et al.*, 2010). The reason for this is the acknowledgment that all SGAs have approximately the same efficacy, and that most are reasonably safe. Systematic reviews and meta-analyses of direct and indirect comparisons of SGAs in the treatment of depression have shown no significant differences in efficacy. Any differences found are small and unlikely to have clinical significance. Equally important, no differences in efficacy were seen in patients with accompanying symptoms or in subgroups based on age, sex, ethnicity, or comorbid conditions. However, despite the similar efficacy, SGAs cannot be considered identical drugs, as there exist clear differences in important areas such as adverse reactions (Gartlehner *et al.* 2007).

In clinical practice, clinicians tend to have a favorite choice for first-line treatment. The most popular one appears to be SSRIs, but many practitioners prefer SNRIs due to their belief that two potential antidepressant mechanisms would work better than one. Having a "favorite pick" has the advantage of saving decision-making time and that the prescribers may be using the medications they are most familiar with, thus reducing the risk of physician errors.

Table 10.1. Some patient characteristics that may be factors in the choice of an antidepressant.

Depressive symptom profile: insomnia or hypersomnia, increased or decreased appetite, normal or impaired concentration and memory, level of energy, etc.

- Tolerability of side effects for individual patients
- Patient's prior history of response to antidepressant treatment
- Family history of response to antidepressant treatment
- Comorbid psychiatric conditions: anxiety disorders, ADHD, pre-menstrual dysphoric disorder (PMDD), anorexia/bulimia, tobacco and substance use, etc.
- Medical conditions: metabolic and endocrine disorders (obesity, underweight, thyroid, diabetes, dyslipidemia), cardiovascular illness (heart conditions, hypertension), central or peripheral neurological illness (seizures, peripheral neuropathy), autonomic disorders (sexual dysfunction, constipation, urinary retention, glaucoma)
- Concurrent medications, both prescribed and OTC, and supplements
- Compliance factors (number of recommended daily doses, tendency to miss doses, cost, health insurance coverage, etc.)

However, this approach ignores the peculiarities of individual patients. Depressed patients present with diverse psychiatric or medical comorbidities, differing medical histories and medical risks, variable tendencies to either express or tolerate medication side effects, histories of treatment response or non-response, and perhaps more importantly, they differ in their symptomatic profiles. They may present with bulimia or anorexia, insomnia or hypersomnia, retardation or agitation, normal or decreased energy, normal or significantly impaired concentration and memory, variable levels of energy or interest, severe or no anxiety, and so on.

Thus, considering the different clinical profiles of antidepressant drugs and the individual profiles of depressed patients, the authors believe that a reasonable approach is for the clinician to try to match the therapeutic actions and type of adverse effects and risks of the drugs with the individual characteristics of a given patient. In Table 10.1, we provide examples of patient factors that should be considered when choosing an antidepressant for the individualized initial treatment of depression.

10.1 Patient Factors to Consider

10.1.1 *Depressive symptom profile*

Fitting the pharmacological profile of the medication to the symptomatic profile of the individual patient may not improve the efficacy of antidepressant treatment. However, it will surely improve patients' medication adherence

Table 10.2. Second-generation antidepressants (SGAs) suggested, according to symptomatic profile.

Symptom	Second-generation antidepressant
Anxiety (generalized, social, panic-like, obsessions and compulsions, etc.)	Start with an SSRI or SNRI (though any SGA other than bupropion will likely help)
Poor attention and memory, lack of energy and initiative, overweight, overeating, oversleeping, retardation, sexual dysfunction	Bupropion or, distant second, an SNRI
Insomnia	Mirtazapine, trazodone
Anorexia	Mirtazapine

and attitude toward treatment by offering them benefits in more areas. In Table 10.2, we list the antidepressants that fit best various individual symptoms of depression.

10.1.2 *Patient's and family histories of response*

If a patient has responded to a medication in the past, that antidepressant ought to be the logical choice, unless there are safety or tolerability issues. An advantage of this approach is that when the individual effective dose is known, a faster titration, targeted on that dose, is possible. Conversely, if there is a history of non-response or adverse reaction, the medication should be avoided. In the former case, naturally, it behooves the prescriber to make sure that effective doses were tried for a long enough period of time, to avoid discarding potentially helpful drugs. Lacking an individual history of response to antidepressants, the family history of response to treatment may be an important factor to consider.

10.1.3 *Comorbid psychiatric conditions*

A clinical presentation of depression accompanied by significant anxiety symptoms favors the choice of an SSRI first and an SNRI as a second option, though any SGA other than bupropion is likely to help. ADHD or other attention problems favor the use of bupropion followed by SNRIs. Tobacco or substance use disorders may favor the use of bupropion. In the presence of aggressiveness and impulse control disorders, an SSRI is probably the best choice. In patients with comorbid psychosis, PTSD-associated depression, and other disorders likely to require multiple psychotropics, we must choose a medication with low risk of drug–drug interactions (DDIs).

10.1.4 *Medical conditions*

In depressed patients with serious cardiovascular conditions, bupropion and SNRIs need to be used with care, and an SSRI is likely the best option. Bupropion should also be avoided in patients with a history of seizures. In associated conditions such as obesity or hypothyroidism where there is low energy, weight gain, and other issues, bupropion could be the best choice. In undernourished or anorexic patients, mirtazapine may help with appetite. Mirtazapine could also be useful in patients with hyperemesis. In diabetes mellitus, with the potential to compromise multiple organs, an SSRI is a safe choice, except in significant neuropathic pain in which case an SNRI, or in severe instances, a TCA could be chosen. SNRIs should be used with care in patients with urinary retention (prostate hypertrophy, prostatitis, and low urinary obstruction), and narrow angle glaucoma. In cancer patients, or in chronic exhausting diseases, bupropion is our first and SNRIs our second choice, which could be better in efforts to preserve or enhance energy. In neuropsychiatric conditions such as Parkinson's disease, dementia, or any illness with cognitive impairment, SSRIs are considered safe, but also bupropion may help with cognition.

A note about depressed patients with Parkinson's disease: some studies suggest that the TCA nortriptyline or SNRIs work better than SSRIs in this population. However, the anticholinergic and cardiovascular effects of nortriptyline should make us cautious as should also the adrenergic side effects of SNRIs.

10.1.5 *Concurrent medications and supplements*

Regarding DDIs between antidepressants and other drugs patients may be using, the most important consideration is that half of all medications marketed in the USA are metabolized by CYP3A4, and antidepressants inhibiting this enzyme should be avoided whenever possible. This warning applies mainly to nefazodone and fluvoxamine. The second most important cytochrome in all of medicine is CYP2D6, and this demands that the prescriber be careful when using its inhibitors that among antidepressants include fluoxetine, paroxetine, duloxetine, and bupropion. The safest SGAs concerning DDIs are sertraline, citalopram/escitalopram, mirtazapine, venlafaxine/desmethylvenlafaxine, trazodone, vilazodone, and milnacipram. The most troublesome, by far, is fluvoxamine.

An important potential DDI is that of antidepressants and the anticancer drug tamoxifen. Many antidepressants carry, in different degrees, the potential to inhibit CYP2D6, which converts tamoxifen, a prodrug, into the active compound endoxifen. Safe options in these patients are venlafaxine (Effexor), an SNRI, which the authors favor because of its broad clinical use and its therapeutic potential in patients with "hot flashes"; desmethylvenlafaxine (Pristiq), a venlafaxine metabolite, more expensive and with pdr dosing recommendations possibly too low for efficacy; mirtazapine (Remeron), a good option in patients with insomnia and low appetite; trazodone (for the treatment of depression we prefer the SR form, Oleptro); vilazodone (Viibryd), a recently introduced SSRI, whose dosing is still uncertain; and milnacipram (Savella), an SNRI, the most expensive of the lot and one that psychiatrists are not as familiar with, as in the USA it has been introduced only for treating fibromyalgia.

Anticonvulsants, especially carbamazepine, may impair the efficacy of several antidepressants by inducing their metabolic enzymes and significantly lowering the levels of medication. Carbamazepine is an inducer for CYP1A2, 2C19, and 3A4, and for conjugation enzymes. Topiramate is an inducer for CYP3A4. Barbiturates and phenytoin are inducers for CYP2B6 and 3A4. Modafinil, approved for narcolepsy but also used to improve alertness and energy, is an inducer for CYP1A2 and 3A4 and may decrease the effect of several antidepressants.

St. John's wort seems to decrease serotonin reuptake and should not be combined with serotonergic antidepressants. It is also an inducer for CYP2C19, 2C9, and 3A4, decreasing the effect of medications metabolized by these enzymes.

10.1.6 *Tolerability of side effects*

Young patients are more reluctant to try antidepressants with a significant chance of sexual side effects. Patients with intellectually demanding jobs are more sensitive to the cognitive and sedative effects of antidepressants such as trazodone or mirtazapine. A good number of patients refuse mirtazapine because of the potential for weight gain.

10.1.7 *Medication adherence*

Antidepressants given once a day have a clear advantage for treatment adherence over those given in divided doses. In patients with a tendency to miss doses, fluoxetine is the best choice. Due to its long half-life, the levels of fluoxetine do not drop abruptly and patients have no discomfort with missed doses or discontinuation.

10.1.8 *Cost and access to medication*

In the USA, the difference in the cost of daily treatment between generic antidepressants, such as generic citalopram, fluoxetine, paroxetine, and sertraline, and "brand-only" antidepressants can be as high as 1:30 or 1:40. This is an important consideration not only for patients without insurance or medication coverage, but also for the growing number of patients with variable copayments, according to the price of medications. Some insurers set a lower cap in the amount, in milligrams or number of tablets, of the most expensive antidepressants, so if patients do not respond to "average" doses, prescribers will have to get prior authorization to be able to increase the dose.

10.2 Second-Generation Antidepressants: Doses and Duration

In Table 10.3, we summarize the dosing issues for SGAs: starting doses, titration, and maximum doses. Regarding the dosing of antidepressant medications, there is a general consensus that, for all of them, it takes at least 2–4 weeks to see the clinical effect of any given dose. Besides this, some studies suggest that treatment response in depression is a gradual process that could be started by week 1 and continued for at least six weeks (Taylor *et al.* 2006).

Because of all of this, when starting patients on antidepressant medications:

(1) To minimize side effects and improve tolerability and acceptance, always start at the low end of the effective dose range.
(2) In patients with significant anxiety, start at an even lower dose, as serotonergic antidepressants may cause an initial exacerbation of anxiety, including panic-like attacks, when given at usual antidepressant starting doses.
(3) The shortest time between dose increases is two weeks. The ideal time is four weeks, but that may seem too slow for very depressed patients or those who are closely monitoring their response to treatment.
(4) Titration with repeated biweekly increases applies mainly to SSRIs. For bupropion, we generally prescribe 150 mg/day, to be increased to 300 mg after 14 days, then reassess the patient after at least 30 days on this last dose to decide about going up to 450 mg. For mirtazapine and trazodone, we usually go slower than usual and allow for a month between dose changes, as both may induce daytime somnolence, a particularly bothersome side effect. For SNRIs, we usually make the first increase in two weeks, and allow for a month before the next one, as increases are proportionally larger than those of SSRIs.

Table 10.3. Suggested starting and maximum adult daily doses (mg/day), and titration process, for initial medication treatment in depression (may differ from doses recommended by manufacturers).[a]

Antidepressant	Starting dose (mg/day)	Titration increases, not sooner than every two weeks (mg/day)	Usual maximum dose (mg/day)	Ceiling dose (mg/day)[b]
Bupropion (once a day, qam, forms)[c]	150	150	450	
Citalopram	10–20	10–20	60	80
Desvenlafaxine (once-a-day)[d]	50			
Duloxetine (once-a-day)	20–30	30	90	120
Escitalopram	5–10	5–10	30	40
Fluoxetine	10–20	10–20 (every 4 weeks)	80	
Milnacipram	25–50 (in 2 doses)	25–50	200 (in 2 doses)	
Mirtazapine qhs	15	15	45	60
Paroxetine	10–20	10–20	60	80
Sertraline	25–50	25–50	200	
Trazodone (once-a-day SR)[e] qhs	150	75	375	
Venlafaxine (once-a-day SR)[f]	75	75	375	450
Vilazodone[g]	40 (10 × 7 days, 20 × 7 days, then 40)			

[a] TCAs and MAOIs are not included as, because of toxicity and side effects, they should be reserved for patients with documented no response to SGAs. Fluvoxamine is also not included as, because of its risky profile for DDIs, it is reserved for OCD. Nefazodone is not included as, due to liver toxicity, it is reserved for patients unresponsive to other SGAs.

[b] Tried when there is partial response at usual maximum dose with no side effects.

[c] Available for one (XL, XR), two (SR), or three (IR) doses/day; one dose in the morning has clear advantage in compliance and convenience, as late doses may delay sleep onset.

[d] The Prescribing Information recommends only 50 mg/day. However, the drug is available in 50 and 100 mg tablets. There is little clinical experience to estimate doses actually needed but, in the authors' opinion, the upper limit is likely to be significantly higher.

[e] Available as immediate- or sustained-release; SR in the evening has clear advantage because of daytime sleepiness with multiple doses.

[f] Available in immediate- and sustained-release forms; once-a-day, XR or SR, has clear advantage in medication adherence.

[g] Recommendations from the Prescribing Information. There is little clinical experience to estimate doses actually needed but, in the authors' opinion, the upper limit is likely to be higher.

For enhanced safety and clarity during titration, we prefer to give the patient written titration instructions, as in the following examples:

Sertraline 50 mg tablets
Half a tablet daily × 14 days
One tablet daily × 14 days
One and a half tablet daily × 14 days
Then, 2 tablets daily
(If there is significant improvement at any dose, stay there until the next visit; if there is significant discomfort, go back to the previous dose.)
or
Bupropion XL
One 150 mg tablet every morning × 14 days
Then, one 300 mg tablet every morning

10.3 Hypnotics and Other Symptom-Specific Medications

It has been shown that treatment of some symptoms associated with depression, such as insomnia or erectile dysfunction, with symptom-specific medications such as hypnotics or phosphodiesterase inhibitors, either alone or in combination with antidepressants, may produce not only an improvement in such symptoms but in core depressive symptoms as well (Fava *et al.*, 2006; McCall *et al.*, 2010; Rosen *et al.*, 2006; Seidman *et al.*, 2001).

Insomnia is a particularly disturbing symptom. It generates great anxiety, as patients spend the night worrying, and it leads to daytime sleepiness and fatigue, with significant functional impairment. All patients with insomnia should be educated about sleep hygiene. If insomnia is severe and a sedating or sleep-inducing antidepressant (mirtazapine, trazodone) is not being used, specific treatment with hypnotic medications should be implemented (see Table 10.4 and Chapter 15). Phosphodiesterase inhibitors are usually useful for the treatment of erectile dysfunction, regardless of whether or not the dysfunction is due to the antidepressant drug, depression itself, or a medical cause such as diabetes.

10.4 Partial Response to Antidepressant Treatment: What to Do?

What to do with partial responders is an important question in the treatment of depression. The vast majority of depressed patients in treatment, including remitters and responders, will still show residual symptoms after treatment completion. A recent three-year prospective study found that depressed

Table 10.4. Medication management of insomnia in the initial treatment of depression.[a]

Medication option[b]	Dose
Use a sleep-inducing antidepressant (mirtazapine, SR trazodone)	As recommended for depression, daily dose given in the evening
Add IR trazodone	Start at low dose 50–100 mg qhs
Add an antihistamine	Diphenhydramine 25–50 mg qhs Hydroxyzine 25–100 mg qhs
Add a benzodiazepine-related hypnotic	Eszopiclone 1–3 mg qhs Zaleplon 5–10 mg qhs Zolpidem 5–12.5 mg qhs
Add a benzodiazepine usually reserved for insomnia	Temazepam 7.5–30 mg qhs
Add other benzodiazepines (when other hypnotics do not work and anxiety seems to be the main cause of insomnia)	Start at lowest strength

[a]Always include sleep hygiene education.
[b]Other than hypnotic antidepressants, all medications should be used *prn* (as needed).

patients still showed on average of two depressive symptoms during remissions. In a recent study, three individual symptoms (cognitive problems, lack of energy, and sleeping problems) appear to dominate the course of depression and were present 85%–94% of the time during depressive episodes and 39%–44% of the time during remissions (Conradi *et al.*, 2010). In the first phase of the STAR*D study, after treatment with the SSRI citalopram, more than 90% of remitters had at least one residual symptom, with the most common residual symptoms being insomnia and appetite/weight changes (Nierenberg *et al.*, 2010).

A good number of patients are satisfied with their treatment response, despite the presence of residual symptoms. However, in cases where residual symptoms still cause significant discomfort or dysfunction, the clinician will have to decide, jointly with the patient, whether to continue the antidepressant for a longer time, add another antidepressant, add "symptom-specific" medications, or switch to another antidepressant.

10.4.1 *Give the antidepressant more time*

As mentioned above, some studies have shown that response in depression is a gradual process that could start by week 1 and continue for at least six weeks

(Taylor *et al.*, 2006). Thus, in patients who, after reaching the upper dose limit, do not remit but show a robust response, a possibility is waiting until the patient completes at least 6–8 weeks on the medication.

10.4.2 *Add another antidepressant*

Adding a second antidepressant seems to enhance the chances of improvement more than switching antidepressants. In the STAR*D study, partial or no responders to an SSRI who were given the SSRI plus bupropion did better than those who switched to another antidepressant (however, this was not a direct comparison) (Trivedi *et al.*, 2006). We recommend adding a second antidepressant only in cases when the response to the first one is not fully satisfactory but worth maintaining. If there is no response at all to the first antidepressant or the response is very poor, we recommend to switch antidepressants and preserve the potential to add more medications in a future step.

We should never combine antidepressants that share the same mechanism of action, because of the risk of toxicity. This also means never combining SSRIs and SNRIs (let us remember that TCAs and MAOIs also increase the amount of free monoamines). Bupropion is an excellent antidepressant to add to SSRIs and SNRIs as it has a unique mechanism and may help residual symptoms such as poor concentration/attention, overeating, or lack of energy. Another advantage of bupropion is that it does not add to the sexual adverse effects of other antidepressants. Mirtazapine, a drug that does not seem to have monoamine reuptake inhibition properties, and trazodone, a drug that at most is a weak serotonin reuptake inhibitor, are also used in combination with SSRIs, SNRIs, or bupropion, especially in patients with insomnia.

10.4.3 *Add symptom-specific medications*

The proposal to use symptom-specific medications in partial responders is not new (Menza *et al.*, 2003). It involves, for example, the use of drugs for insomnia and erectile dysfunction. Sedating drugs should be considered when there is significant anxiety, especially in the form of panic attacks, or when anxiety is a big contributor to insomnia. Phosphodiesterase inhibitors may be useful in men for whom erectile dysfunction is particularly troubling. Low-dose psychostimulants or modafinil may be considered when fatigue or daytime sleepiness causes serious discomfort or dysfunction.

10.4.4 *Switch antidepressants*

Often, the decision to switch in cases of partial response to antidepressants is the patient's. Some patients dislike the idea of taking multiple psychotropic medications, and prefer to switch, even if it means putting at risk the partial response achieved so far. Regarding this situation, we refer the reader to our discussion in the next section.

10.5 No Response to Initial Antidepressant Treatment: What to Do?

There is some evidence showing that even if there is no satisfactory response to a first-line antidepressant, adding a second antidepressant may offer more chances of improvement than switching antidepressants (Trivedi *et al.*, 2006). However, as stated above, in case of no response to the first antidepressant, our preference is to switch antidepressants and thus keep open the option to add new medications in the future. We favor adding a second antidepressant only if the response to the first antidepressant, though unsatisfactory, seems worth maintaining.

A very important observation in the treatment of depression is that failing to respond to one, or even two, antidepressants does not mean a patient is "treatment-resistant." In patients who fail to respond to the first antidepressant, chances of responding to the second antidepressant are still good. Additionally, there is some evidence that, after failure to respond to a first antidepressant, all other antidepressants, including those in the same group as the first one, have similar chances of inducing a response. In the STAR*D study, patients who did not remit with, or tolerate, the SSRI citalopram, showed similar remission rates after switching to bupropion XL, venlafaxine SR, or the SSRI sertraline (Trivedi *et al.*, 2006). However, the standard practice in case of non-response to antidepressant treatment is switching to a medication with a different antidepressant mechanism. In the authors' opinion, a reasonable choice of antidepressant to switch to is the one that best fits the patient's depression symptomatic profile at the time.

10.6 What About Adding Atypical Antipsychotics in the Initial Treatment of Depression?

Two atypical antipsychotics, quetiapine (Seroquel) and aripiprazole (Abilify), have received FDA approval to be used in the adjunctive treatment of major depressive disorder (MDD), "after inadequate response to an antidepressant alone." As discussed above, partial or even poor response to one antidepressant does not mean treatment resistance. There exists a clinical and research consensus that the diagnosis of "treatment-resistant depression" requires failing to respond to multiple antidepressants administered at high enough doses for a reasonable period of time. Thus, treating partial or poor responders to initial treatment as treatment-resistant patients is clearly inappropriate. In the authors' view, antipsychotics may have a role in true "treatment-resistant" or "difficult-to-treat" depressed patients, after more effective and safer options have been exhausted. However, because of their very modest effect and serious acute and chronic side effect profile, antipsychotics should never be used in the initial treatment of unipolar depression.

Thus far, the efficacy documented for atypical antipsychotics in the treatment of unipolar depression seems quite modest in our opinion. In the two studies that led to aripiprazole's approval for depression, the decrease in the outcome measure, the depression scale MADRS, while statistically significant, seems of dubious clinical importance. In the first study, the difference between aripiprazole and placebo in change in the MADRS (where the maximum possible score is 60) was only three points (8.8 *vs.* 5.8, respectively). In the second study, this difference between aripiprazole and placebo was even less than three points (8.5 *vs.* 5.7) (Berman *et al.*, 2007; Marcus *et al.*, 2008). In a recently published study, 225 subjects with MDD were randomized to adjunctive treatment with aripiprazole (2 mg/day × 30 days, then 5 mg/day × 30 days) or placebo. The difference in the number of responders to aripiprazole and placebo, in percentage, was only 5.6%. Grossly, this means an NNT (number needed to treat for benefit from the treatment) of approximately 18. This, as the authors state in the conclusions, is a "marginal efficacy" (Fava *et al.*, 2012). Therefore, we need to balance this modest clinical efficacy in depression with the significant risks and side effect burden associated with antipsychotics. For a discussion of the risks and adverse reactions associated with antipsychotic treatment, we refer the reader to Chapters 3 and 4 on antipsychotic drugs.

10.7 Other Non-Antidepressant Drugs Recently Tried in Depression

Along the years, multiple drugs have been assumed to be useful in patients with depression that do not respond to antidepressants (e.g., lithium, pindolol, thyroid preparations, and pramipexole). Psychiatrists seem to be voting with their feet as these options are tried in fewer and fewer patients. More recently, however, some medications have created interest: buspirone, methylfolate, and ketamine.

10.7.1 *Buspirone*

Buspirone is discussed in more detail in the chapter on medications for anxiety. However, there is some evidence for its efficacy in depression. In the STAR*D study, the "effectiveness" study on treatment of depression, sponsored by the NIMH, patients who did not remit after 12 weeks of treatment with citalopram (mean final dose, 55 mg/day) were randomized to receive augmentation of citalopram with buspirone (286 patients, dose up to 60 mg/day) or sustained-release bupropion (565 patients, dose up to 400 mg/day). The buspirone group and the sustained-release bupropion group had similar remission rates (30.1% and 29.7%, respectively). This finding is not surprising, as buspirone is a serotonergic medication that also seems to have some effects on D_1 and D_2 dopamine receptors (Trivedi *et al.*, 2006).

10.7.2 *Methylfolate (levomefolic acid)*

Folic acid has been tried before in the treatment of depression with disappointing results. However, there is a strong rationale for trying levomefolic acid, the methylated form of folic acid, also known as L-methylfolate or 5-methlytetrahydrofolate (5-MTHF) in depressed patients. Levomefolic acid is the natural and biologically active form of folic acid. When administered to humans as a drug, folic acid needs to be methylated in the body in order to have any activity. This transformation seems to be difficult for a substantial number of people. It has been reported that 10% of patients completely lack the ability to transform folic acid into L-methylfolate and an additional 40% can only transform limited amounts.

A recent publication reports on the use of L-methylfolate as adjunctive therapy in SSRI-resistant major depression. In two randomized, double-blind, parallel-sequential trials, L-methylfolate, added to the SSRI at a dose of 15 mg/day, induced a response rate after 30 days of 32.3% (*vs.* 14.6% for placebo). It is important to notice that the minimum initial effective dose seems to be 15 mg/day, as patients who received only 7.5 mg/day did not show a better response than patients on placebo (Papakostas *et al.*, 2012).

10.7.3 *Ketamine*

Though it will surely take time for glutamatergic agents to be widely available for the treatment of depression, both unipolar and bipolar, this approach seems to be the next big thing in the treatment of mood disorders. Small randomized studies have shown clinical benefits of ketamine in both unipolar and bipolar depressed patients. Ketamine, a noncompetitive antagonist at glutamatergic NMDA receptors, obtained FDA approval for use in anesthesia in 1970, but significant extraneous effects have limited its clinical use and encouraged its abuse. The most dramatic aspect of the antidepressant effect of ketamine is its onset in a matter of hours following IV infusion, making it the first antidepressant without a latency period for the therapeutic effect. This immediate antidepressant effect of ketamine seems to be related to improved neuronal function, especially at the synapses, mediated by increased production of neurotrophic factors such as the BDNF (brain-derived neurotrophic factor).

10.8 Once the Patient Gets Better, How to Stop Antidepressant Treatment?

For decades, it has been a standard recommendation to taper down antidepressant medications, especially serotonergic ones, rather than stop them suddenly, to minimize the discomfort associated with discontinuation syndrome. However, there is another major reason to perform a gradual discontinuation of antidepressant treatment, and this is to diminish risk of a depressive relapse. A study with 398 patients on antidepressants (224 MDD, 75 panic disorder, 62 bipolar II, and 37 bipolar I) compared the time to relapse in patients who discontinued the antidepressant rapidly (over 1–7 days) or gradually (14 days or more). Because the efficacy of antidepressant medications in bipolar disorder is questionable, we are going to consider only the disorders for which antidepressants are considered first-line medications, MDD and panic. In these patients, the time to 50% risk of relapse was 9.10 months with gradual discontinuation (95% CI: 6.84–11.40) and only 3.77 months with rapid discontinuation (95% CI: 1.99–4.54) (Baldessarini *et al.*, 2010).

References

Anderson I, Ferrier I, Baldwin R, *et al.* Evidence-based guidelines for treating depressive disorders with antidepressants: A revision of the 2000 British Association for Psychopharmacology guidelines. *J Psychopharmacol* 2008;22:343–396.

Baghai TC, Blier P, Baldwin DS, *et al.* General and comparative efficacy and effectiveness of antidepressants in the acute treatment of depressive disorders: A report by the WPA section of pharmacopsychiatry. *Eur Arch Psychiatry Clin Neurosci* 2011;261(Suppl. 3):S207–S245.

Baldessarini RJ, Tondo L, Ghiani C, *et al.* Illness risk following rapid versus gradual discontinuation of antidepressants. *Am J Psychiatry* 2010;167:943–941.

Berman RM, Marcus RN, Swanink R, *et al.* The efficacy and safety of aripiprazole as adjunctive therapy in major depressive disorder: A multicenter, randomized, double-blind, placebo-controlled study. *J Clin Psychiatry* 2007;68(6):843–853.

Conradi HJ, Ormel J, de Jonge P. Presence of individual (residual) symptoms during depressive episodes and periods of remission: A 3-year prospective study. *Psychol Med* 2011;41(6):1165–1174.

Fava M, McCall WV, Krystal A, *et al.* Eszopiclone co-administered with fluoxetine in patients with insomnia coexisting with major depressive disorder. *Biol Psychiatry* 2006;59(11):1052–1060.

Fava M, Mischoulon D, Iosifescu D, *et al.* A double-blind, placebo-controlled study of aripiprazole adjunctive to antidepressant therapy among depressed outpatients with inadequate response to antidepressant therapy (ADAPT-A Study). *Psychother Psychosom* 2012;81(2):87–97.

Gartlehner G, Hansen RA, Thieda P, *et al.* Comparative effectiveness of second-generation antidepressants in the pharmacological treatment of adult depression. Comparative Effectiveness Review No. 7. (Prepared by RTI International-University of North Carolina Evidence-based Practice Center) Rockville, MD: Agency for Healthcare Research and Quality, January 2007, Retrieved from www.effectivehealthcare.ahrq.gov/reports/final.cfm

Liebrenz M, Borgeat A, Leisinger R, *et al.* Intravenous ketamine therapy in a patient with a treatment-resistant major depression. *Swiss Med Wkly* 2007;137(15–16):234–236.

McCall WV, Blocker JN, D'Agostino R, *et al.* Treatment of insomnia in depressed insomniacs: Effects on health-related quality of life, objective and self-reported sleep, and depression. *J Clin Sleep Med* 2010;6(4):322–329.

Marcus RN, McQuade RD, Carson WH, *et al.* The efficacy and safety of aripiprazole as adjunctive therapy in major depressive disorder: A second multicenter, randomized, double-blind, placebo-controlled study. *J Clin Psychopharmacol* 2008;28(2):156–165.

Menza M. STAR*D: The results begin to roll in (Editorial). *Am J Psychiatry* 2006;163(7): 1123–1125.

Menza M, Marin H, Opper RS. Residual symptoms in depression: Can treatment be symptom-specific? *J Clin Psychiatry* 2003;64(5):516–523.

Nierenberg AA, Husain MM, Trivedi MH, *et al.* Residual symptoms after remission of major depressive disorder with citalopram and risk of relapse: A STAR*D report. *Psychol Med* 2010;40(1):41–50.

Nutt DJ, Davidson JRT, Gelenberg AJ, *et al.* International consensus statement on major depressive disorder. *J Clin Psychiatry* 2010;71(Suppl. E1):e08.

Papakostas GI, Shelton RC, Zajecka JM, *et al.* L-methylfolate as adjunctive therapy for SSRI-resistant major depression: Results of two randomized, double-blind, parallel-sequential trials. *Am J Psychiatry* 2012;169:1267–1274.

Rosen R, Shabsigh R, Berber M, *et al.* Efficacy and tolerability of vardenafil in men with mild depression and erectile dysfunction: The depression-related improvement with vardenafil for erectile dysfunction study. *Am J Psychiatry* 2006;163(1):79–87.

Rush AJ, Trivedi MH, Wisniewski SR, *et al.* Bupropion-SR, sertraline, or venlafaxine-XR after failure of SSRIs for depression. *N Engl J Med* 2006;354:1231–1242.

Seidman SN, Roose SP, Menza MA, *et al.* Treatment of erectile dysfunction in men with depressive symptoms: Results of a placebo-controlled trial with sildenafil citrate. *Am J Psychiatry* 2001;158(10):1623–1630.

Taylor MJ, Freemantle N, Geddes JR, *et al.* Early onset of selective serotonin reuptake inhibitor antidepressant action. *Arch Gen Psychiatry* 2006;63:1217–1223.

Trivedi MH, Fava M, Wisniewski SR, *et al.* Medication augmentation after the failure of SSRIs for depression. *N Engl J Med* 2006;354:1243–1252.

Trivedi MH, Rush AJ, Wisniewski SR, *et al.* Evaluation of outcomes with citalopram for depression using measurement-based care in STAR*D: Implications for clinical practice. *Am J Psychiatry* 2006;163(1):28–40.

Chapter 11

Benzodiazepines, Buspirone, and Miscellaneous Medications Used in Anxiety Disorders

In this chapter, we discuss a heterogeneous group of drugs used in the treatment of anxiety disorders, when symptoms persist following reassurance, relaxation, and other brief interventions, and when the first line of pharmacological treatment of anxiety, second-generation antidepressants (SGAs), are not sufficient. These alternative anti-anxiety interventions include benzodiazepines, buspirone, antihistamines, some anticonvulsant drugs, and prazosin (for PTSD-associated nightmares). We will also examine briefly the potential anti-anxiety role of other medications such as antipsychotics or beta-blockers. The use of hypnotic drugs for insomnia in these patients will be discussed in Chapter 15.

11.1 Benzodiazepines

The first benzodiazepine, chlordiazepoxide (Librium), was developed in New Jersey at the laboratories of the Swiss company Hoffman-La Roche, and introduced in clinical practice in the USA in 1960. Diazepam (Valium) came shortly after that, in 1963, and soon thereafter, the number of marketed benzodiazepines got in the double digits. Benzodiazepines revolutionized the treatment of anxiety, offering immediate relief, and they became the most widely prescribed group of medications in the 1970s. However, their addictive properties and the development of tolerance to their anxiolytic effect were soon noticed, and benzodiazepine use started to decline from the 1980s onwards. Today, benzodiazepines are more often initiated in emergency or primary care settings than in psychiatric settings, as they help to suppress severe anxiety attacks, including panic attacks, but their prolonged use worries mental health practitioners.

From the perspective of patients and physicians, benzodiazepines can be viewed as "miracle drugs" as they can virtually erase severe anxiety and distress in minutes, bringing "a peace of mind" at least temporarily and helping patients in very disturbing states of mind pause with relief. However, they can also induce dependence, tolerance to the therapeutic effect, and psychomotor impairment. Additionally, after experiencing the "miraculous" rapid onset effect of benzodiazepines, patients are often reluctant to comply with other effective and safe medications that do not work immediately for anxiety disorders, such as antidepressants.

Recently, some research has suggested that benzodiazepines may be a gateway to the use of opiates, a more addictive group of medications. After adjusting for socioeconomic, medical, and substance use variables, a study found that earlier benzodiazepine users were 3.1 times more likely to repeatedly use opiates. "The analyses of the effect of benzodiazepines and chronic pain individually and in combination suggest that use of benzodiazepines is an even stronger predictor of later opioid use than self-reported chronic pain." (Skurtveit *et al.*, 2010) In Table 11.1, we list some pros and cons of benzodiazepines.

Many brand and generic benzodiazepines are marketed in the USA, which is a matter of concern, considering the abuse potential. Here, we will discuss only those that we view as clinically relevant in psychiatric practice. These are:

(1) alprazolam;
(2) chlordiazepoxide;
(3) clonazepam;
(4) diazepam;
(5) lorazepam;
(6) oxazepam;
(7) temazepam; and
(8) triazolam.

11.1.1 *Pharmacology*

The mechanism of action of benzodiazepines is likely to be related to their binding of $GABA_A$ receptors. $GABA_A$ is a large complex receptor coupled to a channel for the chloride ion. GABA is the main inhibitory neurotransmitter in the central nervous system (CNS). Thus, it is not surprising

Table 11.1 Advantages and negative aspects of benzodiazepines.

Advantages	▪ Rapid onset tranquilizing, sedating, hypnotic, anticonvulsant, and muscle-relaxant effects ▪ Immediate action (no latency period) ▪ Wide therapeutic margin (in patients with no respiratory impairment)
Adverse cognitive and motor effects	▪ Psychomotor retardation ▪ Amnesia (anterograde) ▪ Diminished learning ability ▪ Disinhibition ▪ Stimulate a passive style of coping, and interfere with psychotherapy
Risk of tolerance and dependence	▪ Reportedly more likely with fast short-acting benzodiazepines, but possible with all of them ▪ Are benzodiazepines a gateway to opioid use? ▪ Acute toxicity potentiated by alcohol/substance use
Compared to second-generation antidepressants in anxiety	▪ Benzodiazepines are ineffective against depression, a frequent comorbidity ▪ Benzodiazepines are more bothersome and less effective in long-term management of clinical syndromes ▪ Antidepressants are safer in alcohol and substance use disorders ▪ Recurrence of anxiety after stopping medication is faster with benzodiazepines than antidepressants

that benzodiazepines have anti-anxiety, anti-seizure, muscle-relaxant, and hypnotic properties. However, benzodiazepines are only GABA modulators; they enhance the action of GABA but do not "open" the channel by themselves, and do not work in the absence of GABA. $GABA_A$ receptors may bind numerous substances that function as modulators, including, besides benzodiazepines, alcohol, barbiturates, steroids, anesthetics, and pro- and anticonvulsant drugs. Though benzodiazepines are used in other specialties, to induce anesthesia, as antiepileptic drugs, or as muscle relaxants, we will limit the discussion to their actions in anxiety, agitation, insomnia, and alcohol withdrawal.

11.1.1.1 *Pharmacokinetics and drug–drug interactions*

All the benzodiazepines we are discussing here are well absorbed after oral administration. However, the onset of their clinical effect following administration of the drug varies depending on multiple factors such as how fast is the absorption or the entry of the drug into the CNS. The duration of action depends mainly on the half-life of each individual drug, but also on the presence of active metabolites, the most extreme case being diazepam, which has both a long half-life and active metabolites. Alprazolam is practically the only benzodiazepine available in an extended-release preparation. The authors see no advantage in using it instead of an immediate-release benzodiazepine with a longer duration of action, as these have a more predictable absorption. In Table 11.2, we present pharmacokinetic data for some benzodiazepines.

Benzodiazepines are eliminated through oxidation by CYP450 enzymes and/or conjugation:

(1) Alprazolam, clonazepam, diazepam, and triazolam are oxidized by CYP3A4. Chlordiazepoxide has a more complex metabolism, including oxidation by CYP3A4. The effects and toxicity of these benzodiazepines may be increased by CYP3A4 inhibitors, such as valproate, and decreased by CYP3A4 inducers, such as carbamazepine, modafinil, and topiramate.
(2) Lorazepam, oxazepam, and temazepam are not transformed in the body which means they have no active metabolites. They are eliminated through glucuronidation, and their effects may be increased by glucuronidation inhibitors, such as valproate, or decreased by glucuronidation inducers, such as carbamazepine.

Table 11.2 Pharmacokinetics, doses, and available oral forms of the most-used benzodiazepines in the USA.

Action	Drug	Half-life (h)[a]	Oral forms (mg)	Equivalent dose (mg)[b]
Short	Triazolam[c]	4–6	0.125, 0.25 0.25, 0.5, 1, 2	0.25
Intermediate	Alprazolam	8–15	0.5, 1, 2, and XR 0.5, 1, 2, 3	0.5
	Lorazepam	10–20	0.5, 1, 2 (oral or sublingual)	1
	Oxazepam	5–15	10, 15, 30	15–20
	Temazepam	6–16	7.5, 15, 22.5, 30	10–20
Long	Chlordiazepoxide	5–30 (200)[d]	5, 10, 25	10–25
	Clonazepam	20–50	0.5, 1, 2	0.25–0.5
	Diazepam	14–80 (200)[d]	2, 5, 10	5–10

[a] Figures are approximate, as different authors give variable numbers. Half-life increases with age.
[b] Switch is usually to clonazepam, diazepam, or chlordiazepoxide to attenuate withdrawal, because of their long half-life.
[c] Triazolam is still marketed in the USA. However, the higher incidence of cognitive and mood adverse reactions compared to other benzodiazepines, makes its use completely unjustified in outpatient settings (and probably in any setting).
[d] Including active metabolites.

11.1.2 *Adverse effects*

11.1.2.1 *Psychomotor effects*

Benzodiazepines have significant acute and chronic motor and cognitive effects. They may cause excessive sedation, daytime sleepiness, confusion/ disorientation, and memory impairment, and compromise psychomotor performance, posing a risk when driving or operating machinery. Because of all these potential side effects, benzodiazepines significantly increase the risk of falls, especially in the elderly.

The cognitive effects of benzodiazepines are intrinsic to their mechanism of action, and occur in every patient taking them. These effects may significantly affect daily work or academic activities, including intellectual tasks, learning, remembering, driving, and operating machinery. Since many chronic benzodiazepine users are elderly, unemployed, or disabled individuals, this should bring an additional element of worry to clinicians dealing with such cases.

An extensive literature review of clinical research found that benzodiazepines cause a generalized deterioration of cognitive functions, including, in descending order:

- Sensory processing
- Psychomotor speed
- Nonverbal memory
- Visuospatial skills
- Speed of processing
- Problem-solving
- Attention and concentration
- Verbal memory
- General intelligence
- Motor control/performance
- Working memory
- Verbal reasoning

Regarding recovery in cognition after stopping chronic benzodiazepine use, this same meta-analysis concludes: "Data from this study do not support a full recovery, at least in the first 6 months following cessation and suggests that there may be some permanent deficits or deficits that take periods longer than 6 months to completely recover." (Barker *et al.*, 2004)

Triazolam (Halcion). While triazolam is still marketed in the USA and promoted for clinical use, the significantly higher incidence of cognitive and mood adverse reactions compared to other benzodiazepines, including development of severe anxiety, makes its use completely unjustified in outpatient settings (and probably in any setting) in the authors' opinion.

11.1.2.2 *Abuse/dependence*

It is likely that a higher proportion of cases of benzodiazepine abuse and dependence go unnoticed compared to cases addicted to other substances. Benzodiazepine addiction seems to affect more women than men, and is more common in Caucasian young adults that in other ethnic groups. Risk factors associated with benzodiazepine (non-prescribed) use or abuse/dependence include panic, agoraphobic symptoms, and abuse of alcohol, illegal substances, or prescription drugs such as opiates (Becker *et al.*, 2007).

Benzodiazepine withdrawal has similar features to those of alcohol withdrawal, including the escalating, chronological sequence of withdrawal manifestations, and it is a life-threatening medical emergency. Similar to what is done in alcohol withdrawal, benzodiazepine withdrawal is managed with the administration of a long-acting benzodiazepine at a dose high enough to abort the symptoms, with gradual tapering after control is obtained.

11.1.2.3 *Sleep-related behaviors and automatisms*

Similar to other hypnotics, benzodiazepines taken at night may cause these complex risky behaviors that include walking, eating, getting out of home, and trying to drive vehicles. Similar behaviors may occur during the day, in which case we call them automatisms. For a more detailed description of sleep-related behaviors and automatisms, we refer the reader to the section on GABA hypnotics in Chapter 15.

11.1.2.4 *Disinhibition syndrome*

This syndrome, resembling some behaviors seen in alcohol intoxication, includes irritability and impulsivity. This seems more likely to occur in people with history of aggression and impulsivity.

11.1.2.5 *Potential for criminal use*

Because of their sedative potential, benzodiazepines, especially fast-acting ones such as flunitrazepam (Rohypnol) and triazolam (Halcion), are used for criminal purposes, such as rape or robbery.

11.1.3 *Toxicity*

Benzodiazepines are respiratory depressants. In healthy individuals, the therapeutic margin of benzodiazepines (the difference between therapeutic and toxic or lethal doses) is very high. However, in patients with respiratory impairment, including sleep apnea, COPD, and other respiratory ailments, benzodiazepine toxicity grows exponentially. The same steep increase in toxicity and lethality takes place when benzodiazepines are combined with other respiratory depressants, such as alcohol.

Benzodiazepine intoxication is treated with flumazenil, a $GABA_A$ antagonist. Flumazenil has a short half-life, and repeated injections are usually necessary. In patients with benzodiazepine addiction, flumazenil may trigger benzodiazepine withdrawal syndrome.

11.1.4 *Selection and use*

Before discussing the choice of a benzodiazepine for clinical use, we offer a few caveats:

(1) Very short-acting benzodiazepines have no valid use in outpatient psychiatry, and probably not even in any psychiatric setting. In the case of triazolam, the negative side effect profile is compounded by its serious cognitive and mood adverse effects compared to other benzodiazepines.
(2) Very fast-acting benzodiazepines, such as flunitrazepam, have higher potential to be used for criminal purposes than other benzodiazepines.
(3) In our opinion, benzodiazepines should not be considered as first-line treatment for the maintenance treatment of anxiety. They may be used, as sparingly as possible and with decreasing frequency, to supplement long-term treatment with non-addictive medications, such as certain antidepressants.

Regarding the selection of a benzodiazepine for clinical use, some authorities recommend giving preference to longer-acting compounds, such as clonazepam, with the argument that the end of the effect is more gradual and therefore this may probably induce less craving for another dose. We disagree with this recommendation due to clinical and pharmacological reasons, and usually prefer a benzodiazepine with an intermediate half-life, such as alprazolam, lorazepam, oxazepam, or temazepam (though the latter is usually reserved for the treatment of insomnia). The main clinical reason for our preference is that the negative cognitive and motor effects of a benzodiazepine dose tend to persist after the anti-anxiety effect has disappeared, and this period of impairment without benefit is obviously longer for longer-acting compounds. The main pharmacological reason for using benzodiazepines with an intermediate half-life, especially if used once or at the most twice a day, is that they provide more medication-free time or at least lower serum trough levels, and this likely delays the development of dependence or tolerance to the effect. For these same reasons, we see no advantage in using a sustained-release preparation of a benzodiazepine with an intermediate half-life, such as extended-release alprazolam. Another advantage of intermediate half-life benzodiazepines is that several of them have no metabolites (lorazepam, oxazepam, and temazepam), decreasing the variability in the response and the risk in patients with hepatic impairment.

Benzodiazepines with an intermediate half-life are given up to 3–4 times a day. However, long-acting ones could be given twice a day, or even once a day (diazepam and chlordiazepoxide). Ideally, benzodiazepines should not be used on a regular basis but as needed (*prn*) for panic attacks or sudden exacerbations of anxiety symptoms, at the lowest possible end for dose and frequency of administration. Under exceptional circumstances, such as the case of patients presenting with multiple panic or high anxiety attacks per day, regular dosing can be implemented for a limited time, until the effect of other effective interventions for specific anxiety disorders (e.g., SSRI antidepressants or cognitive behavioral therapy [CBT]) becomes apparent).

Dosing should always start at the lowest strength. For panic attacks or severe anxiety attacks, the dose may be increased acutely, two-, three-, or even fourfold, to the one dose that significantly affects the severity of the attacks. Complete suppression of the attacks is not an ideal goal, as it may decrease the motivation to comply with long-term non-addictive treatments (such as SSRIs and CBT). After finding an effective initial dose, we should be wary of further increases. The vast majority of undesirable dose escalations with benzodiazepines probably happen in the initial months of treatment. Patients who have stayed on stable doses for long periods of time seem to fare well (Soumerai *et al.*, 2003). Special care should be exercised to avoid prescribing benzodiazepines to patients with impulse control problems, or a history of alcohol, illegal substance, or prescription drug abuse/dependence.

Placing a patient on high doses of benzodiazepines may be problematic. Benzodiazepine withdrawal is a life-threatening event. For patients taking high doses, prescriptions cannot be suddenly stopped without referral to a hospital, even when the provider is certain the patient is misusing the medication.

Benzodiazepine use must be temporary. Anxious patients should always be started on an antidepressant with anti-anxiety properties, and also psychotherapies such as CBT should be considered. The use of another anti-anxiety agent such as buspirone is also an option. Patients must be educated about the tolerance to the effect and the risk of dependence with prolonged use of benzodiazepines, hence the need to comply with the antidepressant. They also must be warned that there will be no late increases in benzodiazepine dose. We must be parsimonious with renewals of benzodiazepines, giving the patient enough medication until the next visit, but not much more, and keeping good records of refills given.

Patients who come under our care and are already on benzodiazepines often pose special problems, especially if they report being on high doses. Frequently, we cannot verify the reason for the change of provider; there is history or suspicion of frequent provider changes in the past, or the patient is seeing several providers likely to prescribe benzodiazepines (primary care, pain specialist, sleep specialist, neurologist, musculoskeletal specialist, rheumatologist, emergency room provider, etc.). We must be very alert for "red flags" of benzodiazepine misuse, including additional fills for reportedly "lost medication," advanced requests for refills for reasons such as travel, the patient's assertions that there are no refills left when the provider has documented them, frequent visits to the emergency room, or "doctor shopping" behaviors. It is always useful, in case of doubt, to be able to contact the patient's primary medication provider, as well as other specialists who may prescribe benzodiazepines or opiates.

Abrupt termination of benzodiazepine therapy may produce relapse (return of previous anxiety symptoms), rebound (return of increased anxiety symptoms), and withdrawal (similar to alcohol withdrawal, including delirium, seizures, and risk of death). The possibility for these complications seems to be related more to the magnitude of the dose than the duration of therapy. Therefore, tapering down is recommended when stopping benzodiazepines, especially at high doses.

11.1.4.1 *Equivalent doses of benzodiazepines and switching between benzodiazepines*

We are probably more skeptical than most authors regarding the practice of switching between benzodiazepines, usually based on the belief that some of them are less addictive or easier to taper down. Our reasons for this skepticism are multiple: first, other than a 1991 study which found few differences between lorazepam, diazepam, and bromazepam in withdrawal symptoms during tapering, the evidence on this practice is scarce (Murphy *et al.*, 1991); second, a patient unable or unwilling to decrease the dose of a benzodiazepine will likely be unable or unwilling to decrease the dose of another; and third, equivalent doses are imprecise estimates, and the switch adds another element of confusion and delay. Thus, our general recommendation is to gradually decrease the dose of the current benzodiazepine.

A valid reason for switching across benzodiazepines is when tapering the medication in patients taking high doses, a case similar to the treatment/prevention of alcohol withdrawal. In these cases, some providers switch to the equivalent dose of a long-acting benzodiazepine, because the long half-life attenuates the development of withdrawal. The dose of the substitute is then gradually decreased (this could mean hospitalization or giving the patient frequent short-term refills of decreasing amounts). In Table 11.2, we give the equivalent doses for the benzodiazepines we are discussing.

11.1.5 *Indications*

Benzodiazepines are used in generalized anxiety disorder (GAD), panic disorder, social phobia, and PTSD. Though the studies in some disorders have been done mainly with one benzodiazepine (for example, alprazolam for panic disorder), their actions in anxiety seem to be a class effect.

11.1.5.1 *Generalized anxiety disorder*

This is a chronic disorder. For this reason, benzodiazepines should never be the mainstay of treatment. Benzodiazepines can be used, as needed, for severe anxiety attacks or panic-like attacks, temporarily, until the effect of safer medications for the long-term treatment of anxiety is appreciable. If the anxiety attacks persist at the same severity and frequency, this could be an indicator of poor compliance with antidepressants, and lead to a review of treatment. Remember also that benzodiazepines cause motor and intellectual impairment and that the finer the intellectual and motor tasks a patient is expected to perform, the higher the harm he may experience from the medication.

11.1.5.2 *Panic disorder*

This is also a recurrent disorder. It is very heterogeneous regarding frequency of the attacks. In patients experiencing attacks once a day or less often, the use of a middle-acting benzodiazepine, such as alprazolam or lorazepam, poses no special problems. Patients need to start a non-addictive long-term medication, but we have relative control of the doses. Patients who report multiple panic attacks a day are a problem, and we must make clear that multiple dosing with benzodiazepines is a time-limited tool. Panic or anxious patients reporting multiple attacks a day, and showing poor adherence to antidepressants have a bad prognosis regarding tolerance/dependence. A pragmatic solution is getting the patient to take the antidepressant, and giving a small number of benzodiazepine tablets to keep in case they have an attack.

11.1.5.3 *Social anxiety disorder*

Social anxiety disorder (SAD) has very different degrees of severity and occurrence. Patients with daily social anxiety must be started on antidepressants. In patients who are not exposed to anxiety-triggering situations every day, intermittent benzodiazepine use is a possibility. However, we must remember the motor and intellectual impairment intrinsic to benzodiazepines. For activities that involve good motor or intellectual skills, such as taking tests at school, teaching, performing, lecturing, driving, operating machinery, etc., the remedy is probably worse than the illness. Patients who keep reporting daily social anxiety and show poor compliance with antidepressants should raise a red flag for benzodiazepine abuse/dependence.

Anxiety in predictable circumstances. This type of anxiety is akin to social phobia. Benzodiazepines may be very useful when the anxiogenic events do not happen very often and no fine intellectual or motor performance is required in the situation. The best example is fear of flying. However, patients need to be warned and given a low dose to decrease the risk of confusional events during the flight.

PTSD. In this disorder, benzodiazepines are used to decrease the arousal and the anxiety associated with intrusive recollections or cues to the trauma. However, we must bear in mind the high incidence of abuse/dependence in PTSD patients. At the very least, benzodiazepine use in PTSD should be intermittent or time-limited.

Depression. Despite some reports involving alprazolam and clonazepam, benzodiazepines alone have no clinically useful antidepressant effect. This is one of their disadvantages, as depression and anxiety are often comorbid in clinical practice, and antidepressants are effective in both conditions. Besides this, when given alone to depressed patients, benzodiazepines may exacerbate passivity and lack of interest/initiative. However, in depressed patients with severe generalized anxiety, or severe anxiety attacks or panic-like attacks, a well-managed course of benzodiazepines, along with antidepressant treatment, may accelerate and enhance the general response and improve treatment adherence.

Insomnia. For a detailed discussion of the role of benzodiazepines as hypnotic drugs, we refer the reader to Chapter 15.

Alcohol withdrawal. Ultra-long-acting benzodiazepines are the first-line treatment for alcohol withdrawal. Chlordiazepoxide has a theoretical advantage, as its lower lipid solubility leads to a slower decline in the blood levels. However, diazepam is also commonly used.

11.1.6 *Warnings and contraindications*

Benzodiazepines should be used with caution in patients with hepatic, renal, or pulmonary illness.

Benzodiazepines should be used with care in the elderly or patients with cognitive impairment, due to the increased risk of confusion, agitation, delirium, or motor impairment (benzodiazepines are a significant risk for falls).

Benzodiazepines should be used with care in patients taking CYP3A4 or conjugation inhibitors. Conversely, their effects may be decreased in patients taking CYP3A4 or conjugation inducers.

Benzodiazepines should not be combined with alcohol or any respiratory depressant drugs.

As mentioned, abrupt termination of benzodiazepine therapy may produce relapse (return of previous anxiety symptoms), rebound (return of increased anxiety symptoms), and withdrawal (similar to alcohol withdrawal, including delirium, seizures, and risk of death). Therefore, tapering down is recommended when stopping benzodiazepines, especially at high doses.

11.2 Buspirone

Buspirone (Buspar), a non-addictive anti-anxiety drug, was approved by the FDA in 1986. It is a member of the azapirone chemical class, together with gepirone, a medication used in Europe but never introduced in the USA. Buspirone has also shown antidepressant properties. Unfortunately, the expiration of the patent discouraged any further research or application for indications for this medication. It is also regrettable that an extended-release preparation was never developed, since one of the major shortcomings of buspirone is that it has to be administered frequently (up to four times a day).

11.2.1 *Pharmacology*

Buspirone is an anti-anxiety medication with no risk for dependence/ tolerance to the effect. It has a latency period for the onset of the clinical effect, bringing to mind the delayed effect of antidepressant drugs. Buspirone has also shown efficacy in clinical trials in depression, both as monotherapy and as adjunctive treatment, as discussed below. That buspirone has both anti-anxiety and antidepressant properties is not surprising, as it displays high affinity as a partial agonist for the serotonin 5-HT_{1A} receptor, a receptor involved in both anxiety and depression. It also has moderate affinity, as agonist/antagonist, for the dopamine D_2 receptors, and is a weak antagonist at 5-HT_{2C} receptors. The mechanism of action of buspirone, beyond the effect on 5-HT_{1A} receptors, is not completely understood. It has been suggested that buspirone is an agonist/antagonist for dopamine D_2 receptors (agonist for pre-synaptic D_2 receptors, or autoreceptors, antagonist for the post-synaptic D_2 receptors, or heteroreceptors). Some studies have suggested other dopaminergic actions of buspirone, including its antagonizing D_1 receptors.

Buspirone has an extensive first-pass metabolism and only around 4% of an oral dose reaches the general circulation (bioavailability). Food increases the absorption of buspirone. Buspirone has a half-life of approximately 2–12 h. It is metabolized by CYP3A4, and its effects and toxicity are increased by CYP3A4 inhibitors (such as valproate and fluvoxamine) or decreased by CYP3A4 inducers (such as carbamazepine, modafinil, and topiramate).

11.2.2 *Clinical uses*

Buspirone has FDA approval as monotherapy for the treatment of GAD. Less well known are the effects of buspirone in depressive disorders. The antidepressant properties of buspirone as monotherapy have been demonstrated in randomized controlled trials (RCTs), though FDA approval for depression was not pursued. In the large independent STAR*D study on depression, sponsored by the U.S. NIMH, 565 patients with major depression who did not remit with SSRI (citalopram) therapy alone were randomized to augmentation therapy with buspirone (up to 60 mg/day) or sustained-release bupropion (up to 400 mg/day). The buspirone and bupropion groups had similar rates of remission: 30.1% and 29.7%, respectively (Trivedi *et al.*, 2006). Buspirone is, then, an underutilized medication. It is a valid option in the treatment of GAD, as monotherapy or an interesting medication to add in cases of partial response to antidepressants in both depression and anxiety.

Due to its short half-life, buspirone has to be given in several doses a day. The initial recommended daily dose of buspirone is 15 mg (7.5 mg bid), that is titrated at intervals of three days or longer, until a daily dose of 45–60 mg/day (in 3–4 divided doses) is reached (doses of 90 mg/day were used in depression trials). There is a latency period of at least 1–2 weeks for the clinical effects of buspirone to be apparent.

Buspirone is a safe and usually well-tolerated medication. The most commonly reported adverse effects of buspirone involved the CNS or gastro-intestinal system: dizziness, nausea, headache, nervousness, lightheadedness, and excitement. Other reported adverse effects include insomnia, drowsiness, and fatigue.

Rare cases of probable akathisia have been reported with buspirone. Similar to antidepressants, discontinuation symptoms may be seen with buspirone. However, buspirone does not induce dependence/tolerance, nor does it help with benzodiazepine withdrawal.

Buspirone must be used with care in patients with hepatic or renal disease. Caution must be exercised also when using buspirone concomitantly with CYP3A4 inhibitors. CYP3A4 inducers may decrease its effect. It is better not to combine buspirone with monoamine oxidase inhibitors (MAOIs).

11.3 Antiepileptic Drugs

With the exception of the anticonvulsants pregabalin (which appears to have efficacy in GAD and SAD), and gabapentin (for which there is some evidence in SAD), no antiepileptic drug, including lamotrigine, looks very promising for the treatment of anxiety that does not respond to the currently available anti-anxiety medications.

11.3.1 *Pregabalin*

The effectiveness of pregabalin in GAD and SAD has been documented in drug company-sponsored, placebo-controlled RCTs. However, the manufacturer decided to pursue the indication for treatment of fibromyalgia, under the name Lyrica, and the anxiety indication was abandoned (Pande *et al.*, 2003; Feltner *et al.*, 2003). Pregabalin is probably useful in other anxiety disorders, except obsessive–compulsive disorder (OCD), where serotonergic action is practically a must for success. However, we must bear in mind that the efficacy of pregabalin in anxiety was shown at relatively high doses (400–600 mg/day), and that the adverse effects of pregabalin, like those of most medications, are dose-dependent. Thus, at the doses required for the treatment of anxiety disorders, the tolerability is compromised, mainly because of dizziness/somnolence. High cost is also a disadvantage of pregabalin. In our opinion, pregabalin must be tried in anxiety disorders only after other anti-anxiety and antidepressant options have been exhausted.

Despite its being structurally similar to GABA, pregabalin has no effects on the GABA systems. It does not work on GABA receptors or influence GABA release or reuptake. Pregabalin inhibits voltage-gated calcium channels, decreasing late depolarization of the membrane, and reducing the release of excitatory neurotransmitters, such as glutamate.

Pregabalin has a half-life of approximately 6 h. It is eliminated, unchanged, in urine, and has no oxidation or conjugation drug interactions.

Because of its short half-life, pregabalin is administered in two doses a day. In clinical trials on anxiety, pregabalin showed efficacy at doses of 200 mg bid or tid (total daily dose 400–600 mg). For fibromyalgia, the recommended starting daily dose is 150 mg, which may be increased to 300 mg in a week, with a maximum dose of 450 mg/day.

The most common side effects reported with pregabalin are dizziness (roughly 25% more frequent than placebo at high doses), somnolence (roughly 15% more frequent than placebo at high doses), dry mouth, edema (6% *vs.* 2% for placebo), blurred vision, gain of more than 7% body weight (6%–7% more frequent than placebo), and impaired concentration/attention.

Pregabalin should be used with care in patients with impaired renal function or with a history of angiodema. As with all anticonvulsants, it carries a warning regarding suicide and should be tapered down when discontinuing, to decrease the risk of seizures.

11.3.2 *Gabapentin*

Gabapentin has no FDA approval for the treatment of any mental disorder. Despite this, it has an extensive history of clinical use (misuse?) in mental disorders, including the management of severe and chronic illnesses such as bipolar disorder. The only psychiatric disorder in which gabapentin has demonstrated efficacy in RCTs is SAD. However, in that study, relatively high doses of the drug were used (900–3,600 mg/day), which are likely to induce significant clinical sedation (Pande *et al.*, 1999).

Gabapentin is structurally related to GABA, but it has no GABAergic effects. It decreases excitatory neurotransmitter release by its inhibitory effect on calcium channels. It may have antiglutamatergic and sodium channel inhibitory effects. Gabapentin is well absorbed at low to moderate oral doses. It is eliminated unchanged in urine. Its half-life is around 6 h, and it requires multiple daily doses.

The most common serious adverse effects of gabapentin are dizziness (roughly 20% higher than placebo), somnolence (roughly 15% higher than placebo), peripheral edema (6% higher than placebo), ataxia, and cognitive impairment.

Due to its short half-life, gabapentin is given in three doses per day. The usual starting dose is 300 mg in one dose at night, observing for daytime sleepiness the next day. If well tolerated, multiple daily dosing can be started. As mentioned, relatively high doses will be necessary for a clinical effect in anxiety.

Gabapentin should be used with care in patients with impaired renal function. As all antiepileptic drugs, it carries a warning regarding increasing suicidal ideation or behavior. It also should be tapered down when discontinuing, to decrease the risk of seizures.

11.4 Antihistamines

Hydroxyzine's action in GAD has been documented in RCTs, and it has the advantage of having low potential for abuse. However, significant sedation limits its use, especially in high-functioning subjects. Besides this, its anticholinergic adverse effects are a problem, especially in the elderly and cognitively impaired. Hydroxyzine can be a helpful *prn* medication for anxiety peaks and panic-like attacks, in patients in whom, mainly because of history or high risk of addiction, benzodiazepines should be avoided. It may be administered several times a day, up to a tid schedule, always starting low and titrating the dose up. Individual doses fluctuate between 12.5 and 100 mg. It also can be used as one single evening dose for insomnia.

11.5 Prazosin for Nightmares in Post-Traumatic Stress Disorder

In a double-blind crossover study comparing it to placebo in war veterans with chronic PTSD, prazosin (Minipress), at a mean dose of 9.5 mg at bedtime, was superior to placebo for the three primary outcomes: (1) recurring distressing dreams, (2) difficulty falling/staying asleep, and (3) change in overall PTSD severity. Prazosin is an antihypertensive agent that could decrease the excessive noradrenergic output reported in PTSD. Because patients may experience syncope with the initial doses, the medication should be started low (1 mg/day), and gradually increased according to the patient's response and adverse effects, especially syncope and hypotension (Raskind *et al.*, 2003). Using only 1 or 2 mg/day is very likely to be clinically useless, and the provider starting the medication should make sure that the titration process continues after the patient is discharged or transferred.

11.6 Do Antipsychotics Have a Role in Anxiety?

With the exception of OCD, the current evidence does not support a role of antipsychotics in the management of anxiety, not even in the case of difficult-to-treat ("treatment-resistant") anxious patients. Several clinical studies (mainly open-label trials) have suggested efficacy for some atypical antipsychotics in GAD, but placebo-controlled RCTs of atypicals as add-ons in anxiety have been inconclusive. A problem with the use of antipsychotic drugs in non-psychotic disorders is the need for the clear documentation of expected benefits to justify their use given their serious risk for adverse reactions. A review on the use of atypical antipsychotics in treatment-resistant GAD concludes: "Although data suggest efficacy regarding the use of atypical antipsychotics for augmentation of treatment-refractory GAD, more rigorous studies (large, double-blind, placebo-controlled trials) on the safety and efficacy of these agents are needed in order to recommend their use in patients with GAD." (Lorenz *et al.*, 2010) A recent meta-analysis of SGAs in the treatment of GAD is more categorical: "Existing data suggest that SGAs are not superior to placebo as augmentation for refractory GAD." (Lalonde *et al.*, 2011)

11.7 Beta-Blockers

The prescription of beta-blockers in psychiatric settings, which was not infrequent some decades ago, has practically fallen to zero. At those times, these drugs were prescribed for conditions such as performance anxiety ("stage fright") in lecturers or performers, mainly to prevent the bothersome peripheral adrenergic manifestations induced by anxiety (tachycardia, forceful cardiac contractions, dry mouth, tremor, etc.). However, central anti-anxiety actions were also thought likely to play a role, and for this reason, lipophilic beta-blockers, especially propranolol and metoprolol, were then preferred over hydrophilic ones, such as atenolol, for this indication.

Today, other specialists still use beta-blockers for symptoms that we view as part of the anxiety spectrum, especially the so-called *mitral valve prolapse syndrome* (Bachman *et al.*, 2011). Thus, these days, more than prescribing beta-blockers, mental health providers are faced with the decision about continuing or not treatment with beta-blockers started in a different medical environment.

A common problem is that often those patients are afraid to discontinue the beta-blocker, as they see the palpitations and other cardiovascular symptoms as the expression of a serious physical illness. The discussion of the cardiologic validity of mitral valve prolapse syndrome is beyond the scope of this handbook. However, most of mental health authorities now agree that anxiety or panic is not part of the syndrome (Filho *et al.*, 2011). Because of this, our recommendation is to treat the anxiety associated with this syndrome according to the guidelines for the treatment of patients with somatoform disorders, including the proper way to communicate the diagnosis, the education of the patient about the nature of the physical symptoms, and the use of the proper pharmacotherapy for the comorbid mental disorders.

References

Bachmann S, Muller-Werdan U, Huber M, *et al.* Positive impact of the beta-blocker celiprolol on panic, anxiety, and cardiovascular parameters in patients with mitral valve prolapse syndrome. *J Clin Psychopharmacol* 2011;31:783–785.

Barker MJ, Greenwood KM, Jackson M, *et al.* Persistence of cognitive effects after withdrawal from long-term benzodiazepine use: A meta-analysis. *Arch Clin Neuropsychol* 2004;19(3):437–454.

Becker WC, Fiellin DA, Desai RA. Non-medical use, abuse and dependence on sedatives and tranquilizers among U.S. adults: Psychiatric and socio-demographic correlates. *Drug Alcohol Depend* 2007;90(2):280–287.

Feltner DE, Crockatt JG, Dubovsky SJ, *et al.* A randomized, double-blind, placebo-controlled, fixed-dose, multicenter study of pregabalin in patients with generalized anxiety disorder. *J Clin Psychopharmcol* 2003;23(3):240–249.

Filho AS, Maciel BC, Romano MMD, *et al.* Mitral valve prolapse and anxiety disorders. *Br J Psychiatry* 2011;199:247–248.

Lalonde CD, Van Lieshout RJ. Treating generalized anxiety disorders with second generation antipsychotics: A systematic review and meta-analysis. *J Clin Psychopharmacol* 2011;31:326–333.

Lorenz RA, Jackson CW, Saitz M. Adjunctive use of atypical antipsychotics for treatment-resistant generalized anxiety disorder. *Pharmacotherapy* 2010;30(9):942–951.

Murphy SM, Tyrer P. A double-blind comparison of the effects of gradual withdrawal of lorazepam, diazepam and bromazepam in benzodiazepine dependence. *Br J Psychiatry* 1991;158:511–516.

Pande AC, Davidson JR, Jefferson JW, *et al.* Treatment of social phobia with gabapentin: A placebo-controlled study. *J Clin Psychopharmacol* 1999;19(4):341–348.

Pande AC, Crockatt JG, Feltner DE, *et al.* Pregabalin in generalized anxiety disorder: A placebo-controlled trial. *Am J Psychiatry* 2003;160(3):533–540.

Raskind MA, Peskind ER, Kanter ED, *et al.* Reduction of nightmares and other PTSD symptoms in combat veterans by prazosin: A placebo-controlled study. *Am J Psychiatry* 2003;160:371–373.

Skurtveit SS, Bramness J, Salmer R, *et al.* Benzodiazepines predict use of opioids — a follow-up study of 17,047 men and women. *Pain Med* 2010;11(6):805–814.

Soumerai SB, Simoni-Wastila L, Singer C, *et al.* Lack of relationship between long-term use of benzodiazepines and escalation to high dosages. *Psychiatr Serv* 2003;54(7):1006–1011.

Trivedi MH, Fava M, Wisniewski SR, *et al.* Medication augmentation after the failure of SSRIs for depression. *N Engl J Med* 2006;354:1243–1252.

Chapter 12

Medication Treatment of Anxiety Disorders

General Considerations Prior to Starting Drug Treatment

Psychoeducation and reassurance. Following diagnosis, this is a critical first step, particularly for patients presenting bothersome physical symptoms as part of their anxiety syndromes. An important component of psychoeducation is to instruct the patient to avoid anxiogenic substances. Caffeine and nicotine use should be minimized or discontinued, and alcohol use (frequent in anxiety) should be discouraged. Also, patients should be warned about misuse of medications (including over-the-counter ones), and use of illegal substances as well as weight-loss medications and "energy" supplements. Patients should be encouraged to adopt a "healthy" lifestyle and avoid overwork or exhausting social or academic schedules. Sleep hygiene should be instituted and, if necessary, hypnotics can be prescribed on a short-term basis. A "healthy" (low fat, low calorie) well-balanced diet should be encouraged and, ideally, a gradual exercise program should be started.

Importance of psychotherapy/drug combinations. It should be kept in mind that the concomitant use of psychological (e.g., cognitive behavioral therapy [CBT]) and pharmacological interventions significantly increases the chances of success in the treatment of anxiety disorders. However, since in this handbook we focus exclusively on the pharmacological component, we refer the reader to other sources that provide ample coverage of CBT and other psychotherapeutic interventions.

Other Considerations

The principles governing the use of antidepressants in the treatment of anxiety disorders are similar to those described in the case of depressive disorders.

Thus, for a detailed discussion on initial dose, titration, and maximum doses of second-generation antidepressants (SGAs) in anxiety, we refer the reader to Chapter 10. As mentioned in that chapter, serotonergic medications may induce an initial exacerbation of anxiety symptoms, especially jitteriness, anxiety peaks, and even panic-like attacks. It is important to warn patients about this, and make efforts to minimize the chances of this occurrence. Therefore, in patients with anxiety, antidepressants should be started at the lowest possible dose. A good rule of thumb is to use about half of the initial dose used in depression. If paradoxical exacerbation of anxiety occurs during treatment, the dosage may have to be further decreased or discontinued, and to restart the patient on the medication, use half the previous dose of the drug.

Anxious patients are hypervigilant and generally worry more than patients with depression about adverse effects of medications. Openly discussing potential side effects of antidepressants and reassuring the patients about the benign and transient nature of most of these side effects is a critical step in the medication treatment of anxiety disorders.

12.1 Approved and Potential Uses of Antidepressants and Other Medications

The global usefulness of each antidepressant in anxiety disorders has already been examined in the chapter on the respective drugs, and the general efficacy of non-antidepressant drugs in anxiety was discussed in Chapter 11. Following, we list, for each drug or drug group the approved anxiety indications and other anxiety diagnosis in which they could be reasonably tried.

12.1.1 *SSRIs*

The clinical effects of SSRIs on anxiety (and also depressive) disorders are considered a class action, so we will not detail the approved indications of each individual drug. When grouped together, the available SSRIs have FDA-approved indications for the treatment of the following anxiety disorders:

- Generalized anxiety disorder (GAD);
- Panic disorder;
- Social anxiety disorder (SAD);
- Post-traumatic stress disorder (PTSD); and
- Obsessive–compulsive disorder (OCD).

12.1.2 *SNRIs*

Although we address them as a separate class of antidepressants, SNRIs are a more heterogeneous group than SSRIs. SNRIs may differ in their relative inhibition potencies at the serotonin and norepinephrine pumps. Thus, in the case of SNRIs, we are less certain that the effect on individual depressive or anxiety disorders is a class action. Currently, two SNRIs (venlafaxine and duloxetine) have FDA-approved indications for the treatment of the following anxiety disorders:

- Venlafaxine: GAD, panic disorder, and SAD (also reasonable evidence of efficacy in PTSD); and
- Duloxetine: GAD.

12.1.3 *Mirtazapine and trazodone*

While these two drugs are not FDA-approved for the treatment of anxiety, there is reasonable evidence that they are effective for managing certain types of anxiety syndromes and disorders as follows:

- Mirtazapine: SAD, GAD, and PTSD; and
- Trazodone: GAD.

As discussed in the section on antidepressant medications, it should be kept in mind that these two drugs bring additional benefits to anxious patients with insomnia thanks to their sedative and sleep-inducing properties. Also, because of its positive effect on gastrointestinal irritability, mirtazapine helps symptoms such as nausea/vomiting as well as other gastrointestinal symptoms.

12.1.4 *Bupropion*

As discussed in the chapter on bupropion (Chapter 7), even though solid evidence of efficacy of this drug on anxiety disorders coming from double-blind, placebo-controlled, randomized studies is lacking, there are some open clinical reports and anecdotal information suggesting that this agent may be helpful to patients with GAD.

12.1.5 *TCAs and MAOIs*

TCAs and MAOIs have been proven effective for several anxiety disorders, including GAD, panic disorder, SAD, and OCD. However, their narrow therapeutic margin and side effect profile restrict their clinical use to patients with severe depressive syndromes who have not responded to SGAs.

12.1.6 *Benzodiazepines*

Benzodiazepines are effective medications in the acute management of anxiety, including panic disorder and other presentations with acute physical symptoms. However, they are not the mainstay of treatment due to the potential tolerance to their clinical effects that may encourage dose increases, the risk for abuse and dependence, and the psychomotor impairment they may cause. Therefore, their use should be carefully monitored, dosages kept on the low side, and duration of treatment should be limited.

12.1.7 *Antihistamines and anticonvulsants*

Antihistamines (such as hydroxyzine) and anticonvulsants (such as pregabalin or, to a lesser degree, gabapentin) are useful in some cases of GAD and SAD. However, the sedation they produce limits their clinical use, especially in the case of high-functioning patients.

12.1.8 *Antipsychotics*

The evidence for the efficacy of typical and atypical antipsychotics in anxiety disorders is inconclusive and their adverse effect profile is significantly worse than that of other agents currently recommended for treatment of these disorders. Thus, in our view, the use of antipsychotics for anxiety disorders seems unwarranted. The only exception may be difficult-to-treat OCD, where SSRI augmentation with a conventional antipsychotic, haloperidol, or an atypical one, risperidone, has yielded positive results.

12.2 Drug Treatment of Individual Anxiety Disorders

12.2.1 *Generalized anxiety disorder*

In GAD, the first-line treatment should be an SSRI, followed by an SNRI, and either mirtazapine or trazodone as the third line. Buspirone can be also tried after SGAs, either as a single treatment or as an add-on in cases with partial response. Considering its superior risk/benefit profile compared to non-antidepressant medications, bupropion could be tried after other SGAs have failed, mainly as add-on. However, there are no controlled trials supporting bupropion's efficacy on this indication. A tertiary TCA such as clomipramine may be tried next, in view of its strong serotonergic action compared to secondary TCAs, but the use of TCAs is limited by their side effects and toxicity. The anticonvulsant pregabalin is a reasonable choice after both SGAs and TCAs have failed, but the disadvantages are cost and high risk for sedation. Adding hydroxyzine is always a possibility in patients in which we want to avoid benzodiazepines, but sedation is a problem. Despite their clinical efficacy, MAOIs are rarely used in anxiety disorders, except in refractory and very severe cases.

Patients with significant anxiety "peaks" or panic-like attacks may receive benzodiazepines, ideally as needed (*prn*) and using one with a middle half-life. Benzodiazepine use must be reduced and then stopped as the anti-anxiety effect of the antidepressant becomes evident. Complete suppression of the anxiety with benzodiazepines is not the ideal goal, as it may decrease motivation for, and compliance with, antidepressant treatment. Alcohol abuse is fairly common in anxiety disorders, as a tranquilizer during the day and a hypnotic in the evening. Check carefully for alcohol use before prescribing benzodiazepines.

If sleep hygiene, exercise, and elimination of anxiogenic substances do not suffice to improve sleep, or the insomnia is too severe, pharmacological measures can be considered. A benzodiazepine (e.g., temazepam) may be useful when anxiety is clearly the main factor for insomnia. Other options are mirtazapine, trazodone, or hydroxyzine (which possesses some anti-anxiety activity also) or GABA hypnotics (zaleplon, zopiclone, and zolpidem). For a detailed discussion of hypnotic agents, including benzodiazepines and GABA hypnotics, we refer the reader to Chapter 15.

12.2.2 *Social anxiety disorder*

We recommend to start with an SSRI, and consider, in decreasing order, venlafaxine, mirtazapine, or extended-release trazodone, as appropriate treatments in SAD. Benzodiazepines may, in special occasions, prove helpful when the anxiogenic events are infrequent, and no fine motor or intellectual function is needed. When SGAs are not effective or tolerated, a serotonergic (tertiary) TCA may also be tried. Pregabalin may be helpful, but again, sedation and cost are disadvantages. The anticonvulsant gabapentin has showed efficacy in SAD, at doses that may produce sedation. Hypnotics may be used if there is insomnia on the eve of anxiogenic events.

12.2.3 *Panic disorder*

An SSRI or an SNRI should be the first-line treatment for the disorder (not the panic attacks themselves). If these and other SGAs are not effective or tolerated, a tertiary TCA must be tried. Benzodiazepines are very effective medications to abort or suppress panic attacks. In our view, this is another important reason to try to use them more selectively rather than using them as maintenance treatment of panic disorder. In the rare instances when panic attacks occur very far apart, benzodiazepines could become the only treatment. Some patients experience panic attacks during sleep, and in these cases, a benzodiazepine such as temazepam or possibly a GABA hypnotic could be very helpful. Benzodiazepines should be used ideally as *prn* medications. The dose is titrated acutely to the effective dose necessary to abort/suppress the attacks, and further increases should be avoided. Keep in mind that alcohol use is common in patients with panic disorder and this may potentiate the adverse effects of these medications.

12.2.4 *Specific phobias*

Some phobias could be very incapacitating. Examples are agoraphobia, fear of driving, fear of bridges or heights, fear of flying, etc. Antidepressants, combined with psychotherapeutic interventions such as gradual exposure, provide the best chance for success. Benzodiazepines are helpful for reducing anxiety when the subject is exposed to the phobic stimulus. However, regular benzodiazepine administration may decrease the therapeutic effect of exposure treatment and prolong the duration of the disorder.

12.2.5 *Post-traumatic stress disorder*

PTSD is a disorder with a complex and variable symptomatology, for which several medications or medication groups may be helpful. However, probably none of them provides complete relief of PTSD symptoms when given as a single agent. PTSD patients may present depressive symptoms, anxiety features (including free-floating anxiety, panic-like attacks, avoidance, and agoraphobia), intrusive recollections (including flashbacks and nightmares), significant physical manifestations (starting with hyperarousal, and also including cardiorespiratory and other unexplained physical symptoms), dissociation, and even psychotic symptoms. On top of this, abuse of alcohol, drugs, and prescription medications is relatively common. For all these reasons, discussing the comparative efficacy of individual medications or medications groups as a single treatment for PTSD is frequently a moot exercise. Also, while multiple medications have been shown to help alleviate PTSD symptoms, the choice of a first-line medication treatment for the disorder must be judiciously done.

In relation to this, an important review article on the treatment of PTSD states: "The current evidence base of RCTs is unable to demonstrate superior efficacy or acceptability for any particular medication class." However, the same review concludes that some medications are less effective than others: "Nevertheless, the efficacy of medication in PTSD is unlikely to extend to all medications. While there is preliminary evidence that paroxetine is more effective than sertraline in reducing the severity of PTSD symptoms, and although the two mirtazapine trials provide some support for the efficacy of this agent, neither of the bromfaromine, olanzapine and lamotrigine trials demonstrated efficacy with regards to treatment response or symptom reduction." (Stein *et al.*, 2006)

When choosing medications for PTSD, two important considerations are: (1) the symptomatic profile of the individual patient, and (2) the safety and tolerability of the various drugs. For these reasons, SGAs (mainly SSRIs and venlafaxine, but also mirtazapine or extended-release trazodone) are usually recommended for initial treatment. When SGAs are not effective, TCAs may be considered. Insomnia is almost always present, and must be addressed, with sleep hygiene and, if necessary, medication. The anti-adrenergic antihypertensive prazosin (Minipres) has been shown, in RCTs, to help with PTSD-associated nightmares. Bupropion may help in cases where poor concentration, drowsiness, overeating, and low energy are present on top of depressed mood. Antipsychotics should be used if there are psychotic symptoms. Benzodiazepines, despite their extended use, have shown disappointing results in PTSD studies, with poor efficacy not only against intrusive recollections and avoidance, but even against the core symptoms of anxiety. Because of this and the potential risk for drug abuse/dependence in this population, benzodiazepine administration probably should be the exception rather than the rule in the management of PTSD.

12.2.6 *Obsessive–compulsive disorder*

High serotonergic potency seems to be the requirement for drugs to be effective against OCD. Because of this, the TCA clomipramine is often the first choice in OCD treatment. However, several SSRIs seem to be as effective as clomipramine for the treatment of OCD. For this reason, considering their more benign safety profile, SSRIs are often tried first in OCD. It is generally accepted that clinical response in OCD requires SSRI doses at the high end of the spectrum, or even beyond. Considering the paucity of options in the treatment of OCD, cautiously increasing the SSRI dose beyond the usual maximum dose in the absence of significant side effects is a reasonable choice in most cases. A study with sertraline reported benefit in non-responders when the dose was increased up to 400 mg, a dose twice the usual maximum (Ninan *et al.*, 2006). A case report in a severely resistant OCD patient, who had been referred for capsulotomy, documented clinical response when the dose of citalopram was increased to 160 mg, the double of the accepted maximum dosage (Bejerot *et al.*, 1998). Another recommendation, in cases of OCD with partial response, is to give the antidepressant more time to show its effect. However, when response to several SSRIs is unsatisfactory, clomipramine should be the accepted next step.

Regarding augmentation with other types of psychotropic medications, the best results have been reported with the typical antipsychotic haloperidol and with risperidone, the atypical antipsychotic that most closely resembles the typicals.

References

Bejerot S, Bodlund O. Response to high doses of citalopram in treatment-resistant obsessive-compulsive disorder. *Acta Psychiatr Scand* 1998;98(5):423–424.

Bloch MH, Landeros-Weisenberger A, Kelmendi B, *et al.* A systematic review: Antipsychotic augmentation with treatment refractory obsessive-compulsive disorder. *Mol Psychiatry* 2006;11(7):622–632.

Lorenz RA, Jackson CW, Saitz M. Adjunctive use of atypical antipsychotics for treatment-resistant generalized anxiety disorder. *Pharmacotherapy* 2010;30(9):942–951.

Ninan PT, Koran LM, Kiev A, *et al.* High-dose sertraline strategy for nonresponders to acute treatment for obsessive-compulsive disorder: A multicenter double-blind trial. *J Clin Psychiatry* 2006;67(1):15–22.

Ravindran LN, Stein MB. The pharmacological treatment of anxiety disorders: A review of progress. *J Clin Psychiatry* 2010;71(7):839–854.

Stein DJ, Ipser JC, Seedat S. Pharmacotherapy for post traumatic stress disorder (PTSD) *Cochrane Database Syst Rev* 2006;(1):CD002795.

Chapter 13

Medications Used in the Treatment of Mania

Medications with evidence for efficacy in mania include lithium, antipsychotics, valproate (divalproex), carbamazepine, oxcarbazepine, and more recently, tamoxifen. We do not consider that lamotrigine — despite some reports indicating it may have efficacy — has any meaningful role in the treatment of mania. We will discuss this in more detail in the next chapter on bipolar depression. It is also important to be aware that some providers continue to prescribe medications for bipolar patients that do not have a proven antimanic effect, such as is the case with the anticonvulsants gabapentin (Neurontin) and topiramate (Topamax).

13.1 Lithium

The mood-enhancing properties of lithium have been known and utilized for centuries. The first modern evidence-based trial on the efficacy of lithium in mania was done in Australia and published in 1949 (Cade, 1949). Despite the widespread knowledge about its therapeutic value and low cost, lithium has always been an "orphan" drug due to its being a natural element. Therefore, its therapeutic development had to be financed by the Federal Government rather than industry. Possibly due to this, as well as safety concerns related to its narrow therapeutic window and potential toxicity, lithium lost ground to newly developed drugs such as atypical antipsychotics. However, increasing worries about the long-term safety and cost of the atypical antipsychotics have revived the interest in lithium, keeping it as a first-line antimanic agent.

Lithium is a very simple compound; it is a light metallic monovalent cation, and one of the smallest elements, the third, in the periodic table. It is well absorbed, with a reported bioavailability of 80%–100% of a single dose. The absorption of lithium is not negatively affected by the presence of food and actually, it seems to improve when lithium is given with a meal. The time to peak plasma concentration is 1–2 h for the immediate-release form, and 4–5 h for sustained-release forms. However, the elimination half-life, 24 h, with a reported range of 18–36 h, is similar for both immediate- and sustained-release preparations, which makes even the immediate-release forms amenable for once-a-day dosing. Lithium is eliminated unchanged by the kidneys, and its clearance is directly dependent on the glomerular filtration rate (GRF), so it decreases with aging and renal disease.

Multiple neurochemical actions have been reported with lithium, including effects on intracellular second messenger systems (for example, through inositol depletion); enhancing serotonergic and noradrenergic neurotransmission; and inducing changes in the circadian rhythms of the body. However, most authors give central importance to the positive neurotrophic effects of lithium, through inhibition of glycogen synthetase kinase 3 beta (GSK3-β), an enzyme that phosphorylates and inhibits nuclear factors that control cell growth and protection programs. In animals, lithium upregulates neurotrophins, such as brain-derived neurotrophic factor (BDNF), nerve growth factor, neurotrophin-3 (NT-3), as well as receptors to these growth factors in the brain. Lithium also seems to protect neurons against glutamate overcharge, seizures, and apoptosis due to a wide variety of neurotoxins, and stimulate the proliferation of some stem cells, including bone marrow and neural stem cells. However, it is difficult to ascertain the relative relevance of each one of these and other actions for lithium's therapeutic effects, or the sequence in which they occur, if such a sequence really exists.

The antimanic efficacy of lithium has been established in multiple randomized placebo-controlled clinical trials since the 1960s. It has also been established in trials comparing it with typical and atypical antipsychotics as well as anticonvulsant drugs, although these studies usually do not allow us to deduce differences in the antimanic effect. A recent meta-analysis shows lithium to be an effective treatment for mania, with some antipsychotics demonstrating an apparently bigger effect and others a smaller one than lithium, while anticonvulsant drugs show a similar effect (Yildiz *et al.*, 2011). In any case, the consensus among clinicians is that about 75% of patients with mania will show some benefit from lithium treatment, and that, so far, there are no well-established differences in antimanic effects between lithium, antipsychotics, or anticonvulsants.

Besides its antimanic effect, lithium has shown other interesting properties for the treatment of mood disorders. For example, it has demonstrated excellent clinical effects in the treatment of bipolar depression, as we will discuss in the next chapter. Multiple reports (mainly national registry analyses and meta-analyses) suggest that lithium may be protective against suicide in bipolar patients, and even in patients with major depression. Lithium also seems to decrease aggressiveness/impulsivity in bipolar patients, patients with mental retardation, children and adolescents with conduct disorder, and patients with behavioral addictions such as pathological gambling.

13.1.1 *Toxicity*

Lithium has a narrow therapeutic window. The best accepted therapeutic range is a serum level of 0.6–1.2 mEq/L, and it is grossly estimated that serious toxicity starts around 3.0 mEq/L or even lower. The warning symptoms of toxicity are those of delirium or other neurologic symptoms such as nystagmus, ataxia, irritability, and seizures, but the sudden appearance or worsening of systemic symptoms known to be lithium-related should also raise alarm. These include gastrointestinal (nausea/vomiting, diarrhea), renal, muscular (weaknesses, tremor, hypertonia, etc.), and unexplained autonomic changes.

An important observation is that serum lithium levels can be promptly reduced by dialysis. Thus, early intervention with hemodialysis may prevent permanent damage from abnormally high levels. In acute toxicity cases, overdose should be considered, and all the relevant steps taken, including gastric lavage and drug screening.

13.1.2 *Adverse effects*

The most common side effects of lithium are weight gain, tremor, edema, and excessive thirst/increased urinations. The body systems affected by adverse effects of lithium are mainly the central nervous system (CNS), thyroid gland, kidney, and heart.

Neurological. The neurological side effects of lithium cover all the range from mild lethargy, weakness, memory loss, cognitive dulling, and tremor to irreversible neuropathy. Fine tremor is not uncommon with lithium. It may decrease over time but increasing tremor may indicate toxicity. The first option, when there is tremor, is decreasing the dose. For those patients who cannot do it or do not respond, some authors recommend beta-blockers, especially propranolol. However, our preference in the case of significant tremor, is switching medications, as we worry about possible neurotoxicity.

Neurotoxicity, with initial delirium, is usually associated with toxic lithium levels, but some cases have been reported with levels in the therapeutic range. There are reports of lithium-induced EPS (extrapyramidal symptoms), as well as worsening of antipsychotic-induced EPS with lithium therapy. Some reports associate lithium with relapse of antipsychotic-induced neuroleptic malignant syndrome (NMS). There exist also case reports of benign intracranial hypertension (*pseudo tumor cerebri*) associated with lithium.

Thyroid. Thyroid dysfunction with lithium includes both hypothyroidism and hyperthyroidism. However, the last one is exceedingly rare. The figures reported for hypothyroidism associated with lithium therapy are widely variable, with the most recent ones showing less alarming numbers, and even some reports suggesting that the prevalence of hypothyroidism with lithium treatment is not different from that expected in the general population. In the authors' opinion, the risk for hypothyroidism with lithium treatment is real, but very likely the magnitude is lower than that reported in past decades, with some authors putting the risk grossly at 5% of all lithium-treated patients. The risk seems to be significantly higher for females than males, and a study with 209 London patients treated with lithium and followed for a 20-month period, showed that 14.9% of the females and 3.4% of the males had clinically significant hypothyroidism (Kirov, 1998).

Kidney. Patients on lithium may experience defects in urine concentration ability, with resulting polyuria or diabetes insipidus. They may also show edema. Most authors recommend amiloride for the treatment of significant polyuria or diabetes insipidus in patients treated with lithium, as it spares potassium and does not increase lithium levels. If amiloride is not effective, thiazides may be added or substituted for. However, when sodium-depleting diuretics are used, regular lithium and potassium levels are needed. Besides this, using these diuretics is cumbersome, as the dose of lithium should be reduced, and a new titration process started. Very rare cases of nephrotic syndrome have been reported with lithium, which seem to be reversible if the medication is stopped soon. Keep in mind that toxicity due to lithium intoxication, concurrent medical illness, drug–drug interactions, dehydration, and other factors is always a possibility. Some findings suggest that giving lithium once a day may be safer to the kidney than divided dosing, but the rationale for this is unclear.

Cardiac. Conduction defects have been reported with lithium, including sinus bradycardia and sinus dysfunction, atrioventricular (AV) block, and T wave changes. They seem to be reversible with discontinuation of the drug.

However, ECG studies do not seem necessary in patients under age 50 with no history of cardiac illness. In patients with cardiac history or those older than 50 years, a baseline ECG is advised. In patients with pre-existing sick sinus syndrome, a pacemaker should be in place before starting lithium therapy.

Hematological. Lithium may produce benign leukocytosis, something that should be kept in mind to avoid unnecessary worry about elevated white blood cell counts in patients taking the drug.

Skin. Adverse dermatological effects such as acne, psoriasis (new or exacerbation of pre-existing psoriasis), and rash have been reported with lithium.

Weight changes. Weight gain can be significant in some patients on lithium therapy. Patients with polyuria should be advised not to replace lost volume with sugared liquids. Equally, patients need close follow-up of lithium levels when losing weight.

Gastrointestinal. Gastrointestinal irritation, including nausea/vomiting and diarrhea, may happen with lithium. As already mentioned, food may actually improve the absorption of lithium so the drug is better given with meals to decrease gastrointestinal symptoms.

Use in pregnancy. Regarding the use of lithium during pregnancy, the main worry has been the possibility of cardiac teratogenicity, especially the Ebstein anomaly, a rare malformation involving the tricuspid valve and the right ventricle. However, it is clear now that the alarming incidence seen in the initial report in 1975 was due to a reporting bias. In the general population, the Ebstein anomaly seems to be present in 1–5:200,000 births, and recent estimates put the risk for lithium use during pregnancy at 1:1,000–2,000. The use of lithium during pregnancy requires closer follow-up than usual, as the levels are likely to go down with the significant expansion in blood volume and increase in GFR during pregnancy. Then, they will go up with the sudden contraction of blood volume after delivery. Lithium is excreted in the milk in amounts that may cause effects in the nursing child.

13.1.3 *Drug–drug interactions*

Lithium is subject to pharmacokinetic drug–drug interactions in the kidney. Sodium-depleting diuretics (thiazides and loop diuretics such as furosemide), and nonsteroidal anti-inflammatory drugs (NSAIDs) impair elimination and increase lithium levels. These medications can be started in patients on lithium, but the dose of lithium needs to be reduced and a new titration process started. Other types of diuretics such as acetazolamide or amiloride do not seem to affect lithium's elimination. Osmotic diuretics such as mannitol have been reported to increase the elimination and decrease the plasma levels of lithium. ACE (angiotensin-converting enzyme) inhibitors such as lisinopril also reportedly increase lithium levels, though the mechanism is unclear. Caffeine and theophyilline reportedly decrease lithium levels (possibly due to their diuretic effect). Lithium levels may also go up in patients on dietary sodium restriction.

Increased pharmacodynamic toxicity from the combination of haloperidol and other typical antipsychotics and lithium has been reported for decades. However, this association is questioned today as: (1) the recommended doses of typical antipsychotics in past decades were several times higher than those customarily used today; (2) studies combining haloperidol and lithium published in the last 10–12 years have not raised major safety concerns; and (3) studies combining lithium with atypical antipsychotics, both low-to-middle- or high-potency dopamine blockers, have not shown significant additional toxicity from the combination. Thus, it is our opinion that the combination of haloperidol and other high-potency typical antipsychotics with lithium is probably not riskier than the combination of lithium with aripiprazole or other high-potency atypicals.

Increased risk of serotonin syndrome (Section 6.9) has also been suggested from the combination of lithium and serotonergic antidepressants, including SSRIs and SNRIs.

13.1.4 *Dosing*

Lithium is usually given twice per day. However, because of its relatively long (24 h) half-life, all oral lithium preparations, including immediate-release ones, can be given once a day. As mentioned, some evidence suggests that once-a-day dosing could be safer for the kidneys than divided doses.

Some authors recommend starting treatment with a "loading" high dose of lithium. We do not think that the benefits of this practice outweight the risks, and, in healthy adults, we prefer to start with a moderate dose of 600–900 mg/day. On the other hand, the up-titration of the dose can be done faster than most clinicians use, at 5–7-day intervals, according to serum levels. Keep in mind that a lower initial dose and significantly longer intervals between dose changes are required in the elderly and patients with renal disease. The accepted therapeutic range for lithium is 0.6–1.2 mEq/L (or mmol/L). However, we aim for levels in the lower end of this range, around 0.6–0.8 mEq/L, as levels over 0.75 mEq/L do not seem to offer additional benefit. In patients who are clinically stable with subthreshold levels, we may keep the dose constant, as the minimum efficacious level seems to be 0.4 mEq/L.

Once a stable dose has been reached, in healthy adult patients, lithium serum levels should be tested every 3–6 months. Both prior to starting lithium therapy and also at these scheduled intervals, we also request a TSH (thyroid-stimulating hormone) determination, and a "metabolic panel" that includes BUN (blood urea nitrogen), creatinine, glucose, and electrolytes (especially sodium and potassium). In elderly patients, or patients with cardiac conditions, an ECG is a justified addition.

The levels should be tested approximately 12 h after the last dose. Our standard recommendation is to advise the patient to take the evening dosage as usual, and to go to the laboratory early next morning, fasting (because of the metabolic panel), and to avoid taking the morning dose before bloodwork.

13.2 Antipsychotics

The antimanic effects of "typical" antipsychotics like haloperidol and chlorpromazine have been known and utilized for decades. Chlorpromazine, for example, obtained the indication for mania from the FDA in the 1970s. In the USA, most of the atypical antipsychotics have already obtained the FDA indication for the treatment of mania. The antimanic effect of antipsychotics seems to be a class effect, including all typicals and atypicals and even the most recently introduced agents for which there are no published studies in mania yet.

Thanks to intensive promotional campaigns, the "atypical" antipsychotics have become the most widely used antimanic agents in the USA, and some authorities generically call them 'mood stabilizers.' However, this denomination is misleading, as the only antipsychotic with proven effect as monotherapy in both mania and bipolar depression is quetiapine, and several "atypical" antipsychotics have failed randomized trials in the treatment of bipolar depression. Thus, regarding antipsychotics in the treatment of mania, we must keep in mind that: (1) both typical and atypical antipsychotics are effective antimanic agents; and (2) the side effect profile and risks of antipsychotics in bipolar depression are similar to those in schizophrenia, including metabolic and motor side effects, as well as in NMS. To further complicate matters, there is evidence suggesting that patients with mood disorders may be at higher risk in developing EPS from antipsychotics than patients with schizophrenia.

Regarding the description of antipsychotic drugs, to avoid duplication, we refer the reader to both chapters on antipsychotics: Chapter 3 and 4.

13.3 Carbamazepine

Carbamazepine is a potent “narrow-spectrum” anticonvulsant that appears to work primarily through inhibiting the function of voltage-sensitive sodium channels. Carbamazepine has been used in bipolar disorder since the 1970s. However, in recent years, the increasing awareness on the exceedingly high risk for drug–drug interactions with carbamazepine as well as skin and hematologic toxicities has led to a steady decline in its clinical use, particularly by psychiatrists.

Despite the prolonged use of carbamazepine, the evidence of its efficacy as monotherapy in mania is relatively recent, and obtained in studies using total daily doses between 400 and 1,600 mg/day (Weisler *et al.*, 2004; Weisler *et al.*, 2005). Unfortunately, the tolerability of carbamazepine in these trials looks very poor, especially regarding neurological adverse reactions. In the 2004 study by Weisler *et al.*, for example, the completion rate at three weeks for carbamazepine was just 49.5% (*vs.* 44.7% for placebo), and the incidence of neurological adverse reactions was high, including dizziness (carbamazepine 48.5% *vs.* 12.6% for placebo); somnolence (carbamazepine 32.7% *vs.* 15.5% for placebo); and slurred speech (carbamazepine 6.9% *vs.* 0.0% for placebo). In the 2005 study by Weisler *et al.*, the reported rate of ataxia with carbamazepine was 18.9% compared to 0.0% for placebo.

Carbamazepine poses a high risk for metabolic drug–drug interactions. It is a known inducer for several oxidative and conjugation enzymes, which means that it may significantly decrease the effect of many psychotropic drugs and scores of general medications, including contraceptives. Cytochromes whose activity is induced by carbamazepine include CYP1A2, 2C9 and 19, and 3A4. Psychotropic medications whose effect may be reduced by carbamazepine this way include antipsychotics (aripiprazole, clozapine, olanzapine, and quetiapine), antidepressants (citalopram, fluoxetine, mirtazapine, trazodone, and tricyclic antidepressants), anti-anxiety medications (benzodiazepines and buspirone), and methadone. Concerning conjugation, carbamazepine is an inducer of the conjugation enzyme UTG1A4, and may decrease the levels of psychotropics and general medications including asenapin, lamotrigine, valproate (divalproex), and opioid medications. Carbamazepine induces its own elimination, meaning that, especially at the beginning of treatment, relatively stable carbamazepine levels and clinical effects can suddenly decrease.

General medications whose levels and effect can be affected by carbamazepine include oral contraceptives (with risk of unwanted pregnancy), antiretrovirals, antihistamines, clopidogrel, statins, macrolide antibiotics, naproxen and other NSAIDs, propranolol and other beta-blockers, proton-pump inhibitors, steroids, theophylline, verapamil and other calcium channel blockers, and zolmitriptan.

In the USA, carbamazepine carries a warning for serious and sometimes fatal dermatologic reactions, including toxic epidermal necrolysis (TENS) and Stevens–Johnson syndrome (SJS), related to the presence of the HLA-B* allele. The warning puts this risk, in Caucasians, at 1–6 out of every 10,000 new carbamazepine users, and as high as 1:150 in Asian populations. Carbamazepine also carries a warning about aplastic anemia and agranulocytosis, stating that in people using this medication, the risk for these reactions is 5–8 times greater than that for the general population. As with all anticonvulsant medications, carbamazepine now carries a warning about increased suicidality.

Carbamazepine's absorption is reportedly erratic, and is not affected by food. It is metabolized mainly by cytochrome CYP3A4, and the elimination half-life has been reported to be about 24 h. However, because of enzymatic auto-induction, after 2–4 weeks, the half-life decreases to about 8 h.

Side effects and adverse reactions with carbamazepine include several body systems:

Dermatologic. SJS and TENS have already been mentioned above. Carbamazepine also induces benign rashes, but the standard recommendation is discontinuing the medication when reactions involving the skin and mucosal surfaces do appear, as it is difficult to clearly differentiate them. Particularly worrisome is the report that a commonly used analgesic, acetaminophen, increases the risk for serious skin reactions with carbamazepine (Gau *et al.*, 2008). Because of the added potential for skin toxicity, we would not combine carbamazepine with lamotrigine or valproate.

Hematologic. Because of the possibility of rare, but potentially lethal, leukocytopenia and other blood dyscrasias such as thrombocytopenia, patients need to be instructed to report fever, malaise, infections, or abnormal bruising or bleeding. Obviously, we should never combine clozapine and carbamazepine. Carbamazepine's combination with lithium requires care as lithium's hematologic effects may mask carbamazepine-induced leukopenia.

CNS and neurologic. Reports of cognitive "dulling" are not uncommon with carbamazepine. Initial signs of neurotoxicity include drowsiness, dizziness, confusion, ataxia, and diplopia which, according to severity, require discontinuation of the medication or a dose reduction.

Cardiac. Conduction changes have been reported with carbamazepine, especially sinus dysfunction and AV block, not different from those reported with lithium, which would be another reason to worry about the combination.

Gastrointestinal. Nausea/vomiting are commonly experienced at the beginning of therapy. They seem to be less frequent with delayed-release forms. Elevations of liver enzymes, which require follow-up, and rare hepatitis have been reported with carbamazepine. At least one report suggests that carbamazepine potentiates the liver toxicity of acetaminophen.

Renal/electrolytes. Carbamazepine may induce water retention with hyponatremia, and electrolytes need to be checked whenever there are changes in the mental status.

Psychiatric. As with all other anticonvulsants, carbamazepine carries a warning for increased suicide risk.

Use in pregnancy. Reports on the teratogenicity of carbamazepine vary widely, with some reports estimating an incidence of malformations in about 10%–30% of pregnancies exposed to carbamazepine. However, the most reliable recent reports, those of national registries such as the UK Register and the North American Register, give figures in the range of 2%–3%. A recent report also puts the risk of malformations with carbamazepine (and lamotrigine) as monotherapy in the above-mentioned range (2%–3%), and concludes that the elevated figures may have come from polypharmacy, particularly the combination of carbamazepine with valproate (Holmes *et al.*, 2011).

13.3.1 *Dosing*

The usual starting dose of carbamazepine in healthy adults is relatively low, with 200 mg given at bedtime or twice a day to avoid initial neurotoxicity. The dosage is usually increased by 200 mg at regular 4–7-day intervals (could be faster in hospital patients), with an upper limit of 1,800 mg/day, though many clinicians are reluctant to go over 1,200 mg/day. Doses should be divided, even when using sustained-release preparations. Target serum levels employed are those used in the management of epilepsy (4–12 μg/mL), although it remains unclear if these levels really apply to bipolar disorder, as some studies report no correlation between serum levels of carbamazepine and clinical efficacy in bipolar disorder.

13.4 Oxcarbazepine

Oxcarbazepine (Tryleptal) is a carbamazepine analog with less potential than carbamazepine for hetero- and auto-induction of metabolic enzymes and skin or hematologic adverse effects, although it still carries some risk in these areas anyway. Thus, oxcarbazepine may cause failure of hormonal contraception and other drug–drug interactions. In the USA, oxcarbazepine is approved only as an antiepileptic drug, with no indication in bipolar or any other psychiatric disorder. The evidence for the efficacy of oxcarbazepine in bipolar disorder is weak. Studies suggesting efficacy are mainly add-on studies with no placebo comparison, and the best study to date, in bipolar I disorder in children and adolescents, showed no difference between oxcarbazepine and placebo (Wagner *et al.*, 2006). Adverse reactions with oxcarbazepine are basically those of carbamazepine, including hyponatremia. The usual starting dose in adults is 300 mg bid, increasing gradually up to a limit of 2,400 mg/day. However, as there is no conclusive evidence on efficacy, going up to high doses and facing increased risk of adverse effects are not warranted, unless there is an unequivocal clinical response.

13.5 Valproic Acid (Divalproex, Valproate)

The active component in these drugs, valproic acid, is a broad-spectrum antiepileptic drug. It is commercially available as valproic acid, as sodium valproate, or as a mixture of both, called divalproex sodium (Depakote, Depakote ER). Because of intestinal irritation with valproic acid, valproate or divalproex are the preferred forms.

Divalproex is approved in the USA for the treatment of acute manic or mixed episodes in bipolar I disorder. In the past, valproate was often recommended as the first-line drug in rapid cycling bipolar disorder, as some studies showed it superior to lithium, but recent larger studies have shown comparable efficacy. However, with the increasing attention to safety in psychopharmacology, the use of valproate looks more problematic, especially in women, as discussed below.

Valproate/valproic acid seems to increase GABAergic neurotransmission. It also may reduce protein kinase C (PKC), inhibit glycogen synthase kinase 3 (GSK-3), and affect the synthesis of inositol. The relationship of any of these actions with the drug's anticonvulsant or antimanic effect is still unclear. All valproic acid preparations are well absorbed with a bioavailability close to 90% (80% for sustained-release forms). The reported mean terminal half-life for moderate doses of divalproex is 9–16 h. Valproate is eliminated mainly through conjugation (glucuronidation). However, oxidative pathways, including some cytochromes, contribute a large number of metabolites which may produce adverse effects.

Valproic acid may cause significant drug–drug interactions. It is an inhibitor for the conjugation enzymes UGT1A3 and 2B7. The most well-known interaction in this pathway is the potential to increase the toxicity of lamotrigine, but it may affect practically any medication eliminated through conjugation. Valproate is also a weak inhibitor for some cytochromes such as CYP2C9 and probably 3A4.

13.5.1 *Adverse effects*

Minor side effects. Gastrointestinal and neurologic manifestations are relatively common at the onset of treatment including nausea/heartburn, vomiting, diarrhea, sedation, tremor, ataxia, etc., and these symptoms tend to disappear thereafter. However, other riskier or more disturbing side effects of valproate include:

Hepatoxicity. Mild elevations of the liver enzymes in up to 30%–44% of patients have been reported, an effect that requires follow-up to make sure it is not progressing. Clinically significant liver toxicity has been estimated to happen in 1:15,000 (1:800 in children), and includes four types (transient and reversible hepatitis, toxic hepatitis, hyperamonemia, and Reye-like syndrome). Hyperamonemia is being reported with increased frequency, which usually manifests initially by lethargy and confusion. The risk of liver toxicity goes up significantly with co-administration of valproate with other hepatotoxic drugs or substances, including alcohol. Hemorrhagic pancreatitis has also been reported with valproate.

Reproductive system. There is a growing preoccupation about the adverse effects of valproate on the reproductive system. An increased incidence of polycystic ovarian syndrome has been reported in women of fertile age treated with valproate. Valproate has also been shown to induce hormonal alterations in males, for example reducing FSH (follicle-stimulating hormone) levels, but the clinical significance of these changes has not been examined.

Skin. Reported hair loss is not rare with valproate. As with any other anticonvulsant, valproate may cause toxic skin syndromes.

Hematologic. Thrombocytopenia and platelet dysfunction may occur with valproate, and rare agranulocytosis has been reported. Thus, the appearance of ecchymosis must raise alarm, and patients must have full CBC (complete blood count), including platelet count, and bleeding time before surgery.

Neurologic/cognitive. These are common, including asthenia, sedation, somnolence, dizziness, memory problems, ataxia, tremor, nystagmus, diplopia, amblyopia, and blurred vision.

Psychiatric. As all other anticonvulsants, valproate carries a warning for increased suicide risk.

Use in pregnancy. Valproate is significantly more teratogenic than other antiepileptic drugs. The most reliable reports put the incidence of major malformations with valproate at about 10% of pregnancies, with a relative risk of 7.3. Because of this, and the reproductive adverse effects, many experts question the use of valproate for psychiatric indications in women of childbearing age.

13.5.2 *Dosing*

In healthy adults (valproate should never be used in patients with liver disease), valproate is usually started at 500–1,000 mg/day, in divided doses or one dose at bedtime (for sustained-release preparations). Some providers use a "loading" strategy, giving initial doses up to about 2,000 mg. We do not advise this, as the benefits of this strategy are not clearly proven, and the risks are relatively high. The dose is increased gradually, according to tolerance and serum levels. Though some authors emphasize that the correlation of serum levels and antimanic effect is not clear, at least one study suggests that there is a linear relationship between serum levels and the antimanic effect of valproate, and that the target level for the best effect in acute mania is above 94 μmol/mL (Allen *et al.*, 2006). In general, the accepted therapeutic range of serum levels is 50–150 μg/mL. Determinations of serum levels should be accompanied by testing of liver enzymes (LFT) and CBC with platelet count. In patients on stable doses, these laboratory assessments should be performed at least every six months.

13.6 Tamoxifen

Despite some initial reports from open studies that suggested its efficacy on mania, FDA approval has not been sought as tamoxifen is now available in generic form, and therefore there is limited commercial incentive to promote its use. Perhaps the most important clinical study of tamoxifen in mania was published in 2007. In this small-sized, double-blind, placebo-controlled three-week trial, 63% of tamoxifen patients responded compared to 13% of placebo patients (Zarate *et al.*, 2007). Following that report, at least two other studies have shown efficacy for tamoxifen in mania: a double-blind, placebo-controlled three-week trial enrolling 66 patients (Yildiz *et al.*, 2008), and a double-blind, randomized, placebo-controlled trial of tamoxifen as adjunctive treatment to lithium (Zohreh *et al.*, 2011). The rationale for trying tamoxifen as a treatment for mania relates to its activity on the PKC pathway, a system that has been thought to be potentially involved in bipolar disorder. Tamoxifen is an anti-estrogen drug, widely used in the treatment of breast cancer and other neoplasms. It is also a prodrug, transformed by the cytochrome CYP2D6 into its active form, endoxifen.

References

Allen MH, Hirschfeld RM, Wozniak PJ, *et al.* Linear relationship of valproate serum concentration and optimal serum levels for acute mania. *Am J Psychiatry* 2006;163(2): 272–275.

Bebchuk JM, Arfken CL, Dolan-Manji S, *et al.* A preliminary investigation of a protein kinase C inhibitor in the treatment of acute mania. *Arch Gen Psychiatry* 2000;57:95–96.

Cade JF. Lithium salts in the treatment of psychotic excitement. *Med J Aus* 1949;2(10): 349–352.

Gau SS, Chao PF, Lin YJ, *et al.* The association between carbamazepine and valproate and adverse cutaneous drug reactions in patients with bipolar disorder: A nested matched case-control study. *J Clin Psychopharmacol* 2008;28(5):509–517.

Holmes LB, Mittendorf R, Shen A, *et al.* Fetal effects of anticonvulsant polytherapies — different risks from different drug combinations. *Arch Neurol* 2011, doi:10.1001/archneurol.2011.133

Kirov G. Thyroid disorders in litihium-treated patients. *J Affective Disord* 1998;50(1):33–40.

Wagner KD, Kowatch RA, Emslie GJ, *et al.* A double-blind, randomized, placebo-controlled trial of oxcarbazepine in the treatment of bipolar disorder in children and adolescents. *Am J Psychiatry* 2006;163(7):1179–1186.

Weisler RH, Kalali AH, Ketter TA, *et al.* A multicenter, randomized, double-blind, placebo-controlled trial of extended-release carbamazepine capsules as monotherapy for bipolar disorder patients with manic or mixed episodes. *J Clin Psychiatry* 2004;65:478–484.

Weisler RH, Keck PE Jr, Swann AC, *et al.* Extended-release carbamazepine capsules as monotherapy for acute mania in bipolar disorder: A multicenter, randomized, double-blind, placebo-controlled trial. *J Clin Psychiatry* 2005;66:323–330.

Yildiz A, Guleryuz S, Ankerst DP, *et al.* Protein kinase C in the treatment of mania — a double-blind, placebo-controlled trial of tamoxifen. *Arch Gen Psychiatry* 2008;65(3): 255–263.

Zarate CA, Singh JB, Carlson PJ, *et al.* Efficacy of a protein kinase C inhibitor (tamoxifen) in the treatment of acute mania: A pilot study. *Bipolar Disord* 2007;9:561–570.

Zoreh A, Rezai F, Salehi B, *et al.* Double-blind, randomized, placebo-controlled 6-week study on the efficacy and safety of tamoxifen adjunctive to lithium in acute bipolar mania. *J Affective Disord* 2011;129:327–331.

Chapter 14

Medications Used in Bipolar Depression, Mixed States, and Rapid Cycling

The effectiveness of current pharmacological options for the treatment of all forms of depression in bipolar patients is very limited. For this reason, even though this is a psychopharmacology textbook, we will briefly discuss electroconvulsive therapy (ECT), a key choice for this indication. ECT offers such significant advantages over available medications in managing the "riskier" cases of bipolar depression, that ignoring this therapy in any discussion of bipolar depression would be a glaring omission.

14.1 Electroconvulsive Therapy

A recently published algorithm proposes, as the first step in the initial evaluation of depressed bipolar patients, to ponder the following question: "*Is electroconvulsive therapy urgently indicated?*" As per the authors of this algorithm, "ECT is urgently indicated in patients with severe suicidality, catatonia, insufficient oral intake, and medical conditions (e.g., pregnancy) that may limit the use of psychotropics." They conclude: "When rapid response is essential, ECT is the treatment of choice." They also postulate that in patients with a history of medication-refractory bipolar depression, despite the comparatively low response rates in this population (about 50%), ECT may still be viewed as a treatment of "first resort" because of the morbidity and mortality associated with prolonging the course of illness with medication options that will likely be ineffective (Ansari *et al.*, 2010).

ECT has a long, eventful history in the treatment of severe depression, including bipolar depression. Here, we will discuss only the most recent evidence and will do so briefly. A North American multicenter study sponsored by the NIMH, that included 220 patients with unipolar and bipolar depression, confirmed once again that ECT has comparable efficacy in unipolar and bipolar depression and found that the remission and response rates and numbers of individual treatments for both groups were equivalent. In this study, 78.8% of unipolar depressives and 80.0% of bipolar depressives responded to the treatment (had at least a 50% reduction in their HAM-D scores) (Bailine *et al.*, 2010). Another recent study of ECT, including 130 patients, 17 with MDD (major depressive disorder), 46 with bipolar I, and 67 with bipolar II disorder, reports a 67.4% response rate for bipolar I depression and 79.1% for bipolar II depression (Medda *et al.*, 2009). Regarding the speed of response to ECT, results from at least two other studies have suggested that depressed bipolar patients respond to ECT faster than depressed unipolar ones (Daly *et al.*, 2001; Sienaert *et al.*, 2009).

ECT *vs.* drug treatment. So far, there are no good prospective comparative studies of the efficacy of ECT compared with medications in bipolar depression. However, in the near future, we may get the definitive study in this area as a prospective, randomized, controlled six-week trial examining the efficacy of ECT compared to pharmacological treatment in bipolar depression, is currently under way (Kessler *et al.*, 2010).

Mixed states. Results from multiple studies have supported the efficacy of ECT in mixed bipolar states. A recent study comparing the response to ECT in medication-resistant bipolar I patients with MDD ($N = 46$) to those with mixed states ($N = 46$), found no statistically significant differences in response (50% or higher decrease in HAM-D scores) between the two groups with response rates of 69.6% for bipolar depression and 66.0% for mixed states, and remission (HAM-D scores ≤ 8) rates of 26.1% and 30.0%, respectively (Medda *et al.*, 2010).

Rapid cycling patients. Regarding rapid cycling patients, a recent study on a small sample of patients with bipolar I and II disorder with a rapid cycling course that had no response to previous treatments, reported that all patients improved during ECT treatment administered monthly. Eight (56%) of the patients did not relapse during the two-year follow-up period, and the rest relapsed only an average of once per year. Sick days decreased 13-fold from 304 to 24 days per year (Minnai *et al.*, 2011).

ECT and anticonvulsants. A recent study of ECT in patients on or off anticonvulsant drugs, showed that patients on anticonvulsants experienced a symptomatic improvement similar to those who were not on these medications. However, patients on anticonvulsants required a significantly higher number of ECT sessions to achieve this improvement (Virupaksha *et al.*, 2010).

14.2 Lithium

Despite the relative neglect of lithium as primary therapy in recent years, the largest number of positive randomized controlled trials (RCTs) in bipolar I depression have focused on this drug (eight trials targeting lithium and only one or two targeting other medications) (Keck and McElroy, 2009). Two recent studies also suggest that lithium is useful in bipolar depression both in the young (Lefpfiker *et al.*, 2007) and the aged (Patel *et al.*, 2006). To this numeric advantage, we must add the many years of experience in the use of lithium, and the fact that it is by far the most proven medication in the long-term management of all phases of bipolar disorder. As mentioned in the previous chapter on the treatment of mania, lithium also seems to exert an anti-suicidal effect. Because of all of these positive factors, starting or optimizing therapy with lithium seems to be the best first step in treating depressed bipolar patients, after ruling out the need for ECT. Additional advantages of lithium in bipolar depression are that it may be combined with anticonvulsant, antipsychotic, and antidepressant medications, and that it may be useful also in mixed states and rapid cycling.

14.3 Quetiapine

Quetiapine is the only antipsychotic with an FDA-approved indication as monotherapy for bipolar depression in the USA. Its clinical efficacy is supported mainly by three large studies: (1) a double-blind, placebo-controlled trial of quetiapine monotherapy (Calabrese *et al.*, 2005); (2) a double-blind, placebo-controlled trial of quetiapine and lithium monotherapy (Young *et al.*, 2010); and (3) a double-blind, placebo-controlled study of quetiapine and paroxetine monotherapy (McElroy *et al.*, 2010). In the eight-week comparison with lithium, quetiapine clearly separated from placebo during the trial while lithium did not. However, it would be worth re-examining the titration of lithium and revisiting the issue in a longer trial, as inspection of the graphics shows a growing separation of lithium from placebo in the last two weeks of the trial, especially in the case of bipolar I patients. Regarding the effect of quetiapine on specific symptoms of depression, we quote again from the above-mentioned algorithm article: "Of note, however, in terms of depressive symptoms as measured by MADRS scores, impressive improvements were noted primarily in sleep and appetite scores, with much less robust improvements in primary depressive symptoms, such as apparent sadness, pessimistic thoughts, and suicidal thoughts." (Ansari *et al.*, 2009)

Quetiapine can be combined with lithium, anticonvulsants, and antidepressants, although the increased risk for side effects from these combinations should be kept in mind. The combination of olanzapine and fluoxetine is also approved for bipolar depression, but the difficulty in titrating the dose for each drug separately according to clinical response or change in specific symptoms is a limiting factor for clinical use.

With quetiapine being the only antipsychotic recommended for monotherapy in bipolar depression, an important question to be raised is what to do with depressed bipolar patients taking other antipsychotics, either typical or atypical, that have been well tolerated and have proven effective for preventing mania. We do not recommend antipsychotic combinations for this indication, except in extreme cases of treatment resistance. In our opinion, the decision about switching these patients to quetiapine or trying other options, such as lithium, is to be made on a case-by-case basis, considering, for example, the history of response to and the adverse reactions of different agents.

14.4 Lamotrigine

In the USA, the FDA-approved psychiatric indication for lamotrigine (Lamictal) is the "maintenance treatment of bipolar I disorder." Lamotrigine is not approved for the treatment of bipolar depression. There are multiple reports and studies suggesting efficacy of lamotrigine in bipolar depression, but the quality of many of these studies is questionable, and conclusive proof is still lacking. Good-quality RCTs show no statistically significant differences between the drug and placebo. This was actually the case with five double-blind, placebo-controlled trials of lamotrigine in the treatment of acute bipolar depression, sponsored by GSK, the manufacturer of Lamictal. An analysis of these studies concludes: "Lamotrigine did not differ significantly from placebo on primary endpoints [17-item HAM-D in Studies 1 and 2; MADRS in Studies 3, 4 and 5]." In one study (Study 1), lamotrigine significantly separated from placebo on some secondary measures of efficacy (Calabrese *et al.*, 2008). Even more significantly, the large NIH-sponsored effectiveness study of bipolar disorder, STEP-BD, did not find any significant differences between lamotrigine, inositol, and risperidone when these were used for open-label augmentation in treatment-resistant bipolar depression (Nierenberg *et al.*, 2006).

Because of the above, we consider lamotrigine to be a third- or fourth-line intervention, after ECT, lithium, and quetiapine, in bipolar I depression, and a fourth- or fifth-line intervention in bipolar II depression, after all of the above plus antidepressants.

Another negative aspect of lamotrigine is that the Prescribing Information includes a "black box warning" to alert on life-threatening, serious skin reactions, including Stevens–Johnson syndrome, toxic epidermal necrolysis, and/or rash-related death. The frequency of these serious skin reactions is largely dependent upon the use of initial high doses or fast titration schedules. It is not an allergic or idiosyncratic reaction, and seems to be due to the accumulation of a toxic metabolite. The best way to prevent these reactions is a slow dose titration. We start at 25 mg/day and increase the daily dose by 25 mg at weekly intervals. This way, it takes almost two months to reach the "target" dose, that in psychiatry is estimated to be in the range of 200–400 mg/day.

Lamotrigine is eliminated by conjugation in the liver. The elimination half-life after repeated doses of lamotrigine has been reported to be about 25 h, which would make it suitable for once-a-day dosing. However, it is usually given twice a day. Conjugation inducers, most of which are antiepileptic drugs, reduce the half-life and serum levels of lamotrigine. On the other hand, valproate and other conjugation inhibitors increase the half-life and serum levels of lamotrigine and with them the risk of toxicity. Despite the existence of guidelines to titrate the dose of lamotrigine, in patients on valproate, from a very low initial dose, we never use the combination and do not recommend using it.

14.5 Valproate

During the 21st century, at least four RCTs have examined the efficacy of valproate compared to placebo in bipolar depression, with an indication of efficacy. However, the size of the studies is small, with a total of only 142 subjects, and we still need larger studies to confirm or disprove the findings (Smith *et al.*, 2010). Valproate, then, would be in the same category as lamotrigine, but its significant side effect/adverse reaction burden, which seriously limits the possibility of concomitant use, especially with antipsychotics or other anticonvulsants, puts it behind lamotrigine in our list of recommendations.

14.6 Antidepressants

The controversy on the efficacy of antidepressants in depressed bipolar patients and their risk for switch into mania has been going on for half a century, and many guidelines now omit antidepressants altogether or consider them a last-ditch possibility. The issue of antidepressant-induced "switches" into mania has likely been magnified in the past by the use of data that did not control for the "switch" that is a natural part of the illness itself, and therefore the overall risk of "switch" with antidepressants seems to be lower than previously reported, although, clearly, the risk is still there. Additionally, some studies in the USA and Great Britain suggest that SNRIs are more likely than SSRIs to induce manic "switches," and that bupropion has the lowest risk for this. Studies also suggest that bipolar II patients are at lower risk of antidepressant-induced "switch" than bipolar I patients, and that bipolar II patients tend to "switch" into hypomania rather than mania (Altshuler *et al.*, 2006).

Recently, the STEP-BD effectiveness trial reported no benefit with the addition of antidepressants (paroxetine and bupropion) to mood stabilizers in bipolar depression, even though they did not report separate analyses by bipolar subtype. Interestingly, the STEP-BD also concluded that antidepressants did not increase the risk of affective switch in this population (Sachs *et al.*, 2007). Another analysis of STEP-BD data reported no significant differences in outcomes among depressed bipolar patients who continued or discontinued antidepressants. From these analyses, the authors of that report also concluded that type II bipolar disorder did not predict enhanced antidepressant response (Ghaemi *et al.*, 2010). A recent meta-analysis also concludes that "although antidepressants were found to be safe for the acute treatment of bipolar depression, their lack of efficacy may limit their clinic utility." However, the authors of that report add that "further high-quality studies are required to address the existing limitations in the literature" (Sidor *et al.*, 2011).

On the other hand, some studies have suggested that antidepressants may be useful as monotherapy in bipolar II depression. A randomized open-label study, comparing venlafaxine with lithium monotherapy in a 12-week trial in bipolar II depression, concluded that there was "a suggestion of efficacy" for antidepressant monotherapy with a low hypomanic switch rate (Amsterdam *et al.*, 2008). Another study followed bipolar II patients who had recovered from a major depressive episode during initial open-label fluoxetine monotherapy. They were then randomly assigned to 50-week treatment with double-blind monotherapy with fluoxetine, lithium, or placebo. The fluoxetine group had the longer mean time to relapse, 249.9 days, versus 156.4 days for the lithium group, and 186.9 for the placebo group. There were no differences among groups regarding hypomanic symptoms (Amsterdam *et al.*, 2010).

Thus, even though we do not recommend using antidepressants in bipolar I patients, we also believe that with such paucity of good options, we should not completely rule out antidepressant use in depressed bipolar II patients. In treating these patients, however, we offer the following pointers: (1) do not use antidepressants in depressed bipolar patients who are experiencing a mixed state, or are rapid cyclers; (2) ideally use antidepressants as adjuncts to an antimanic agent (remember that we do not consider lamotrigine a good antimanic agent); however, the authors have good experience with antidepressants as monotherapy in depressed bipolar II patients who could not tolerate antimanic agents; (3) use a very careful titration upwards, starting at half the initial antidepressant dose or even lower; (4) if there is a mood response but tolerable hypomanic symptoms appear, we may try decreasing the antidepressant dose rather than stopping the medication altogether; and (5) if no clear response is seen in a reasonable period of time, make sure you discontinue the antidepressant before taking other steps.

14.7 Ketamine in Bipolar and Treatment-Resistant Depression

Even though it will likely take some time for glutamatergic agents to be widely available for the treatment of both unipolar and bipolar depression, reports on ketamine's promising clinical effects appear to forecast that this approach could become the next "highlight" in the treatment of mood disorders. Small randomized studies with ketamine, a glutamate NMDA noncompetitive receptor antagonist used in anesthesia, have shown benefits in both depressed unipolar and bipolar patients (Diaz-Granados *et al.*, 2010; Zarate *et al.*, 2012). The most dramatic aspect of the antidepressant effect of ketamine is that the onset of its clinical effect comes very quickly, within 24 h after the infusion, making it the first antidepressant without a latency or "lag" period for its therapeutic effect. This immediate antidepressant effect of ketamine seems to be related to improved neuronal function, especially at the synapses, mediated by increased production of neurotrophic factors such as BDNF.

Even more recently, a study at Mount Sinai and Baylor, on 72 medication-free patients with treatment refractory depression, randomly administered a single 40-min infusion of either ketamine or midazolam, showed 24-h response rates of 63.8% for ketamine and 28% for midazolam, with depression scale decreases of 16.5 and 8.8, respectively (MADRS scores). These differences were all statistically significant (Morrough *et al.*, presented at the 2013 meeting of the Anxiety Disorders Association of America).

14.8 Pharmacological Treatment of Mixed States and Rapid Cycling Bipolar Disorder

We have already discussed the possible benefit of ECT in bipolar patients with mixed states and rapid cycling. Here, we will briefly outline medication options for these clinical subtypes. For a relatively long period of time, valproate was preferred to lithium in the management of rapid cycling bipolar disorders. However, this was not supported by a large (254 patients), long-term (20-month), randomized comparison of lithium and divalproex in the maintenance treatment of rapid cycling bipolar disorder. The results showed no statistically significant differences between lithium and valproate in the relapse rate into any type of mood episode (56% and 50%, respectively), relapse into depression (4% and 29%, respectively), and relapse into mania (19% and 22%, respectively) (Calabrese *et al.*, 2005).

Because of the above, in our opinion, the pharmacological approaches to the treatment of bipolar depression with concurrent manic symptoms (mixed states), and of rapid cycling bipolar disorder, are basically the same, already stated in the case of bipolar depression, with some caveats:

(1) Give even more weight to the possibility of ECT in the initial steps.
(2) For initial therapy, consider lithium first, quetiapine second, and valproate third.
(3) Avoid lamotrigine as monotherapy.
(4) Do not expect antipsychotics, other than quetiapine, to be effective as monotherapy. As stated in a recent review article: "With the exception of quetiapine, the extant evidence seems to suggest that the atypical antipsychotics tend to be unimodal and exert better antimanic than antidepressant effect among rapid cyclers when they are efficacious (primarily treating and preventing mania)." (Muzina, 2009)
(5) Avoid antidepressants.

References

Altshuler LL, Suppes T, Black DO, *et al.* Lower switch rate in depressed patients with bipolar II than bipolar I disorder treated adjunctively with second-generation antidepressants. *Am J Psychiatry* 2006;163(2):313–315.

Amsterdam JD, Shults J. Comparison of short-term venlafaxine versus lithium monotherapy for bipolar II major depressive episode: A randomized open-label study. *J Clin Psychopharmacol* 2008;28:171–181.

——. Efficacy and safety of long-term fluoxetine versus lithium monotherapy of bipolar II disorder: A randomized, double-blind, placebo-substitution study. *Am J Psychiatry* 2010;167:792–800.

Ansari A, Osser DN. The psychopharmacology algorithm project at the Harvard South Shore Program: An update on bipolar depression. *Harvard Rev Psychiatry* 2010;18(1): 36–55.

Bailine S, Fink M, Knapp R, *et al.* Electroconvulsive therapy is equally effective in unipolar and bipolar depression. *Acta Psychiatr Scand* 2010;121:431–436.

Calabrese JR, Huffman RF, White RL, *et al.* Lamotrigine in the acute treatment of bipolar disorder depression: Results of five double-blind, placebo-controlled clinical trials. *Bipolar Disord* 2008;10:323–333.

Calabrese JR, Keck PE, Macfadden W, *et al.* A randomized, double-blind, placebo-controlled trial of quetiapine in the treatment of bipolar I or II depression. *Am J Psychiatry* 2005;162:1351–1360.

Calabrese JR, Shelton MD, Rapport DJ, *et al.* A 20-month, double-blind, maintenance trial of lithium versus divalproex in rapid-cycling bipolar disorder. *Am J Psychiatry* 2005;162(11):2152–2161.

Daly JJ, Prudic J, Devanand DP, *et al.* ECT in bipolar and unipolar depression: Differences in speed of response. *Bipolar Disord* 2001;3:95–104.

Diazgranados N, Ibrahim L, Brutsche NE, *et al.* A randomized add-on trial of an *N*-methyl-D-aspartate antagonist in treatment-resistant bipolar depression. *Arch Gen Psychiatry* 2010;67(8):793–802.

Ghaemi SN, Ostacher MM, El-Mallak RS, *et al.* Antidepressant discontinuation in bipolar depression: A systematic treatment enhancement program for bipolar disorder (STEP-BD) randomized clinical trial of long-term effectiveness and safety. *J Clin Psychiatry* 2010;71(4):372–380.

Keck PE, McElroy SL. Treatment of bipolar disorder. In: Schatzberg AF, Nemeroff CB, eds. *Textbook of Psychopharmacology*. 4th ed. American Psychiatric Publishing, Inc., Arlington, 2009.

Kessler U, Vaaler AE, Schoyen H, *et al.* The study protocol of the Norwegian randomized controlled trial of electroconvulsive therapy in treatment resistant depression in bipolar disorder. *BMC Psychiatry* 2010;10:16.

Lepfiker E, Iancu I, Horesh N, *et al.* Lithium therapy for unipolar and bipolar depression among the middle-aged and older adult patient subpopulation. *Depress Anxiety* 2007;24(8):571–576.

McElroy SL, Weisler RH, Chang W, *et al.* A double-blind, placebo-controlled study of quetiapine and paroxetine as monotherapy in adults with bipolar depression. *J Clin Psychiatry* 2010;71(2):163–174.

Medda P, Perugi G, Zanello S, *et al.* Response to ECT in bipolar I, bipolar II and unipolar depression. *J Affective Disord* 2009;118:55–59.

——. Comparative response to electroconvulsive therapy in medication-resistant bipolar I patients with depression and mixed state. *J ECT* 2010; 26(2):82–86.

Minnai GP, Salis PG, Oppo R, *et al.* Effectiveness of maintenance electroconvulsive therapy in rapid-cycling bipolar disorder. *J ECT* 2011;27(2):123–126.

Muzina DJ. Pharmacologic treatment of rapid cycling and mixed states in bipolar disorder: An argument for the use of lithium. *Bipolar Disord* 2009;11(Suppl. 2):84–91.

Nierenberg AA, Ostacher MJ, Calabrese JR, *et al.* Treatment-resistant bipolar depression: A STEP-BD equipoise randomized effectiveness trial of antidepressant augmentation with lamotrigine, inositol, or risperidone. *Am J Psychiatry* 2006;163:210–216.

Patel NC, DelBello MP, Bryan HS, *et al.* Open-label lithium for the treatment of adolescents with bipolar depression. *J Am Acad Child Adolesc Psychiatry* 2006;45(3):289–297.

Sachs GS, Nierenberg AA, Calabrese JR, *et al.* Effectiveness of adjunctive antidepressant treatment for bipolar depression. *N Engl J Med* 2007;356:1711–1722.

Sidor MM, MacQueen GM. Antidepressants for the acute treatment of bipolar depression: A systematic review and meta-analysis. *J Clin Psychiatry* 2011;72(2):156–167.

Sienaert P, Vanstelaad K, Demyttenaere K, *et al.* Ultra-brief pulse of ECT in bipolar and unipolar depressive disorder: Differences in speed of response. *Bipolar Disord* 2009;11:418–424.

Smith LA, Cornelius VR, Azorin JM, *et al.* Valproate for the treatment of acute bipolar depression: Systematic review and meta-analsyis. *J Affective Disord* 2010;122:1–9.

Virupaksha HS, Shashidhara B, Thirtalli J, *et al.* Comparison of electroconvulsive therapy (ECT) with or without anti-epileptic drugs in bipolar disorder. *J Affective Disord* 2010;127:66–70.

Young AH, McElroy SL, Bauer M, *et al.* A double-blind, placebo-controlled study of quetiapine and lithium monotherapy in adults in the acute phase of bipolar depression (EMBOLDEN I). *J Clin Psychiatry* 2010;71(2):150–162.

Zarate CA Jr., Brutsche NE, Ibrahim L, *et al.* Replication of ketamine's antidepressant efficacy in bipolar depression: A randomized controlled add-on trial. *Biol Psychiatry* 2012; 71(11):939–946.

Chapter 15

Medications Used in the Treatment of Insomnia

Probably, no mental symptom demands a more cautious anamnesis and evaluation of the complaint itself, and a more thorough review of possible causal or contributing factors, than insomnia. The diagnosis must be made carefully, as patients often have a misconception of what insomnia is. In the USA, and likely in other countries, advertising has created the false impression that we should sleep uninterruptedly through the night, and even short awakenings to evacuate are reported as insomnia. In clinical practice, many of our patients feel they should be able to fall asleep instantly at a set time disregarding the length of the preceding wake time. Thus, patients who complain of a long sleep latency tend to be those going to bed early after sleeping late into the day, and many of these patients have a normal or even prolonged total sleep time.

After a reliable diagnosis of insomnia has been established, we must rule out secondary insomnia, caused by a medical condition (for example, obesity, sleep apnea, respiratory and heart conditions, and neuromotor conditions such as restless legs syndrome or Parkinson's disease), use of stimulant medications, substance abuse, or just poor sleep hygiene. Not uncommonly, poor sleep hygiene is a significant contributing factor for insomnia. This includes, for example, lack of exercise or strenuous exercise close to bedtime, consuming heavy meals or stimulant drinks in the late afternoon or in the evening, or getting involved in engaging activities (such as internet surfing or electronic games) at night.

15.1 General Rules

(1) Education in sleep hygiene should always be part of the treatment and must, ideally, precede the pharmacotherapy of insomnia. Although a

detailed discussion of sleep hygiene exceeds the objectives of this handbook, the authors emphasize the need to educate insomniac patients in this regard, whether as the sole initial approach or used in combination with hypnotic medications.

(2) Always first consider safer medications with low potential for abuse. This means, for example, antihistamines or trazodone. An additional reason to try these medications first, even if evidence from large randomized trials in insomnia is lacking for them, is the fact that studies on the pharmacotherapy of insomnia usually show a high placebo response.

(3) If insomnia is related to a mental disorder, try to manage it with the medications intended for the main disorder. This means, for example, using mirtazapine or trazodone in depressed patients; using a sedating antipsychotic in psychotic or manic patients; or using mirtazapine, trazodone, or a benzodiazepine at night in anxious patients.

(4) Regarding dosing, with all hypnotic medications, but especially with GABA receptor agonists: (i) start at a low dose and go up gradually according to response; (ii) try a short-acting medication first, especially when the problem is initial insomnia or awakenings shortly after falling asleep; (iii) make sure that the period between medication-taking and the time when patients are getting up is long enough for the effect to dissipate, avoiding daytime sleepiness/impairment; (iv) because of variations in individual effects, patients should also be instructed to try the hypnotic medication first during the weekend or on the night preceding an off-work day; and (v) always instruct the patient to periodically check the need for the medication, withholding it and observing if insomnia reappears.

(5) Due to the negative balance when we compare the clinical need for the drug with the risky adverse effect profiles of certain drugs, the authors do not consider that chloral hydrate, tricyclic antidepressants, antipsychotics, and antiepileptic drugs should ever be used as primary medications for insomnia (the exception being the use of a relatively safe and well-tolerated antiepileptic drug, such as gabapentin, at night, in patients in which significant neuropathic pain is a factor for insomnia).

15.2 Antihistamines as Hypnotics

In the USA, antihistamines are the most commonly used hypnotic drugs. They are the hypnotic component in widely used over-the-counter (OTC) preparations, such as the "PM" or "NIGHT" versions of many analgesics and cold medications. It is obviously safer to prescribe the antihistamine as monotherapy rather than let the patient use combinations. Antihistamines are preferred for the initial treatment of insomnia whenever there is a worry about dependence/addiction. Main problems are daytime sleepiness ("hangover"), which can be usually corrected by taking the medication early into the evening, and anticholinergic side effects, which are more problematic in the elderly. In the USA, the antihistamines most often used as hypnotics are diphenhydramine (Benadryl, usual nightly dose 25–50 mg), and hydroxyzine (Vistaril, usual nightly dose 25–100 mg). However, because of the long elimination half-life reported for hydroxyzine (20–25 h), which likely increases the chances of next-day impairment, diphenhydramine should be the preferred choice of an antihistamine as a hypnotic.

Diphenhydramine reportedly has an elimination half-life of 5–11 h, a time to maximum concentration (T_{max}) of 2–2.5 h, and is metabolized mainly by CYP2D6, 1A2, 2C9, and 2C19. Several studies of variable quality have shown sleep-improving effects of diphenhydramine in different populations, though the effect seems to be more marked on sleep maintenance than on sleep onset, probably reflecting the relatively long T_{max} time (Glass *et al.*, 2008). It is probably not a good idea to prescribe simultaneously diphenhydramine during the day and also as a hypnotic at bedtime, because studies of daytime dosing have reported a decrease of the sedating effect after less than a week of treatment.

15.3 Sedating Antidepressants (Trazodone and Mirtazapine)

As discussed in Chapter 10 on the treatment of depression, these two medications should be considered in depressed (or anxious) patients with significant insomnia. For use as an add-on to other psychotropic medications, trazodone should be preferred because of its better tolerability and less liability for weight gain, short T_{max} (1–2 h for the immediate-release form), and significantly shorter half-life (4–9 h) that minimizes the risk of daytime impairment. Immediate-release trazodone is obviously preferred, and the dosage should start at 50 mg qhs and be titrated, according to response and tolerability, up to a maximum of 300 mg qhs. For the adverse effects of trazodone, including priapism, see Chapter 8.

15.4 Melatonin Receptor Agonists

15.4.1 *Melatonin*

The release of melatonin by the pineal gland during the daily period of darkness is one of the physiological events triggering and maintaining sleep. This hormone binds melatonin receptors, especially MT_1 and MT_2. It is available as an OTC oral preparation. Melatonin is metabolized mainly by CYP1A2 and 2C19 and, after oral administration, the reported half-life of melatonin fluctuates between 1–4 h, with a T_{max} of approximately 30 min. Interestingly, the sleep-enhancing effects of melatonin do not correlate with the serum levels. Evidence seems to show that the timing of sleep enhancement with melatonin depends on other factors different from the dose, such as the time of administration. Due to this lack of a dose–response or serum level–response relationship, it has been difficult to determine the dose of melatonin needed for sleep enhancement, and the doses used in studies fluctuate widely from 0.3–75 mg. However, 2 mg seems to be the dose recommended most often. In any case, the effect of melatonin seems to be more marked on sleep onset than on sleep maintenance or duration. Despite its generally benign profile, melatonin may induce side effects, including headache and sedation/psychomotor slowing in the day.

15.4.2 *Ramelteon*

Ramelteon (Rozerem) is a prescription hypnotic which, unlike benzodiazepines and related hypnotics, is not subject to especial control in the USA. Ramelteon is an agonist at the melatonin MT_1 and MT_2 receptors, with a receptor binding profile similar to that of melatonin. Like melatonin, there is no close correlation between dose/levels and effect, but an oral dose of 8 mg has been used in studies and recommended in the U.S. FDA-approved Prescribing Information for ramelteon. According to the Prescribing Information, a dose of 16 mg did not offer additional benefit, but increased the incidence of adverse effects (fatigue, headache, and daytime sedation). The most consistent therapeutic finding in studies with ramelteon has been decreased sleep latency with no consistent effect on total sleep time or sleep maintenance. Thus, ramelteon seems to be indicated mainly in delayed sleep onset, including jet lag and shift sleep problems.

Ramelteon is metabolized primarily by CYP1A2 with minor contributions by other isoenzymes, and it undergoes significant first-pass elimination, with an absolute oral bioavailability of only 1.8%. The reported half-life is 1–2.6 h. However, ramelteon has active metabolites with lower affinity for melatonin receptors but significantly longer half-lives, which means increased receptor exposure.

Ramelteon seems to be a relatively safe medication with no potential for abuse/dependence/tolerance to the effect. According to the Prescribing Information, the incidence of adverse effects such as somnolence, fatigue, and dizziness is practically similar to that with placebo. However, as is also the case with other hypnotics, ramelteon carries a warning for cognitive and behavioral effects, including hallucinations and sleep-related behaviors. Hormonal changes have been reported with long-term use of ramelteon, including moderate prolactin elevations in women (but not in men) and abnormal morning cortisol levels in elderly patients. The clinical significance of these changes and the relationship with ramelteon therapy is still unclear.

15.5 GABA Receptor Agonists

15.5.1 *Benzodiazepines*

Benzodiazepines were the most widely prescribed medications for insomnia until the introduction of the semi-selective GABA agonists such as zolpidem, zopiclone, and zaleplon. Benzodiazepines should be used for short-term management of insomnia, and should be considered only for patients with apparent low risk for drug abuse, in which anxiety seems to be an important factor for insomnia. Though all benzodiazepines are good hypnotic agents, some of them have been customarily prescribed for insomnia in the USA and Europe, mainly temazepam, estazolam, flurazepam, quazepam, and triazolam. Out of this list and due to pharmacokinetic and safety reasons, the authors only recommend temazepam. In our opinion, there is no justification, to prescribe benzodiazepines with long half-lives, such as flurazepam (40–250 h), quazepam (20–120 h), and estazolam (10–30 h), for the treatment of insomnia. Regarding triazolam, as mentioned in Chapter 11, the authors consider its use unjustified in any setting, due to the significantly higher incidence of cognitive and mood adverse reactions compared to other benzodiazepines.

Temazepam has significant advantages for use as a hypnotic, including its rapid onset and intermediate duration of action (6–16 h), as well as elimination by conjugation with no active metabolites. Besides this, at least in the USA, temazepam is marketed in a wide range of solid oral strengths and a 10 mg/5 mL solution, which facilitate dose titration. The usual starting dose in adults is 7.5–15 mg qhs.

A special consideration in patients who need these medications during the day for symptoms of anxiety, and who also require treatment for insomnia, the authors often use other benzodiazepines with intermediate action, such as alprazolam and lorazepam. In these cases, we simply order, 1 h before bedtime, a dose similar to that taken during the day, with the instruction to duplicate it if ineffective for insomnia. Because of their long half-lives, the authors do not think that commonly used, long-acting benzodiazepines such as clonazepam, chlordiazepoxide, and diazepam should be utilized for the treatment of insomnia.

All benzodiazepines carry significant potential for abuse/dependence, sleep-related behaviors (discussed in detail in the following section, on GABA hypnotics), daytime sedation, motor and cognitive impairment, and dangerous interactions with alcohol, a substance often used to induce sleep. For a thorough description of the risks associated with benzodiazepine use, the reader should consult Chapter 11. The U.S. Prescribing Information for temazepam carries some warnings similar to those of GABA hypnotics, including severe anaphylactic reactions of the mouth and upper airways.

15.5.2 *GABA hypnotics*

In the USA, GABA hypnotics include zolpidem (Ambien), zaleplon (Sonata), and eszopiclone (S-zopiclone, Lunesta). Except for the fact that the dose is just one half, eszopiclone is similar to the zopiclone used in other continents. As is also the case with benzodiazepines, these hypnotic drugs act as allosteric modulators of GABA activity by binding GABA receptors. However, while benzodiazepines demonstrate comparable affinity for GABA receptor subtypes α_1, α_2, α_3, and α_4, zolpidem and zaleplon have higher affinity for the α_1 subtype and zopiclone for the α_2 and α_3 subtypes. At low and moderate doses, the GABA hypnotics show mainly a hypnotic effect. At higher doses, however, they affect cognition and mood and may induce tolerance to the hypnotic effect, abuse/dependence, and a withdrawal syndrome similar to benzodiazepines.

The absorption of benzo-derivated hypnotics is faster on an empty stomach, so they should be administered ideally far from the last meal of the day, close to bedtime. All three medications are metabolized mainly by CYP3A4, and are subject to interactions with CYP3A4 inhibitors and inducers, for example grapefruit. The reported half-lives for immediate-release oral forms are 2.6 h for zolpidem, 6 h for S-zopiclone, and 1 h for zaleplon. Reportedly, only eszopiclone has active metabolites, although the activity of these metabolites is significantly lower than that of the parent compound. Likely related to its shorter half-life, the clinical action of zaleplon is significantly shorter, approximately 4 h, than that of zolpidem and S-zopiclone, approximately 7–8 h.

15.5.2.1 *Clinical effects*

In randomized clinical trials, zolpidem and eszopiclone have shown benefit for both decreasing sleep latency (initial insomnia) and the number/duration of awakenings (sleep maintenance). Zaleplon has shown benefit in decreasing the sleep latency (initial insomnia) possibly due to its short half-life and also, as a consequence of this (even though this is not mentioned in the U.S. Prescribing Information), it is considered permissible to repeat the dose of zaleplon in the middle of the night, if several hours remain until the planned wake time.

15.5.2.2 *Dosing and timing*

- Short-acting forms should be preferred, whenever possible.
- Start at a low dose and titrate up as needed.
- For better action, GABA hypnotics should be taken on an empty stomach.
- Patients should take the dose of GABA hypnotics (and any hypnotic medication) when they are ready to go to bed.

The last recommendation should be emphasized. Patients who stay involved in any behaviors after taking the medication, especially engaging in demanding behaviors such as surfing the internet, watching TV, working, playing games, or interpersonal interactions may stay awake and enter into a confusional state with unusual perceptions (hallucinations) and/or automatic behaviors. For the same reason, patients should not try to force sleep with hypnotics at a time different from their usual bedtime, or in a location other than home, such as during long flights or when traveling by other means. The risk for these abnormal mental states goes up when hypnotic agents are combined with any other sedative medication or substance, including alcohol.

The recommended daily dose of immediate-release zolpidem (Ambien) is 5 or 10 mg. The recommended daily dose of extended-release zolpidem (Ambien CR) is 6.25 or 12.5 mg (it should be tried only after immediate-release forms have been ineffective). Sublingual zolpidem (Intermezzo), available in 1.75 and 3.5 mg tablets, is FDA-approved to be taken when there is difficulty going back to sleep in the middle of the night, if at least 4 h remain until the planned time of wake (though in this case, zaleplon is likely a better option).

The recommended daily dose of zaleplon (Sonata) is 5–10 mg, although a dose of 20 mg is accepted in the U.S. Prescribing Information in some cases. Zaleplon is more useful when the problem is sleep initiation or waking up shortly after going to sleep, or in patients who need to wake up after a short time. It does not seem to significantly help with sleep maintenance (awakenings during the night). However, as mentioned, some providers allow repeated doses during the night.

The recommended daily dose of eszopiclone (Lunesta) is 1–3 mg. As mentioned above, eszopiclone helps with both sleep onset and sleep maintenance.

15.5.2.3 *Tolerance to the hypnotic effect*

There is some debate regarding the issue of tolerance to the sleep-enhancing effect of GABA hypnotics. Multiple case reports document dose escalation that in some cases leads to dependence and a withdrawal syndrome similar to that of benzodiazepines, including seizures. In clinical practice, we periodically find patients who report having to increase the dose to reach the same hypnotic effect, and we have also observed patients who start abusing these medications by taking them during the day.

15.5.2.4 *Unintended overdose*

A usually ignored risk of GABA hypnotics (and other hypnotics) is accidental overdose. Once patients get sedated and/or confused, they may take additional doses of the medication without being fully aware of the fact. Thus, some patients who overdose on hypnotics deny suicidal intent but cannot explain the overdose. Others, who reliably deny taking more medication than prescribed, run out of medication sooner than expected, and often blame the pharmacist for "shortchanging" them in the amount of medication dispensed.

15.5.2.5 *Adverse effects and risks*

The risk for daytime sedation, psychomotor impairment, confusion/disorientation, and hallucinations exist for all GABA hypnotics. However, the duration of action, depending on the elimination half-life, is obviously a critical factor. Thus, the incidence of sedation or hallucinations seems to be relatively low with zaleplon and relatively high with extended-release zolpidem (see Table 15.1).

On 10 January 2013, the FDA sent a Drug Safety Communication regarding zolpidem and daytime impairment. In that document, the FDA

Table 15.1 Relationship between adverse mental reactions and half-life for GABA hypnotics (percentages from the U.S. Prescribing Information for the three medications).

Adverse reaction	**Ambien CR 12.5 mg**	**Lunesta 3 mg**	**Sonata 20 mg**	**Placebo**
Somnolence	15%	8%	6%	1–3%
Hallucinations	4%	3%	1%	0–<1%

recommends that the bedtime dose of zolpidem be lowered because of data showing that blood levels in some patients may be still high enough the morning after use to impair activities that require alertness, including driving. According to the warning, women appear to be more susceptible to this risk because they eliminate zolpidem from their bodies more slowly than men. Thus, the dose of zolpidem for women should be lowered from 10 to 5 mg for immediate-release products and from 12.5 to 6.25 mg for extended-release products. For men, the FDA recommends that healthcare professionals also consider prescribing the lower doses, 5 mg for immediate-release products and 6.25 mg for extended-release products (FDA, 2013).

The warning on zolpidem raises questions about other GABA hypnotics, especially eszopiclone and sublingual zolpidem. Eszopiclone has a longer elimination half-life than zolpidem and, unlike zolpidem, it has active metabolites. All this suggests that there is a risk for next-day impairment similar to, or higher than that of zolpidem. Sublingual zolpidem, although administered at a lower dose, is sometimes administered up to 4 h before wake time, which also poses the question of daytime impairment.

An important aspect of daytime impairment with hypnotic medications is driving impairment. In healthy adults, a comparison of zopiclone 7.5 mg (equivalent to 3.75 mg of eszopiclone), ramelteon 8 mg, and placebo found that both ramelteon and zopiclone significantly impaired driving performance, cognition, memory, and psychomotor performance the morning following bedtime administration relative to placebo. In contrast to zopiclone, ramelteon produced no balance impairments (Mets *et al.*, 2011). In healthy elderly patients, a comparison of temazepam 20 mg, zopiclone 7.5 mg (equivalent to 3.75 mg of eszopiclone), and placebo found that temazepam 20 mg is unlikely to impair driving 10 h or more after bedtime administration in healthy elderly subjects under 75 years of age, while zopiclone 7.5 mg moderately impaired driving at least until 11 h after administration (Leufkens *et al.*, 2009). Another comparison of zolpidem and zopiclone with placebo after a single administration at night in aged subjects found that compared to placebo, both zopiclone 7.5 mg and zolpidem 10 mg significantly impaired several measures of simulated driving performance (Bocca *et al.*, 2011).

15.5.2.6 *Sleep-related behaviors*

These are complex behaviors that patients perform at night while not being fully awake and which they usually do not remember the next day. When the same type of behavior follows the ingestion of the drugs during the day, because of abuse or error, they are called automatisms. Commonly reported sleep-related behaviors include:

- sleep-walking;
- sleep-driving;
- making and eating food;
- cleaning behaviors;
- having sex;
- conversations and other interpersonal interactions; and
- phone conversations and electronic communications.

Sleep-related behaviors have generated abundant news in the mass media and psychiatric and forensic publications. Dramatic sleep behaviors reported include shooting others, para-suicidal behavior, and a case of self-inflicted gunshot to the head (Chopra *et al.*, 2012; Daley *et al.*, 2011; Gibson *et al.*, 2011). In some legal cases involving murder, the defense invoked the involuntary intoxication with GABA hypnotics. Apparently, and unfortunately for patients, if they were made aware of the risk of intoxication by the prescriber, the intoxication is not then considered involuntary (Daley *et al.*, 2011).

Information on the frequency of sleep behaviors with hypnotic agents and other psychotropic drugs is scarce. Sleep-related behaviors may apparently happen with any hypnotic agent, including OTC antihistamines and benzodiazepines, and even non-hypnotic psychotropic medications. However, the incidence seems to be highest in the case of GABA hypnotics. A study of spontaneous adverse event reports associated with zolpidem use in Australia from 2001–2008 states: "We conclude that zolpidem's adverse drug reaction reports have higher odds for parasomnia, amnesia, hallucinations and perhaps suicidality compared to either all other drugs or hypnotics, even before the media publicity cluster. However, the extant literature and the limitations of these spontaneously reported adverse drug reaction data do not allow us to conclude that these events are causally related to zolpidem." (Ben-Hamou *et al.*, 2011)

References

Ben-Hamou M, Marshall NS, Grunstein RR, *et al.* Spontaneous adverse event reports associated with zolpidem in Australia 2001–2008. *J Sleep Res* 2001;20:559–568.

Bocca ML, Marie S, Lelong-Boulouard V, *et al.* Zolpidem and zopiclone impair similarly monotonous driving performance after a single nighttime intake in aged subjects. *Psychopharmacology* 2011;214(3):699–706.

Budhiraja LB, Parthasarathy S. Sedating medications and undiagnosed obstructive sleep apnea: Physician determinants and patient consequences. *J Clin Sleep Med* 2005;15:1(4): 367–371.

Chopra A, Selim B, Silber MH, *et al.* Para-suicidal amnestic behavior associated with chronic zolpidem use: Implications for patient safety. *Psychosomatics* 2012, doi: 10.1016/j.psym.2012.10.012

Daley C, McNiel DE, Binder RL. "I did what?" Zolpidem and the courts. *Am Acad Psychiatry Law* 2011;39:535–542.

Food and Drug Administration. Drug Safety Communication: Risk of next-morning impairment after use of insomnia drugs; FDA requires lower recommended doses for certain drugs containing zolpidem, 10 January 2013, Retrieved from www.fda.gov/downloads/Drugs/DrugSafety/UCM335007.pdf

Gibson CE, Caplan JP. Zolpidem-associated parasomnia with serious self-injury: A shot in the dark. *Psychosomatics* 2011;52:88–91.

Glass JR, Sproule BA, Hermann N, *et al.* Effects of 2-week treatment with temazepam and diphenhydramine in elderly insomniacs: A randomized, placebo-controlled trial. *J Clin Psychopharmacol* 2008;28(2):182–188.

Huedo-Medina TB, Kirsch I, Middlemass J, *et al.* Effectiveness of non-benzodiazepine hypnotics in treatment of adult insomnia: Meta-analysis of data submitted to the Food and Drug Administration. *BMJ* 2012;345:e8343.

Krystal AD. Antidepressants and antipsychotic drugs. *Sleep Med Clin* 2010;5(4)571–589.

Leufkens TRM, Vermeeren A. Highway driving in the elderly the morning after bedtime use of hypnotics. *J Clin Psychopharmacol* 2009;29(5):432–438.

Mets MAJ, de Vries JM, de Senerpont Domis LM, *et al.* Next-day effects of ramelteon (8 mg), zopiclone (7.5 mg), and placebo on highway driving performance, memory functioning, psychomotor performance, and mood in healthy adult subjects. *Sleep* 2011;34(10): 1327–1334.

Rishi MA, Shetty M, Wolff A, *et al.* Atypical antipsychotic medications are independently associated with severe obstructive sleep apnea. *Clin Neuropharm* 2010;33:109–113.

Shirani A, Paradiso S, Dyken ME. The impact of atypical antipsychotic use in obstructive sleep apnea: A pilot study and literature review. *Sleep Med* 2011;12:581–597.

Chapter 16

Medications Used in the Treatment of Attention Disorders

Attention deficit hyperactivity disorder (ADHD) is generally seen as a disorder of childhood. However, contrary to the extended popular belief, ADHD does not "disappear" as patients become adults. The estimated prevalence of ADHD in adults in the USA has been estimated to be 4.4%, a percentage that is not too far from that estimated in children aged 5–12 years (6%–9%) (Dopheide *et al.*, 2010). However, a diagnosis of ADHD is rarely made in adults using primary care or mental health services and therefore, the great majority of adult patients with ADHD remain untreated.

As with other psychiatric conditions, the therapeutic approach to ADHD should start with educating the patient and the family about the disorder and providing strategies to help patients and their families deal with the symptoms and complications of this disorder. Regarding specific interventions, the efficacy of pharmacological treatment has been established in randomized controlled trials (RCTs), and it should be the first-line treatment for the disorder. In addition, as is also the case with other disorders, non-pharmacological strategies are a desirable complement (not an alternative, in our opinion) to approved medications. Because of the potential for abuse and dependence, pharmacological treatment with stimulant medications needs to be carefully monitored.

16.1 Stimulant Medications (Psychostimulants)

Here, the term 'stimulant medications' refers to amphetamines and methylphenidate, the cornerstone of ADHD treatment.

Amphetamine was first synthesized in 1887 in Germany. It was soon found that the addition of a methyl group to the amphetamine molecule increased its potency. In today's practice, methamphetamine (especially, the D-isomer) is the prevailing compound. Since the 1930s, amphetamine and related compounds have been tried with some success in management of heterogeneous disorders such as narcolepsy, fatigue, asthma, obesity, and depression.

Methylphenidate was synthesized in 1944, clinically introduced in the 1950s, recognized as a stimulant in 1954, and proposed for the treatment of attention disorders in the 1960s. As in the case of amphetamine, methylphenidate was also tried in diverse conditions, such as chronic fatigue, lethargic and depressive states, including those associated with tranquilizing agents and other drugs, agitation in the elderly, depression, and narcolepsy.

In the USA, stimulant medications are controlled substances and are classified as Schedule II drugs. When used in large amounts, or taken via intranasal or intravenous routes, stimulants have high potential for abuse and dependence. In the brain, stimulants appear to work mainly by affecting the release of dopamine and norepinephrine, two neurotransmitters that play key roles in cognition, decision-making, impulse control, mood, appetite, sleep, and motor activation. However, the exact mechanism of action and the specific mechanisms underlying the cognitive and behavioral improvements observed with stimulant treatment of ADHD are not clearly understood. For both amphetamines and methylphenidate, it has been shown that different isomers exert differential activities. Besides this, at least in the case of methylphenidate, one isomer (L-methylphenidate) has significantly higher first-pass elimination than the other, with resulting serum levels that could be one-tenth of those of D-methylphenidate. For these reasons, the proportion of the two isomers in pharmaceutical preparations has clinical importance.

16.1.1 *Pharmacokinetics and drug–drug interactions*

Both amphetamines and methylphenidate are well absorbed after oral administration. The half-lives of both types of stimulants are short, about 3–6 h for amphetamines and 2–4 h for methylphenidate. Because of this short half-life, immediate-release preparations need to be administered several times a day. An interesting pharmacokinetic observation regarding the action of stimulant medications is that their clinical effect seems to be more pronounced when plasma levels are rising than when they are steady, which would also support the use of divided dosages.

Amphetamines are eliminated through several routes, with approximately 30% excreted unchanged, another part deaminated, and a minimal amount metabolized by CYP2D6. However, rare cases of severe toxicity with stimulants have been reported in poor metabolizers for CYP2D6 substrates who are given stimulants simultaneously with CYP2D6 inhibitors. Thus, it is probably a safe practice to avoid the combination of amphetamines with CYP2D6 inhibitors such as fluoxetine, paroxetine, or duloxetine. In this context, we must also remember that bupropion, a second-line medication for ADHD, is an inhibitor for CYP2D6. Thus, when we combine stimulants with bupropion, it is probably safer to use methylphenidate rather than amphetamines.

Methylphenidate is eliminated through de-esterification by carboxylesterase 1 (CES1) into the inactive metabolite ritalinic acid. However, some substances, especially alcohol, seem to change the metabolism of methylphenidate, leading to increased production of active metabolites, such as ethylphenidate, that may increase the risk of toxicity. Thus, the combination of methylphenidate and alcohol should be specifically discouraged.

One of the oral forms of amphetamine is a prodrug called lysdexamphetamine (Vyvanse), a combination of L-lysine and D-amphetamine, which is transformed by active hydrolysis in the intestine back to D-amphetamine. Even though this preparation may theoretically have a lower abuse potential than other stimulants, the introduction of an additional metabolic step to get to the active compound *in vivo* introduces another source of biological variability for the clinical effect. There is a transdermal system for methylphenidate (Daytrana), which is a patch delivering a mixture of the two isomers. Despite the skin absorption that eludes the first-pass clearance in the liver, the reported relative biovailability of the two isomers is similar to that of oral preparations, with the D-isomer being responsible for most of the clinical effect. The patch has a slower onset of action than oral preparations and its practical advantage is the ability to stop the stimulant effect by removing the patch. For ongoing use of the patch, it is recommended to remove it less than 9 h after it was applied, in order to prevent the cumulative absorption of high amounts of medication.

The combination of all stimulant medications with monoamine oxidase inhibitors (MAOIs) is contraindicated, based on the general assumption that increasing the levels of free dopamine and norepinephrine while inhibiting their metabolism may lead to increased toxicity.

16.1.2 *Adverse effects*

In addition to the risk for abuse/dependence, another safety issue related to the use of stimulant drugs is their cardiovascular risk. However, despite significant increases in blood pressure and heart rate, according to a recent report, the rates of sudden death in young patients taking stimulants do not appear to be much higher than what would be expected in the case of unexposed subjects (Schelleman *et al.*, 2011). Another recent study reports on 529 children, ages 7–9, who were randomized for 14 months to stimulant medication, behavioral therapy, the combination of the two, or community treatment "as usual," and then followed for up to 10 years. Results of this study showed an increased heart rate during treatment but not thereafter, and no increased risk for pre-hypertension or hypertension in children taking stimulants (Vitiello *et al.*, 2011). However, on 9 February 2006, the Drug Safety and Risk Management Advisory Committee of the FDA had voted to recommend a warning describing the cardiovascular risks of stimulant drugs. This warning states that sudden death has been reported with usual doses of CNS stimulants in children and adolescents with structural cardiac abnormalities or other serious heart problems, and sudden death, stroke, and myocardial infarction have been reported in adults taking CNS stimulants at usual doses. It concludes that stimulant drugs should not be used in patients with known structural cardiac abnormalities, cardiomyopathy, serious heart rhythm abnormalities, coronary artery disease, or other serious heart problems.

The adverse reactions/side effects of stimulant medications include:

Neurologic. Most of adverse effects of stimulants are related to the hyperstimulation of the CNS, including insomnia and appetite suppression that occur even at therapeutic doses, as well as worsening of tics. Other CNS effects, usually seen at higher doses, include headache, irritability, changes in arousal (hyperactivity and anxiety followed by exhaustion), and mood changes (elation followed by depressed mood and increased sensitivity). In children, there is concern about the possible effect of stimulants on growth. While there appears to be a negative but moderate effect in this regard, the issue is unsettled. For a more detailed discussion of this issue, we refer the reader to a child/adolescent psychopharmacology source.

Cardiovascular. We have already discussed possible cardiovascular risks earlier in this chapter. Briefly, stimulants may induce elevations in blood pressure, which if mild and treatable, do not require discontinuation of the drug. Tachyarrhythmias are rare but require careful attention.

Gastrointestinal. These include gastric discomfort and abdominal pain.

Acute toxicity. This may occur in medication abusers, after accidental overdose, or due to substance or drug–drug interactions. It is an exaggeration of the cardiovascular and CNS effects already described. Patients show physical adrenergic signs such as an increased pulse and blood pressure or dry mouth and pupillary dilatation, mood lability, irritability and agitation, stereotyped behaviors, motor signs such as bruxism, and paranoia and other delusions. The final stages involve hypertension, tachycardia, arrhythmias, hyperthermia, frank psychosis, delirium, seizures, and even death. Treatment is symptom-specific, including cooling measures for hyperthermia, benzodiazepines for seizures/agitation, anti-adrenergic agents for cardiovascular symptoms, and antipsychotics for psychosis/delirium.

Chronic toxicity. This is related mainly to chronic drug abuse, and frequently takes the form of a paranoid psychosis ("amphetamine psychosis"), with ideas of reference, mistrust, and paranoid delusions, and different types of hallucinations, such as tactile hallucinations ("bugs crawling under the skin").

Withdrawal. Rather than pharmacological withdrawal, abrupt stopping of high-dose stimulants produces a rebound syndrome characterized by a lack of energy, overeating, oversleeping, and depression that can include suicidal tendencies. Stimulants are strongly reinforcing and drug cravings are usually severe. Thus, abusers stopping these medications have little chance of maintaining sobriety when followed in an outpatient setting, and may require instead close supervision in residential inpatient settings.

16.1.3 *Clinical use*

Before starting stimulant medications, patients should have a comprehensive medical and family history and a detailed physical examination, especially looking for cardiovascular pathology. They also need a thorough psychiatric evaluation, especially looking for the presence of, or increased risk for, substance abuse. Except for cases with cardiac pathology suggested by the history or the physical exam, it does not seem necessary to administer ECG tests to patients who are going to be started on stimulants. Stimulants may be used on stable hypertensive patients without cardiac pathology, but these patients require careful regular monitoring of cardiovascular parameters.

Despite the similar mechanism of action of the two classes of stimulants, some patients may be more or less responsive to either amphetamines or methylphenidate. Therefore, a trial of stimulants should ideally include using both types of drugs sequentially before switching to a different group of medications. Stimulants may increase blood pressure and heart rate, and these parameters should be closely monitored.

In the USA, there are many different preparations of stimulant medications available, including immediate- and sustained-release tablets or capsules, immediate- and sustained-released solutions, and a transdermal form. Some existing presentations may include complex mixtures of substances, salts, or unusual drug strengths that seem intended to discourage switching to another stimulant or to prevent the development of generic copies. However, because there is a significant difference in price, it is important for the prescriber to consider the more cost-effective preparations available in the market, especially for uninsured patients or patients with limited medication coverage.

Stimulant medications available in the USA include:

(1) D-amphetamine
- Immediate release (Dexedrine, Dextrostat)
- Sustained release (Dexedrine Spansules)
- Oral solution (LiquADD)

(2) D-amphetamine + amphetamine (two salts of each)
- Immediate release (Adderall)
- Sustained release (Adderall XR)

(3) D-amphetamine prodrug
- D-amphetamine + lys-D-amphetamine (Vyvanse)

(4) Methylphenidate
- Immediate release (Ritalin, Methylin)
- Oral solution (Methylin)
- Sustained release (Concerta, Medadate CD, Methylin ER, Ritalin SR, Ritalin LA)
- Sustained-release liquid (Quillivant XR)
- Transdermal (Daytrana)

(5) Dexmethylphenidate
- Immediate release (Focalin)
- Sustained release (Focalin XR)

Stimulant medications should be started at a low dose and titrated up at regular intervals until there is no further clinical improvement in ADHD symptoms and side effects are tolerable. The recommended adult doses for the stimulant medications listed above are:

(1) D-amphetamine, immediate release: start with 5–10 mg qd or bid, maximum daily dose 40–60 mg (in several doses).

(2) D-amphetamine, sustained release: start with 10 mg qd, maximum daily dose 40–60 mg (in one or several doses).
(3) Lysamphetamine: start with 30 mg qd, maximum dose 70 mg qd.
(4) Methylphenidate, immediate release: start with 5 mg qd, bid, or tid, maximum dose 40–80 mg (in several doses).
(5) Methylphenidate, sustained release: start with 10–20 mg qd, maximum dose 40–80 mg (in one or several doses).
(6) Methylphenidate, transdermal: start with 10 mg patch, maximum dose 30 mg patch (not to wear for >9 h).
(7) Dexmethylphenidate, immediate release: start with 2.5 mg bid, maximum dose 20 mg bid.
(8) Dexmethylphenidate, sustained release: start with 5 mg qd, maximum dose 40 mg.

16.2 Atomoxetine

Drugs with norepinephrine reuptake inhibition properties (such as secondary TCAs) have been used in the treatment of attention disorders for decades. Atomoxetine (Strattera) is a serotonin–norepinephrine reuptake inhibitor (SNRI) approved in the USA for the treatment of ADHD. Medications in this group are considered antidepressants, and an analog, reboxetine, has been long in use in Europe for the treatment of depression. Atomoxetine's clinical effect on ADHD appears to be inferior to that of stimulant medications. However, the fact that atomoxetine is not under special control as stimulants are and it has no risk for abuse/dependence, is a big advantage and many providers try it first not only in patients at increased risk for abuse/dependence but also in average patients. However, atomoxetine carries a warning for increased suicidality, which seems to be a more serious possibility in the case of young patients.

Atomoxetine is well absorbed after oral administration, and its absorption does not seem to be affected by food. The reported half-life is 5 h, and it is metabolized mainly by CYP2D6 in the liver.

The side effects/adverse reactions of atomoxetine are basically those of adrenergic medications, including hyperarousal and nervousness, insomnia, pulse and blood pressure increases, dry mouth, mydriasis and exacerbation of glaucoma, decreased appetite, nausea, urinary retention, constipation, impairment of sexual function, and menstrual abnormalities. Rare but serious cases of hepatitis have been reported. Post-marketing reports include QT prolongation, syncope, and seizures, but the relationship of these conditions with the medication is unclear. Atomoxetine should not be combined with MAOIs, and its combination with adrenergic medications, both psychotropic (TCAs and SNRIs) and general/cardiovascular (dopamine, dobutamine, bronchodilators, and vasoconstrictors used in cold medications) should be either avoided or used with extra care.

The recommended dose of atomoxetine in adults is 20–100 mg/day, in one or two doses.

16.3 Bupropion

As mentioned in Chapter 7, bupropion is considered to be a weak inhibitor of norepinephrine and dopamine reuptake. Although there is no formal FDA approval for bupropion's use in ADHD, it has been used in patients with deficits of attention for many years with good clinical results. The doses and titration of bupropion are very similar in depression and ADHD, although in ADHD some providers prefer to use the immediate-release forms, administered in several doses, starting at 75–100 mg administered in a twice-per-day schedule. Nevertheless, a significant number of providers simply use the same sustained-release forms they use in depression.

16.4 Modafinil

The efficacy of modafinil in pediatric ADHD was supported by at least three RCTs. However, the FDA advisory committee rejected the application for the ADHD indication due primarily to worries about safety (skin toxicity). Thus, in the pediatric clinical trials, two patients developed erythema multiforme/Stevens–Johnson Syndrome (EM/SJS), three patients developed early prodromal EM/SJS, and seven patients developed symptoms suggestive of prodromal EM/SJS. In adult ADHD, a randomized, double-blind, placebo-controlled crossover study of modafinil and D-amphetamine showed no difference in effect between the two drugs. However, that study was too small (21 completers), and too brief (two weeks for each treatment with a four-day washout period) for the results to be reliable (Kumar, 2008).

16.5 α_2-Adrenergic Agonists (Guanfacine and Clonidine)

As mentioned above, adrenergic pathways may be involved in alertness/attention, and noradrenergic medications have long been used in the treatment of ADHD. The potential mechanism of action of guanfacine and clonidine in ADHD is still unclear, but it may be related to the enhancement of working memory through improvements of neuronal connectivity in the prefrontal cortex. Guanfacine and clonidine seem to have a smaller clinical effect than stimulants, atomoxetine, and bupropion on ADHD, but they may bring advantages over the other medications for managing aggressive behaviors, tics, and sleep. A clinical advantage for guanfacine is its higher selectivity for α_{2A} receptors compared with clonidine, which may result in less sedation and dizziness. Therefore, here, we will focus only on guanfacine and will provide a brief outline of the evidence and pointers for its clinical use.

Guanfacine is FDA-approved for the treatment of ADHD in children and adolescents. In adult ADHD, efficacy has been "suggested" by results from small-scale RCTs comparing guanfacine to stimulants. A crossover trial showed that more patients preferred amphetamines to guanfacine, possibly because of a more positive impact of amphetamines on "motivation." The authors of that report argue that "in addition to attention problems, a defect in motivation toward delayed rewards is also believed to be a core deficit of ADHD. DAMP may have an effect on these (delayed) reward systems in a way that guanfacine does not." (Taylor *et al.*, 2001)

Guanfacine is available in immediate- and sustained-release preparations (Tenex and Intuniv, respectively). The reported half-lives are almost the same for both forms, 16 h for immediate-release and 18 h for sustained-release guanfacine. Thus, even the immediate-release formulation can be given once a day. The dosing recommendation is for all patients to start with a dose of 1 mg once daily and adjust it in increments of no more than 1 mg per week. The maximum recommended dose is 4 mg/day.

A significant factor limiting guanfacine's use is the frequency of side effects, especially those affecting the CNS and cardiovascular system. The warnings for guanfacine include hypotension, bradycardia, and syncope. It has to be used with caution in patients at risk for hypotension, bradycardia, heart block, or syncope (e.g., those taking antihypertensive medications). Blood pressure and heart rate need to be monitored prior to initiation of therapy, and periodically while on therapy. Sedation is very common, with some studies reporting somnolence in about 40% of patients. Guanfacine has additive effects with other CNS depressant drugs, and patients should be cautioned against driving or operating machinery until they know how they respond to the medication. Other common side effects of guanfacine are fatigue, nausea, and lethargy.

References

Dopheide JA, Pliszka SR. Attention-deficit-hyperactivity disorder: An update. *Pharmacotherapy* 2009;29(6):656–679.

Kumar R. Approved and investigational uses of modafinil: An evidence-based review. *Drugs* 2008;68(13):1803–1839.

Schelleman H, Bilker WB, Strom BL, Kimmel SE, *et al.* Cardiovascular events and death in children exposed and unexposed to ADHD agents. *Pediatrics* 2001;127(6): 1102–1110.

Taylor FB, Russo J. Comparing guanfacine and dextroamphetamine for the treatment of adult attention-deficit/hyperactivity disorder. *J Clin Psychopharmacol* 2001;21(2):223–228.

Vitiello B, Elliott GR, Swanson JM, *et al.* Blood pressure and heart rate over 10 years in the multimodal treatment study of children with ADHD. *Am J Psychiatry* 2012; 169(2):167–177.

Chapter 17

Medications Used in the Treatment of Dementia

One of the most poignant questions regarding the use of psychotropic medications in general practice applies to the treatment of cognitive problems in elderly populations. The question is: does the "statistically significant" change in symptom scales documented in clinical trials (efficacy) actually correspond to real benefits in the daily functioning and life activities of these patients (effectiveness)?

In 1996, the acetylcholinesterase (AchE) inhibitor donepezil (Aricept) was approved in the USA for the treatment of mild to moderate Alzheimer's disease (AD). After a long hiatus, two other AchE inhibitors followed. These were rivastigmine (Exelon) introduced in 2000, and galantamine (Reminyl) introduced in 2001. The last medication of this kind to be approved in 2003 was memantine (Namenda), an antagonist of glutamate NMDA receptors, for the treatment of moderate to severe AD. It is important to notice that memantine has not showed benefits over placebo in the case of milder to moderate AD. All these medications are relatively expensive, with the exception of generic donepezil, already available in the USA.

Soon after the introduction of these medications, mental health specialists began questioning their clinical significance. Even in clinical trials, where the effect is measured in change in clinical scales and not in real-life outcomes, the number needed to treat for these medications (number of patients that must be treated for one to show the effect) was in the double digits, which means a very marginal effect. Then, in 2004, the results of the AD2000 study were published. This was a study involving 565 community resident patients with mild to moderate AD, who were randomized to donepezil or placebo for 12 weeks. Four hundred and eighty-six patients who completed this phase were re-randomized to long-term double-blind treatment with donepezil or placebo. The primary outcomes measured were two real-life outcomes: entry into institutional care, and loss of a predetermined number of activities of daily living (progression of disability). No significant differences were found in these outcomes across the two treatment groups. At three years, 42% of patients on donepezil were institutionalized, versus 44% on placebo ($p = 0.4$). Similarly, the progression of disability at three years was 58% for donepezil versus 59% for placebo ($p = 0.4$). There were no significant differences between donepezil and placebo in behavioral/psychological symptoms, course of illness, formal care costs, unpaid caregiver time, adverse events, or deaths. No differences were seen either between the 5-mg and the 10-mg doses of donepezil (AD2000 Collaborative Group, 2004). Also, a large 12-week trial found that donepezil was not more effective than placebo in treating agitation in patients with AD (Howard *et al.*, 2007).

Thus, despite multiple positive studies mainly sponsored by industry, the most recent publications are not very encouraging about the usefulness of medications now available for the treatment of dementia.

In any case, the publication of AD2000 fanned the flames of the debate. In 2005, the UK National Institute for Health and Clinical Excellence (NICE) withdrew the recommendation for the clinical use of donepezil. However, the issue is a minefield, due mainly to the expectations of patients and families. Later, NICE revised its guidelines to suggest that donepezil be used in moderate-stage patients for whom the evidence is strongest. Currently, NICE recommends AchE inhibitors in patients with mild to moderate AD, and memantine for people with moderate AD who are intolerant or have a contraindication to AChE inhibitors, or individuals with severe AD. For all medications, NICE established the condition that only specialists in the care of dementia should initiate treatment (NICE, 2011).

17.1 Side Effects

The main side effects of AChE inhibitors are cholinergic: gastrointestinal (diarrhea, vomiting, anorexia, and nausea), neurologic (insomnia, hallucinations, dizziness, and fatigue), muscular (muscle cramps and fasciculation, and CPK elevations), bradycardia, worsening of COPD and bronchial obstruction, and urinary dysfunction. AChE inhibitors should not be used in patients with bradycardia. Memantine is usually well tolerated, with the main side effects being observed in the CNS (confusion, somnolence, and hallucinations).

17.2 Pharmacokinetics

AChE inhibitors are well absorbed after oral administration. Donepezil and galantamine are metabolized mainly by CYP3A4. Rivastigmine is eliminated primarily via cholinesterase-mediated hydrolysis. Donepezil has a longer half-life (70 h versus 7 h for galantamine and 1.5 h for rivastigmine), and therefore donezepil is the only one that can be given once a day in the form of immediate-release preparations. The half-life of memantine has been reported to be 60–80 h and its elimination is mainly through the kidneys (at least half of memantine is excreted unchanged in urine), with the rest metabolized by non-CYP enzymes.

17.3 Pointers for Clinical Use

Regarding the clinical use of FDA-approved medications in the treatment of dementia, we list below several recommendations:

(1) The decision to use these medications should be made in a case-by-case basis. Cost/benefit is always a question. For example, in the case of uninsured patients or patients with high copay rates, we need to ask whether or not the financial stress that this will pose to the individual or the family justifies the relatively weak clinical benefits.
(2) To start treatment, give preference to AChE inhibitors over memantine as the latter has a more questionable benefit in mild AD. Among AChE inhibitors, donepezil is favored for its longer half-life, better tolerability, and lower cost in generic form.
(3) Do not encourage unrealistic expectations; educate patient and family about the illness and also about the effect of the medications.
(4) If there is no appreciable clinical effect, discontinue the medications.
(5) In patients with severe dementias, significant functional deterioration, or poor quality of life, who are unlikely to derive clinical benefits, the authors recommend not to start any of these medications or consider stopping them if the patient is already on them.

References

AD2000 Collaborative Group. Long-term donepezil treatment in 565 patients with Alzheimer's disease (AD2000): Randomized double-blind trial. *Lancet* 2004;363:2010–2015.

Howard RJ, Juszczak E, Ballard CG, *et al.* Donepezil for the treatment of agitation in Alzheimer's disease. *N Engl J Med* 2007;357(14):1382–1392.

UK National Institute for Health and Clinical Excellence. Donepezil, galantamine, rivastigmine and mementine for the treatment of Alzheimer's disease, March 2011, Retrieved from www.nice.org.uk/nicemedia/live/13419/53619/53619.pdf

Chapter 18

Medications Used in Smoking Cessation and Alcohol Use Disorders

In this chapter, we describe those medications that are commonly prescribed for the treatment of addictions in primary care or outpatient psychiatry settings. This refers primarily to medications used for managing smoking cessation (nicotine dependence) and alcohol use disorders. The treatment of other types of substance use disorders generally requires more intensive or specialized interventions, including hospitalization. Regarding their drug management, we refer the reader to specialized publications on the treatment of addictions.

18.1 Medications Used in the Treatment of Nicotine Dependence (Smoking Cessation)

Prior to discussing specific medications used for treating tobacco use and dependence, a caveat is needed. Psychological interventions, especially counseling on smoking cessation, significantly increase the chances of success of pharmacotherapy in the treatment of nicotine addiction. Thus, a quality intervention for smoking cessation should always involve a behavioral/psychological component in addition to pharmacotherapy.

For a succinct but complete description of combined interventions for smoking cessation, we refer the reader to:

Fiore MC *et al.* A clinical practice guideline for treating tobacco use and dependence: 2008 update. *Am J Prev Med* 2008;35(2):158–176.

For a useful, brief description of counseling in smoking cessation, we refer the reader to:

Tonstad S. Smoking cessation: How to advise the patient. *Heart* 2009; 95:1635–1640.

Medications used in the treatment of nicotine dependence in the USA include nicotine replacement therapies (NRTs), as well as vareniciclin and bupropion. Other drugs that have shown efficacy for smoking cessation, such as clonidine and nortriptyline, are not widely used, mainly due to their safety profile.

18.1.1 *Varenicline*

Varenicline (Chantix) is a partial agonist/antagonist for nicotinic cholinergic receptors ($\alpha_4\beta_2$). It blocks nicotine from binding the receptor but also stimulates the receptor to induce the release of dopamine, thus decreasing craving. Varenicline has good oral absorption, and is eliminated unchanged in the urine. It has a half-life of approximately 17 h.

Varenicline seems to be the most efficacious among current pharmacotherapy interventions for smoking cessation. In acute trials, varenicicline more than doubles the chances of abstinence as compared with placebo. According to a recent Cochrane review (Cahill *et al.*, 2012), the pooled RR (relative risk) for continuous or sustained abstinence at six months or longer for varenicline at standard dosage versus placebo was 2.27 (95% CI: 2.02–2.55); the pooled RR for varenicline versus bupropion at one year was 1.52 (95% CI: 1.22–1.88); and the RR for varenicline versus NRT for point prevalence abstinence at 24 weeks was 1.13 (95% CI: 9.94–1.35).

The most frequent adverse event with varenicline in clinical trials is nausea (16% for 0.5 mg bid and 30% for 1 mg bid, versus 10% for placebo), while the most common psychiatric mental adverse effect is insomnia (19% for 0.5 mg bid and 18% for 1 mg bid, versus 13% for placebo).

Warnings and precautions with varenicline include:

- Angiodema and hypersentivity reactions.
- Serious skin reactions, which are reportedly rare.
- Cardiovascular events, which tend to occur mainly in patients with cardiovascular disease. However, an important consideration in the pharmacotherapy of smoking cessation is that the magnitude of the cardiovascular risk associated with smoking justifies the use of medications that may pose at least a moderate cardiovascular risk as is the case with varenicline or bupropion. Obviously these agents should be avoided in patients with serious or unstable cardiac conditions.
- Agitation, hostility, depressed mood, and suicidal thinking have been also associated with varenicline. A recent review of the FDA's Adverse Event Reporting System (AERS) found a substantial, statistically sigificant increased risk of reported depression and suicidal/self-injurious behavior with varenicline. Bupropion also showed an increase, but it was smaller. The review

> concludes: "The findings for varenicline, combined with other problems with its safety profile, render it unsuitable for first-line use in smoking cessation." (Moore *et al.*, 2011)

Varenicline comes in 0.5- and 1-mg tablets to be taken twice a day (bid). The 1-mg bid dosage provides higher rates of success for smoking cessation, but also significantly increases the risk for adverse effects compared to the 0.5-mg bid dose. Thus, some providers prefer to stay on the 0.5-mg bid dosage for long-term treatment.

18.1.2 *Bupropion*

For a detailed discussion of bupropion, including adverse effects, warnings, and contraindications, we refer the reader to Chapter 7. Here, we will only highlight that, besides the actions of the drug that were described in that chapter, bupropion seems to be also a noncompetitive antagonist for several nicotinic receptors — the ones involved in nicotine's addiction. The recommended dose of sustained-release bupropion for smoking cessation is 150 mg in the morning for three days, which can be increased to 150 mg twice a day. Patients should start taking the medication 1–2 weeks before the scheduled date to quit smoking.

An important consideration in the pharmacotherapy of smoking cessation is whether or not the magnitude of the cardiovascular risk associated with smoking justifies the use of medications with potential cardiovascular risks such as the case with varenicline or bupropion. We believe that in most instances, this use is amply justified since the cardiovascular liability of these agents is rather modest. However, they should not be used in patients with serious or unstable cardiac conditions.

18.1.3 *Nicotine replacement therapy*

While used for a long time in Europe, sublingual nicotine tablets were never introduced in the USA. Preparations available in the USA for NRTs include:

- nicotine gum;
- nicotine lozenges;
- nicotine inhaler;
- nicotine nasal spray; and
- nicotine patch.

The main concern with the use of NRTs in the past was the possibility of increasing the risk for acute cardiovascular events. While this concern has dissipated with the growing clinical use of these agents, NRTs should be used with care in patients' post-myocardial infarction, and those with serious arrhythmias or unstable angina pectoris. It should be emphasized again that the high cardiovascular risk brought about by smoking justifies the use of smoking cessation therapies despite their low to moderate cardiovascular risk.

18.1.3.1 *Nicotine gum*

Nicotine gum is an OTC medication, available in 2- and 4-mg pieces. The 4-mg piece is recommended for heavy smokers (25 or more cigarettes per day). The recommendation is to use one piece every 1–2 h for the first six weeks (no more than 24 pieces per day). The gum should be used for up to 12 weeks. Most patients need 10–15 pieces per day.

An important point to be brought up here is that patients need to be educated about the proper way of using the gum. Patients should be instructed to chew on the piece of gum until there is a mild "tingling" or "peppery" taste, indicating nicotine release. The patient then "cheeks" the piece of gum for several minutes before chewing again. This cycle provides time for buccal absorption and should be repeated for 30 min per piece or until the taste dissipates. Patients should avoid eating or drinking anything besides water for 15 min before and after using the gum. The most common adverse effects of nicotine gum are mouth soreness, hiccups, jaw ache, and gastric discomfort, most of which can be minimized with the proper "cheeking" technique.

18.1.3.2 *Nicotine lozenges*

Nicotine lozenges are an OTC medication available in 2- and 4-mg pieces. These are recommended for patients who smoke their first cigarette within 30 min of, or more than 30 min after waking, respectively. No more than 20 lozenges should be used per day. The lozenges should be used for up to 12 weeks.

Lozenges should be allowed to dissolve in the mouth rather than chewing or swallowing them. Although their absorption is buccal, as in the case of nicotine gum, lozenges are simpler to use and may yield better treatment adherence. Also, similar to what was stated above in the case of the nicotine gum, patients should avoid eating or drinking anything besides water for 15 min before and after using the lozenge. The most common adverse effects of lozenges are nausea, hiccups, and heartburn. Patients on the 4-mg piece may experience headache and coughing.

18.1.3.3 *Nicotine nasal spray*

This is a prescription-only device. Nicotine spray delivers nicotine more rapidly than other NRTs. Each spray contains 0.5 mg, and one dose involves one spray per nostril (total 1 mg). Nicotine spray produces higher peak nicotine levels than other NRTs and has the highest dependence potential. Thus, more patients use it for longer periods or at higher doses than recommended. The minimum recommended treatment is 8 doses/day with a maximum limit of 5 doses/h or 40 doses/day. The recommended duration of therapy is 3–6 months. Most patients use initially 12–16 doses per day. Nicotine spray causes local nose irritation in most patients, but this is usually transient. The spray should not be used in patients with severe airway disease.

18.1.3.4 *Nicotine inhaler*

This is also a prescription-only device. It consists of a plastic container for a cartridge with cotton impregnated with 10 mg of nicotine. Although called an "inhaler," the vapor is absorbed mostly across the oral mucosa. It provides lower arterial levels of nicotine than cigarettes or other NRTs. However, the need for frequent puffing to deliver substantial amounts of nicotine mimics some of the behaviors of smoking. The usual recommended dosage is 6–16 cartridges per day. The recommended duration of therapy is six months, with gradual tapering during the last three months. Adverse effects include irritation of oral cavity and throat, and cough.

18.1.3.5 *Nicotine patch*

Patches can be both an OTC or a prescription-only medication. They usually come in strengths that deliver 21, 14, or 7 mg/24 h. There is also a patch delivering either 22 or 11 mg/24 h. Instructions in the package about application should be closely followed. If the patch causes vivid dreams or interferes with sleep, the patient may need to wear the patch only while awake (16 h each day). However, nicotine may continue to be absorbed through the skin for several hours after the patch is removed. Treatments of eight weeks or even shorter periods seem to be as efficacious as those for longer periods. A standard recommendation is using the 21 mg/day patch for four weeks, then the 14 mg/day one for two weeks. However, treatment can be individualized based on such factors as the amount smoked, degree of dependence, etc. An important consideration is that dosages of the patch are less flexible than those of other NRTs, and that many patients are actually underdosed with the standard patch doses. Thus, use of doses higher than 21 mg/day are appropriate for smokers who fail single-dose patch therapy or whose nicotine withdrawal symptoms are not relieved with standard therapy. Individualized initial patch doses can be 7–14 mg (for patients smoking <10 cigarettes per day); 14–21 mg (for patients smoking 10–20 cigarettes per day); 21–42 mg (for patients smoking 21–40 cigarettes per day); and >42 mg (for patients smoking >40 cigarettes per day).

Up to half the patients using nicotine patches experience local skin reactions. If these are clinically significant, topical corticosteroids may be used. It is recommended that the location of the patch be rotated among different areas.

18.2 Medications Used in the Treatment of Alcohol Use Disorders

18.2.1 *Disulfiram*

Disulfiram (Antabuse) was approved in the USA for the treatment of alcohol use disorders in 1949. Disulfiram works by blocking the second step in the metabolism of alcohol, inhibiting the enzyme aldehyde dehydrogenase which catalyzes the oxidation of acetaldehyde to acetic acid. The elevated blood levels of acetaldehyde resulting from this inhibition cause a very uncomfortable reaction, usually lasting from 10 min to an hour (average half an hour), with uncomfortable feelings of heat and flushing of the skin, especially in the chest and head, throbbing headache, difficulty breathing, blurred vision, anxiety, palpitations, and decreased blood pressure. The most severe reactions may include also sweating, nausea, vomiting, dizziness, and confusion. Reported deaths related to disulfiram are usually the result of high doses of the drug combined with significant amounts of alcohol. However, some deaths have occurred even with low doses of disulfiram combined to a single drink.

In the risk-averse American medical culture, disulfiram is clearly underutilized. In motivated individuals who accept supervised administration and have reasonably good impulse control, it could be a useful intervention. Few comparisons have been made between disulfiram and the newer drugs approved for alcohol dependence. However, disulfiram seemed to show some superiority in a recent randomized, multicenter, open-label, comparative trial of disulfiram, naltrexone, and acamprosate in alcohol-dependent patients. In this two-and-a-half-year trial, an initial 12-week continuously supervised medication treatment period was followed by a targeted medication period up to 52 weeks (during which patients were provided medications that they could take when they perceived their propensity to drink was high), and then a 67-week follow-up period (during which patients could continue on the medication). The study included 243 outpatients. All three study groups showed marked reduction in drinking, from baseline to the end of the study. During the supervised phase, disulfiram was more effective in decreasing heavy drinking days (HDDs) and average alcohol consumption, and increasing time to first drink, as well as the number of abstinent days. During the targeted medication period, there were no significant differences between the groups in time to first HDD and days to first drinking, but the abstinent days were significantly more frequent in the disulfiram group (Laaksonen *et al.*, 2008).

Disulfiram is well absorbed orally. It has a short half-life, but because it is an irreversible inhibitor of the enzyme aldehyde dehydrogease, the effects are long-lasting. The potential for an interaction with alcohol persists for at least two weeks after the last dose of disulfiram. Disulfiram is also an inhibitor for CYP2E1, which is involved in the metabolism of anesthetic agents and acetaminophen, so care should be exercised in the administration of these medications. Inhibition of other metabolic enzymes has been described with disulfiram, but they require very high concentrations of the drug and are very rare.

Side effects of disulfiram include drowsiness, lethargy, and fatigue. Serious adverse reactions include optic neuritis, peripheral neuropathy, and hepatotoxicity. They are rare but patients on disulfiram must be monitored regularly for visual changes, signs of neuropathy, and liver toxicity.

Patients on disulfiram should avoid taking not only alcoholic drinks, but also alcohol-containing foods (vinegar, sauces, etc.), or medications and even topical preparations containing alcohol (aftershave lotions). The FDA's warning for disulfiram reads: "Never give disulfiram to a patient in a state of alcohol intoxication or without the patient's full knowledge. The patient should not take disulfiram for at least 12 hours after drinking. A reaction may occur for up to 2 weeks after disulfiram has been stopped."

The usual dose of disulfiram in the USA is 250–500 mg/day. However, some patients may require doses of 1 g/day or higher to reach a level of activity sufficient for an interaction with alcohol.

18.2.2 *Naltrexone*

Naltrexone (Revia) was approved for use in alcohol dependence in the USA in 1994 (it had been approved for opioid dependence in 1984). Naltrexone is an opioid antagonist, and appears to decrease the euphoriant actions of alcohol by blocking the opioid reward system to the "priming" effects of alcohol. Naltrexone seems to affect diverse aspects of alcohol use, including alcohol intoxication, alcohol reinforcing properties, craving for alcohol, and tendency to continue drinking.

Naltrexone is well absorbed after oral administration, but undergoes extensive first-pass metabolism (something avoided with intramuscular administration). Elimination is mainly through the kidneys, but the liver also seems to play a role in the metabolism of naltrexone, and for this reason, caution is recommended when administering naltrexone to patients with both renal and hepatic impairment.

Naltrexone has a very modest effect in alcohol-dependent patients, with a more visible effect on decreasing HDDs than on abstinence rates. This can be exemplified in the results of the COMBINE study, a North American 11-center, 16-week trial in 1,383 recently alcohol-abstinent volunteers. In this trial, eight groups of patients under medical management received naltrexone, acamprosate, both medications, or placebo, with or without a combined behavioral intervention (CBI). A ninth group received CBI only (no pills). Compared to placebo, the results were statistically significant for practically all the interventions except acamprosate. However, it must be noted that the net clinical results were relatively modest for all interventions. There were no differences in percentage of days abstinent through treatment, and in percentage of HDDs, the difference with placebo for the best treatments was around 5%. These effects dissipated shortly after stopping the intervention (Anton *et al.*, 2006).

The potential benefits of naltrexone are obviously affected by treatment compliance. For this reason, the approval of an injectable form of naltrexone (Vivitrol) for monthly administration, could improve clinical results. The six-month trial that led to FDA's approval showed that, compared with placebo, 380 and 190 mg of long-acting naltrexone resulted in a 25% and 17% decrease, respectively, in HDDs (Garbutt *et al.*, 2005).

The adverse effects of naltrexone are mainly gastrointestinal, with the most worrisome being the risk of liver toxicity. Because of this, the medication should not be started in intoxicated patients or patients in acute withdrawal. Initial liver function testing is advisable to avoid prescribing naltrexone in patients with elevated enzyme levels. Follow-up monitoring is not considered necessary, unless symptoms warrant it, as, in general, treatment with naltrexone may decrease enzyme levels. Other side effects are headache, irritability, weakness, and joint and muscle pain.

Contraindications to the use of naltrexone, besides significant hepatic disease, include opioid use or withdrawal. Reasonable certainty must exist that there has been no opioid use in the previous 7–10 days and, if there is any doubt, a naloxone challenge test must be performed before starting naltrexone.

The FDA-recommended dose of oral naltrexone is 50 mg/day. The standard recommendation is starting at 25 mg/day, and then increased by 25 mg every 3–7 days, to a maximum dose of 150 mg/day, according to the patient's tolerability and report of effect. For injectable naltrexone, the FDA-recommended dose is 380 mg every four weeks.

18.2.3 *Acamprosate*

Acamprosate, an amino acid derivative, appears to increase inhibitory GABA neurotransmission and affect in complex ways the process of excitatory neurotransmission, such as that for glutamate. The effect of acamprosate in alcohol dependence seems to be even more modest than that of naltrexone. A meta-analysis of 12 studies estimates a number needed to treat for benefit to be around 10 (95% CI: 7–15) (Bouza *et al.*, 2004). Recent comparative studies of acamprosate with naltrexone and/or behavioral interventions, have reported a lack of significant effects of acamprosate on alcohol dependence (Morley *et al.*, 2006; Anton *et al.*, 2006).

The main side effects of acamprosate are gastrointestinal (diarrhea, nausea, flatulence, and vomiting), neurologic (insomnia, headache, and confusion), sexual dysfunction, and pruritus.

The recommended dose of acamprosate is two 333-mg tablets given three times a day, a dosing schedule that poses serious compliance problems. Acamprosate is eliminated by the kidneys and therefore should be used with care, or not at all, in patients with renal problems.

References

Anton RF, O'Malley SS, Ciraulo DA, *et al.* Combined pharmacotherapies and behavioral interventions for alcohol dependence: The COMBINE study: A randomized controlled trial. *JAMA* 2006;295:2003–2017.

Bouza C, Magro A, Munoz A, *et al.* Efficacy and safety of naltrexone and acamprosate in the treatment of alcohol dependence: A systematic review. *Addiction* 2004;99:811–828.

Cahill K, Stead LF, Lancaster T. Nicotine receptor partial agonists for smoking cessation. *Cochrane Database Syst Rev* 2012;(4):CD006103.

Fiore MC, Jaen CR, Baker TB, *et al.* A clinical practice guideline for treating tobacco use and dependence: 2008 update. *Am J Prev Med* 2008;35(2):158–176.

Garbutt JC, Kranzier HR, O'Malley SS, *et al.* Efficacy and tolerability of long-acting injectable naltrexone for alcohol dependence: A randomized controlled trial. *JAMA* 2005; 293:1617–1625.

Laaksonen E, Koski-Jannes A, Salaspuro M, *et al.* A randomized, multicentre, open-label, comparative trial of disulfiram, naltrexone and acamprosate in the treatment of alcohol dependence. *Alcohol Alcohol* 2008;43(1):53–61.

Moore TJ, Furberg CD, Glenmullen J, *et al.* Suicidal behavior and depression in smoking cessation treatments. *PLoS One* 2011; 6(11):e27/06.

Morley KC, Teesson M, Reid SC, *et al.* Naltrexone versus acamprosate in the treatment of alcohol dependence: A multi-centre, randomized, double-blind, placebo-controlled trial. *Addiction* 2006;101:1451–1462.

Srisurapanont M, Jarusuraisin N. Naltrexone for the treatment of alcoholism: A meta-analysis of randomized controlled trials. *Int J Neuropsychopharmacol* 2005;8:267–280.

Tonstad S. Smoking cessation: How to advise the patient. *Heart* 2009;95:1635–1640.

Chapter 19

Drug–Drug Interactions

In the traditional sense, a drug–drug interaction (DDI) means that a drug modifies the effects, either therapeutic or adverse, of another. However, in our current environment, mental health prescribers need to worry not only about the potential interactions of psychotropic medications with other prescription drugs, but also with the many substances that people ingest in their daily quest to deal with psychological distress, improve mental or physical function, or change their mood. This heterogeneous mix includes over-the-counter (OTC) drugs, food supplements, substances of abuse, other psychotropic drugs or hormones used without medical prescription, and even the growing market of special drinks and foods loaded with psychoactive compounds.

There is good consensus among health experts that the vast majority of DDIs go undetected, so that clinical estimates are generally unreliable. A recent publication, extrapolating from the incidence of DDIs in emergency room visits and hospital admissions, estimated that in the USA, DDIs are causing 74,000 emergency room visits and 195,000 hospital admissions per year (Percha *et al.*, 2013). When we take into account that OTC drugs and food supplements can also interact with prescription drugs, the number of potential DDIs gets even higher.

In the USA, the risk for DDIs grows almost on a daily basis with the parallel increase in the number of medications taken by Americans. According to data from the U.S. National Center for Health Statistics (NCHS), from 2007–2010, the percentage of the total U.S. non-institutionalized population taking at least one prescription drug in the last 30 days was 47.5%, the percentage taking three or more prescription drugs 20.8%, and the percentage taking five or more prescription drugs 10.1%. These figures increase as people age. Thus, for people 65 years of age and over, the percentage taking at least one medication was 90.4%, the percentage taking three or more medications 66.4%, and the percentage taking five or more medications 39.8% (NCHS, 2011).

Regarding the risk of DDIs in the elderly, a prospective 16-week cohort study among consecutive new patients aged 65 years and older, admitted to a community hospital, who were taking >5 drugs on average, estimated that the prevalence of potential CYP-mediated DDIs in this population was 80%. In this study, the probability of at least one CYP-mediated DDI was 50% for patients taking 5–9 drugs, 81% for patients taking 10–14 drugs, 92% for patients taking 15–19 drugs, and 100% for patients taking 20 or more drugs. The addition of each medication to a five-drug regimen conferred an additional 12% risk of a potential CYP-mediated DDI after adjusting for age and sex (Doan *et al.*, 2013).

DDIs are a growing source of concern in most countries, and algorithms to detect them are increasingly used by pharmacies and drug providers in the USA. They are also being incorporated into the electronic medical records now mandated for all American healthcare providers. However, the interactions included in these databases are in most cases limited to those DDIs related to the CYP450 (cytochrome) oxidation system. Thus, other important DDIs such as those in non-CYP metabolic pathways, interactions in phase II drug metabolism (conjugation), or pharmacodynamic DDIs (when the effects of a medication directly add to, or interfere with the effects of another) are not systematically addressed.

Generally, DDIs are divided into *pharmacokinetic* (those that change the transit of a drug through the body), and *pharmacodynamic* (those that change the effect of a drug at the point of action). Clinically, both types of interactions may cause increased drug effects and toxicities, or decreased effectiveness of the "target" drug(s). In the following sections, we will review the different types of DDIs, and will devote additional time to discuss the types of DDIs that are more commonly observed in medical settings nowadays. To exemplify the ubiquity and heterogeneity of DDIs, in Table 19.1, we list 10 of the most frequent or serious DDIs involving psychotropic drugs.

19.1 Pharmacokinetic Drug–Drug Interactions

Pharmacokinetic DDIs may take place in multiple organ systems during the transit of a drug through the body, including its absorption, distribution to the various body compartments, metabolism, and excretion from the body.

Table 19.1 Ten relevant DDIs involving psychotropic drugs.

1. **Inhibitors/inducers of CYP1A2 combined with clozapine (and olanzapine).** CYP1A2 inhibitors (such as fluvoxamine or ciprofloxacine) may increase the levels of clozapine (and olanzapine) to toxic levels. Drugs that induce CYP1A2 (such as carbamazepine and modafinil), or nutritional and environmental inducers of CYP1A2 (such as broccoli, brussels sprouts, different types of cabbage, char-grilled meat, and smoke from tobacco) may decrease the effect of clozapine and olanzapine; inversely, after their discontinuation, the levels of clozapine and olanzapine may increase to toxic values.
2. **Contraception failure with CYP3A4 inducers.** Inducers of CYP3A4, 5, and 7, the cytochrome that metabolizes estradiol, especially carbamazepine and topiramate, may decrease the effect of birth control pills and result in pregnancy.
3. **Therapeutic failure of the anti-estrogen tamoxifen with CYP2D6 inhibitors.** CYP2D6 inhibitors block the conversion of the prodrug tamoxifen to the active compound endoxifen. The safest antidepressants to use in patients taking tamoxifen are mirtazapine, venlafaxine, trazodone, and, possibly, vilazodone.
4. **Toxic levels of multiple substrates of conjugation with the addition of valproate.** Valproate has the potential to inhibit multiple conjugation enzymes, leading to toxicity of conjugation substrates including lamotrigine, 3-OH benzodiazepines (lorazepam, oxazepam, and temazepam), opioids, acetaminophen, and NSAIDs.
5. **Pharmacodynamic (GABA) toxicity of alcohol plus benzodiazepines or GABA hypnotics.** This is a dangerous interaction in any patient, but even more in patients with respiratory impairment. Remember that alcohol is an anxiolytic and a hypnotic agent frequently abused by patients with anxiety.
6. **Renal interactions leading to decreased excretion of lithium.** Thiazide and loop diuretics (but not potassium-sparing diuretics), NSAIDs and, probably, ACE inhibitors may increase lithium levels.
7. **Interactions with methadone.** Methadone poses many more risks for DDIs than most providers generally think. It is metabolized mainly by CYP3A4, but other cytochromes may also contribute, especially CYP1A2. Thus, toxicity with methadone has been described with the concomitant use of CYP3A4, 5, or 7 inhibitors or upon discontinuation of CYP1A2 or CYP3A4, 5, or 7 inducers. High levels of methadone are particularly risky because of the high potential for QT prolongation, a potential risk that many providers tend to ignore (indeed, many methadone clinics do not routinely require ECGs at pre-treatment or during regular follow-up, which in our view should be a standard precautionary measure).
8. **Cumulative toxicity leading to QT prolongation.** Let us remember here that among the multiple risk factors for QT prolongation, the most important one is taking several medications with this potential concurrently. QT-prolonging drugs are found in practically all areas of medicine. Among psychiatric medications with this potential, we already mentioned methadone above. Regarding antipsychotics, the ones posing the highest risk are thioridazine and ziprasidone, but all of them, both typical and atypical, have the potential for QT prolongation, especially when used at high doses. Among antidepressants, tricyclics pose a very high risk, but it has been observed that some of the newer antidepressants may also be risky (e.g., citalopram, escitalopram, and, possibly, fluoxetine).

(*Continued*)

Table 19.1 (*Continued*)

9. **Interactions with supplements.** St. John's wort is the "prize winner" here! It may not only cause toxicity when added to serotonergic medications, but induces P-glycoprotein and CYP3A4, 5, and 7, which creates the potential to decrease the effect of most medications marketed in the USA.
10. **Interactions with food.** The potential of grapefruit to inhibit CYP3A4 and P-glycoprotein in the intestinal lining and liver is by far the riskiest one, as it may cause toxic elevations in the levels of most medications marketed in the USA.

Table 19.2 Psychotropic drugs primarily eliminated through the kidney.

- Gabapentin (Neurontin)
- Lithium
- Memantine (Namenda)
- Milnacipram (Savella), mainly renal elimination as the parent drug or glucuronide
- Paliperidone (Invega), 60% eliminated unchanged in urine (paliperidone is the active metabolite of risperidone; thus, risperidone's elimination is also partially dependent on the kidney)
- Pregabalin (Lyrica), 90% excreted unchanged in urine
- Topiramate (Topamax), 70% eliminated unchanged in urine

19.1.1 *DDIs during absorption of psychotropic medications*

Cholesterol-binding resins, such as cholestyramine (Questran, Cholestid) or laxatives based on fiber such as psyllium (Metamucil), may sequester medications, especially ions such as lithium, directly in the intestinal lumen, thus preventing their absorption. Therefore, patients should be warned to take oral medications far apart from these compounds.

On the other hand, naringin and other compounds present in grapefruit and other citric juices, inhibit the activity of the oxidation enzyme CYP3A4 in the intestinal lining, significantly increasing the absorption of medications metabolized by this cytochrome, and increasing the risk for toxicity.

19.1.2 *DDIs during excretion of psychotropic medications*

The most common DDIs during the excretion phase of drugs occur in the kidney, when a drug increases or decreases the excretion of another. The outstanding example of this in psychopharmacology is the inhibition of the renal excretion of lithium by thiazides and loop diuretics, as well as NSAIDs (see Chapter 13). In Table 19.2, we offer a list of psychotropic drugs primarily excreted in the urine, which makes them more susceptible to DDIs at the kidney level.

19.1.3 *DDIs involving transport proteins*

Drug interactions in this area have few practical applications in clinical psychiatry, but are critical in other specialties, such as oncology. However, the knowledge of DDIs in this system is growing fast and therefore a review of transport protein-related DDIs will hopefully prepare the reader to assimilate the steady flow of information that will be coming in the near future.

Defense systems in the body include multiple transporters that pump "toxic" substances out of the organism (for example, back in the intestinal lumen) or out of body compartments such as the CNS. The most well-known of these "defensive" protein transporters is P-glycoprotein, also called MDR1 (multidrug resistance protein 1) or ABCB1 (ATP-binding cassette B1 protein). In the intestinal lining, for example, P-glycoprotein works in tandem with CYP3A4 to decrease the entry of many substances, including medications, into the bloodstream. Immediately following enteric absorption, within the intestinal epithelial cell, CYP3A4 oxidizes these compounds, while P-glycoprotein pumps them back into the intestinal lumen. At the brain–blood barrier (BBB), protein transporters provide an additional level of protection for the brain from exogenous substances, such as drugs. There, P-glycoprotein, other MDRs, and proteins of the ABC transporters, work to keep medications out of the CNS, pumping them back into the general circulation. It is known that the CNS levels of the antipsychotic risperidone are affected by changes in the activity of these transporters. Some substances, including several drugs, are inhibitors or inducers for MDR proteins, and through this mechanism they may decrease or increase the efflux of drugs that are substrates of the transporter proteins. Loperamide, an opioid derivative used in the treatment of diarrhea, is normally kept out of the CNS by efflux transporters. However, when administered concurrently with P-glycoprotein inhibitors, loperamide enters the CNS and causes typical opiate mental effects. St. John's wort, a herb commonly used for depression, is an inducer of P-glycoprotein, and decreases the effects of psychotropic medications which are substrates for this transporter. Milk thistle, another herb used for hepatic and biliary problems, is an inhibitor of P-glycoprotein. Grapefruit juice, which inhibits CYP3A4, is also an inhibitor of P-glycoprotein, and has significant potential to cause toxicity by CYP3A4 and P-glycoprotein substrates.

19.1.4 *DDIs involving inhibition or induction of oxidative CYP450 enzymes*

This is the type of DDI that receives most attention and which is the most frequently detected these days. As mentioned in Chapter 1, the cytochromes are not the only oxidative enzymes of pharmacological relevance in humans. However, the cytochromes constitute the largest oxidative system and are the main area for potential DDIs to appear. The activity of CYP450 oxidative enzymes, also called cytochromes, can be inhibited or increased ("induced") by medications or other environmental compounds. Inhibition of a metabolic enzyme leads to increased levels and elevated effect, and therefore a higher risk of toxicity for its substrates. Induction of a metabolic enzyme leads to elevated levels and effects for its substrates. Often, the inhibitor or inducer is a substrate for the affected enzyme, but this is not always the case. For example, bupropion, metabolized by CYP2B6, is an inhibitor for CYP2D6. Certain drugs may also be inhibitors or inducers for several enzymes. For example, fluvoxamine, metabolized by CYP1A2, is an inhibitor, besides this enzyme, for 2C9, 2C19, and 3A4; fluoxetine, metabolized mainly by CYP2D6, also inhibits 2C19 and 3A4.

The cytochromes are heme-containing proteins, and they are fairly abundant in nature. Cytochrome enzymes are microsomal bodies, located in the endoplasmic reticulum; they convert most lipid-soluble compounds to more easily excreted water-soluble polar forms. Close to 700 of these enzymes have been identified in different species. In humans, they are present in the liver and other organs (gut, brain, lungs, skin, etc.). However, only the P450 in families 1, 2, and 3 appear to be responsible for the metabolism of drugs, and therefore are potential sites for DDIs. Even more, out of the estimated 20 CYP450 enzymes in families 1, 2, and 3, less than a dozen are quantitatively relevant in the metabolism of pharmaceuticals.

The most important CYP450 in all of medicine is CYP3A4. It is said that approximately half of the medications currently available in the USA are metabolized by CYP3A4, including most of macrolide antibiotics, antiretrovirals, antihistamines, calcium channel blockers, HMG-CoA reductase inhibitors (cholesterol-lowering medications), anticancer agents, and a good number of other miscellaneous medications. The second most important CYP enzyme in all of medicine, and the most important in psychiatry, is CYP2D6, which metabolizes a significant number of psychotropic drugs, and most of beta-blockers, opioid analgesics, antiarrhythmics, and several other medications. In decreasing order of importance, we list CYP2A6, 2B6, 2C19, 2C8/9, and 2CA1/2.

In Table 19.3, the psychotropic substrates and the most relevant general medicine substrates for CYP450 enzymes are presented. In Tables 19.4 and 19.5, we list the most relevant inhibitors and inducers for these enzymes. However,

Table 19.3 Psychotropic and general substrates for CYP450 enzymes (cytochromes).

1A2	2B6	2C9	2C19	2D6	3A4,5,7
Psychotropics					
Clozapine (main)	Bupropion	Fluoxetine	Citalopram	Amphetamines	AcHO inhibitors
Cyclobenzaprine	Methadone		Fluoxetine	Aripiprazole	Aripiprazole
Fluvoxamine			Methadone	Atomoxetine	Benzos:
Mirtazapine			Tertiary TCAs (main)	Chlorpromazine	Alprazolam
Olanzapine (main)				Citalopram	Clonazepam
Tertiary TCAs				Codeine	Diazepam
				Duloxetine	Midazolam
				Fluoxetine (main)	Triazolam
				GHB	Buprenorphine
				Haloperidol (main)	Hypnotics:
				Hydrocodone→ (active)	Zaleplon
				Metoclopramide	Zolpidem
				Mirtazapine	S-zopiclone

(*Continued*)

Table 19.3 (*Continued*)

1A2	2B6	2C9	2C19	2D6	3A4,5,7
				Oxycodone	Buspirone
				Paroxetine	Carbamazepine
				Perphenazine	Citalopram
				Risperidone	Haloperidol (minor)
				Secondary TCAs (main)	Marijuana (THC)
				Tertiary TCAs (minor)	Mirtazapine
				Tramadol	PCP and ketamine
				Venlafaxine	Quetiapine
					Risperidone (minor)
					Sertraline
					Trazodone
					Vilazodone (main)

(*Continued*)

Table 19.3 (*Continued*)

1A2	2B6	2C9	2C19	2D6	3A4,5,7
Other drugs and supplements (misc.)					
Caffeine	Cyclophosphamide	Angiotensin II blockers	Beta-blockers	Tamoxifen→endoxifen	Antiretrovirals
Lidocaine	Efavirenz	Oral hypoglycemics	Chloramphenicol		Antihistamines
Melatonin		NSAIDs	Clopidogrel		Ca channel blockers
Naproxen		Torasemide	Cyclophosphamide		Statins
Ondansetron		S-warfarin	Indomethacine		Immune modulators
Propanolol			Nelfinavir		Macrolide antibiotics
Theophylline			Progesterone		Phosphodiesterase inhib
Verapamil			Propranolol		Steroids
Zolmitriptan			Proton pump inhib		
			R-warfarin		

Table 19.4 Main inhibitors for CYP450 enzymes (cytochromes).

1A2	2B6	2C9	2C19	2D6	3A4,5,7
Fluvoxamine		Fluvoxamine	Fluoxetine	Bupropion	Fluvoxamine
	Thiothepa		Fluvoxamine	Duloxetine	Nor-fluoxetine
Amiodarone	Ticlopidine	American ginseng		Fluoxetine	Valproate
Cimetidine		Amiodarone	Modafinil	Paroxetine	
Ciprofloxacin		Fenofibrate	Topiramate	(Citalopram?)	Amiodarone
Interferon		Fluconazole		(Sertraline?)	Azole-antifungals
		Isoniazide	Cimetidine		Camellia Sinensis
		Lovastatin	Indomethacine	Goldenseal	Cimetidine
		Phenylbutazone	Ketoconazole		Grapefruit juice
		Sulphometoxazole	Proton pump inhibitor		HIV antivirals
		Zafirlukast	Ticlopidine		Macrolide antibiotics (not azythromycin)
					Ca channel blockers
					Starfruit juice

Table 19.5 Main inducers for CYP450 enzymes (cytochromes).

1A2	2B6	2C9	2C19	2D6	3A4,5,7
Carbamazepine	Phenobarbital	Carbamazepine	Carbamazepine	Dexamethasone	Barbiturates
Modafinil	Phenytoin	Secobarbital		Rifampicin	Carbamazepine
			Ginkgo biloba		Modafinil
Insulin	Metamizole	Phenytoin	Northindrone		Oxcarbazepine
Nafcillin	Rifampicin	Rifampicin	Prednisone		Phenytoin
Methylcholantrene			St. John's wort		Topiramate
Omeprazole			Rifampicin		
St. John's wort					Glucocorticoids
					Metamizole
Smoke/tobacco					Rifampicin
Brussel sprouts					
Grilled meat					Echinacea?
					St. John's wort?

considering the high percentage of psychiatric patients who also take non-psychotropic medications, a comprehensive source to look up for relevant DDIs is essential to the proper practice of clinical psychopharmacology these days. Multiple databases for DDIs are accessible on the web, including mobile devices. A resource we highly recommend is the "Cytochrome P450 Drug Interaction Table," by Flockhart DA, available at http://medicine.iupui.edu/clinpharm/ddis/.

19.1.5 *DDIs involving inhibition or induction of conjugation enzymes (phase II metabolism)*

The conjugation system, an important elimination pathway, usually is not as amply recognized as it deserves. Different from oxidative enzymes (phase I metabolism), conjugation enzymes do not chemically modify the substrates, but bind them to soluble compounds, facilitating elimination. Conjugation enzymes catalyze the transfer of sugars, especially glucuronic acid, to a variety of molecules, both endogenous and xenobiotics, to make them more hydrophilic and more easily excreted. Many of the substances conjugated to sugars by this system are the products of the oxidative enzymes, so very often conjugation is simply viewed as a continuation of the oxidative metabolic reactions. However, conjugation is the only elimination pathway for numerous active drugs that are not oxidized, or for metabolites of oxidized drugs with pharmacological activity. Thus, DDIs at this level may lead to serious clinical consequences.

The conjugation enzymes, uridine-5-diphospho-glycosyltransferases, also called uridine-5-diphospho-glucuronosyltransferases, or UGTs, are expressed in many tissues, but DDIs related to them are most likely to occur in the intestine, liver, and kidneys. For conjugation, UGTs require a cofactor, uridine-5-diphospho-glucuronic acid (UDPGA), to yield glucuronic acid.

In Table 19.6, we list the main substrates, inhibitors, and inducers for conjugation enzymes. However, the reader must keep in mind that conjugation is a less specific process than oxidation. The UGTs are less compartmentalized than oxidative enzymes. Once a conjugation substrate has saturated the preferred enzyme, the saturation process may extend to other UGTs. Another process by which conjugation substrates may inhibit the whole system is exhausting the required cofactor, UDPGA.

Valproic acid is the conjugation inhibitor causing most DDIs in psychiatry, but alcohol, NSAIDs, and acetaminophen are also risky, especially when used at high doses. On the other hand, conjugation may also be "induced" (increased), which leads to a faster elimination and lower levels of conjugation

Table 19.6 Main substrates, inhibitors, and inducers for conjugation enzymes.

Psychotropic substrates	Inhibition	Inducers
3-OH benzodiazepines (UGT2B7) Lorazepam Oxazepam Temazepam	• Any substrate has the potential to saturate the enzyme and competitively inhibit the elimination of other substances metabolized by the same enzyme	**Anticonvulsants** Carbamazepine Phenobarbital Phenytoin
Antipsychotics Asenapine (UGT1A4, also Oxidation by CYP1A2)		**Estrogen** Ethynylestradiol (reduces concentration of lamotrigine by 40%–65%)
Antidepressants Desmethylvenlafaxine (which UTG?, minor oxidation through CYP3A4)	• Glucuronidation enzymes are less compartmentalized than CYP ones, and inhibition may extend to other enzymes	
Mood stabilizers Lamotrigine (UGT1A4) Valproate (UGT1A6 and 2B7 major, but also 1A3, 1A4, and 1A9)	• Another mechanism in which a substrate may inhibit the whole glucuronidation system is by exhausting the cofactor, glucuronic acid	
Opioids (UGT2B7) Dihydrocodeine Hydromorphone Morphine Nalmefene Nalorphine Naloxone Naltrexone Norbuprenorphine Acetaminophen (UGT1A6)		
NSAIDs (UGT2B7) Naproxen		

(*Continued*)

Table 19.6 (*Continued*)

Psychotropic substrates	Inhibition	Inducers
Ketoprofen		
Ibuprofen		
Fenoprofen		
Zomepirac		
Diflunisal		
Indomethacin		

substrates. The most frequent conjugation inducer causing DDIs in psychiatry is carbamazepine, a drug that may also induce several cytochromes, and plays havoc with plasma levels and clinical effects of numerous psychotropic and non-psychotrophic drugs.

19.2 Pharmacodynamic DDIs Involving Psychotropic Drugs

As mentioned earlier, pharmacodynamic DDIs occur when a medication directly increases or decreases the effects of another. A "positive" (additive) pharmacodynamic interaction occurs when medications with similar actions are given concurrently, which obviously increases the risk for adverse effects and toxicity. In the section on antidepressants, the risky interaction between MAOIs and other antidepressant drugs has been already discussed. Another frequent and usually overlooked "positive" (additive) pharmacodynamic DDI occurs when antipsychotic medications are used simultaneously with the antinausea/GERD medications metoclopramide (Reglan) and prochlorperazine (Compazine), which are actually antipsychotic drugs. Antidepressants with different approved indications are sometimes prescribed simultaneously by different specialists. The SNRIs duloxetine (Cymbalta) and milnacipram (Savella), FDA-approved for the treatment of fibromyalgia, are sometimes prescribed by rheumatologists and other non-psychiatrists to patients who are also taking tricyclics, SSRIs, or SNRIs. Another common pharmacodynamic DDI contributing to adverse effects is the combination of antipsychotic drugs with anticholinergic effects and anticholinergic medications used to prevent or treat EPS, such as benztropine or trihexyphenidyl.

A "negative" pharmacodynamic DDI occurs when medications with opposite effects are taken simultaneously. For example, it is not unusual for elderly patients with dementia, taking acetylcholinesterase inhibitors in efforts to improve cognition, to be prescribed anticholinergic drugs to decrease urinary frequency, or antipsychotic drugs with anticholinergic effects, such as clozapine or quetiapine, all of which may impair cognition. Another example of a "negative" pharmacodynamic DDI involving psychotropic drugs is the co-administration of dopamine blockers, such as antipsychotic drugs, and dopaminergic agents used in the treatment of Parkinson's disease, such as L-DOPA or pramipexole.

19.3 Drug–Drug Interactions due to Cumulative Toxicity

A dramatic example of cumulative toxicity involving psychotropic medications is the causation of malignant arrhythmias (torsades de pointes) by a wide array of medications, including antipsychotics, tricyclic antidepressants, antihistamines, antibiotics, and antiarrhythmic drugs. Several other factors also weigh in the risk for malignant arrhythmias, including pre-existent QT prolongation, female gender, electrolyte disturbances (especially hypokalemia), concomitant cardiovascular disease, and substance abuse. However, the most important variable is the number of QT-prolonging medications given simultaneously. In the section on antipsychotic medications, we have discussed this cumulative toxic effect in more detail. What follows is a list of miscellaneous agents with potential for QT prolongation and malignant arrhythmia:

- Antipsychotics (all the medications in this group increase the risk)
- Tricyclic antidepressants (all the medications in this group increase the risk)
- Antiarrhythmic drugs (all the medications in this group increase the risk)
- Antihistamines: astemizole and terfenadine
- Anti-infectives: erythromycin, clarythromycin, and pentamidine (and probably azythromycin)
- Antimalarials: halofantrine and chloroquine
- Gastric motility drugs: metoclopramide, cisapride, and domperidone
- Opiate agonists: methadone
- Supplements: licorice and *zhigancao*

19.4 Drug–Drug Interactions Related to Food Supplements and Substances of Abuse

As mentioned at the beginning of this chapter, in the face of a possible DDI, we also need to consider food supplements, OTC drugs, and substances of abuse among the possible sources for these effects. To facilitate this task, in

Table 19.7, we list some DDIs involving food supplements, and in Table 19.8, the metabolic pathways for some substances of abuse. Among supplements, we want to emphasize the multiple risks for DDIs related to the use of St. John's wort, a natural substance favored by many individuals with mood disorders. We also need to warn about the risks posed by black cohosh, a supplement that is increasingly being promoted for "women's health."

Table 19.7 DDIs with herbal supplements.

Herbal supplement	Effect
Betel nut	Contains arecoline, a cholinergic alkaloid (enhance effects of cholinergic drugs or antagonize anticholinergics)
Black cohosh	Affects the production of pro- and anticoagulant factors in the liver, likely may cause bleeding or thrombosis
Ephedra	Contains ephedrine and related alkaloids (potentiates caffeine and stimulants)
Gingko bilova	Induces CYP2C19; decreases platelet adhesion (enhances effects of aspirin, anticoagulant meds); vasodilator (may cause priapism when combined with risperidone)
Kava	Inhibits CYP2E1; potentiates sedatives, blocks D receptors and may cause EPS and exacerbate PD
Psyllium	Prevents lithium ionization and absorption
Yohimbine	Can cause hypertension with serotonergic/noradrenergic antidepressants)
St. John's wort	• Induces CYP3A4, 2E1, and 2C19 • Induces P-glycoprotein • Some DDIs reported with St. John's wort: o Immunusuppresants: treatment failure (cyclosporine and tacrolimus) o Hormonal therapy: treatment failure (ethynylestradiol and other steroids) leading to pregnancy o CV drugs: treatment failure (coumadin, digoxin [P-glycoprotein substrate], nifedipine, verapamil, simvastatin and atorvastatin) o Antiretrovirals: treatment faiure (indinavir and nevirapine) o Anticancer drugs: treatment failure (imatinib and irinotecan) o CNS drugs: treatment failure (benzodiazepines, anticonvulsants and methadone); serotonergic syndrome with antidepressants

Table 19.8 Metabolism of substances of abuse.

- Amphetamines, including "ecstasy": CYP2D6
- Buprenorphin: CYP3A4, and to a lesser extent 2C8, to buprenorphine (active metabolite eliminated by glucuronidation)
- Cocaine: plasma and hepatic esterases (induces CYP3A4 in lab animals, induces P-glycoprotein)
- Codeine: CYP2D6 to a potent metabolite, or glucuronidation (unchanged codeine)
- GHB (gamma-hydroxybutyrate): CYP2D6
- Heroin: plasma esterases to morphine
- Hydrocodone: CYP2D6 to a more potent metabolite hydromorphone (eliminated by glucuronidation)
- Marijuana (THC and its metabolites): CYP3A4 and, to a lesser extent, 2C9
- Methadone: CYP2B6 and 2C19 (CYP3A4 and others?)
- Morphine: glucuronidation
- Oxycodone: CYP2D6
- PCP and ketamine: CYP3A4

Appendix: DDI Review Questions

(Answers at the end)

1. A very risky antibiotic to use in patients taking olanzapine (Zyprexa) or clozapine (Clozaril) is:

   (A) Amoxicillin
   (B) Azithromycin
   (C) Ciprofloxacin
   (D) Levofloxacin
   (E) None of them
   (F) All of the above

2. According to the Prescribing Information for aripiprazole (Abilify), when carbamazepine is co-administered, one should:

   (A) Observe the patient for emerging EPS
   (B) Double the dose of aripiprazole
   (C) Decrease the dose of aripiprazole
   (D) No need to worry

3. A patient, stable on depot risperidone (Risperdal Consta), is hospitalized for gastrointestinal symptoms, and prescribed IV liquids, loperamide, and metoclopramide. He shows sudden spasms of the neck. You should:

    (A) Recommend to speed up the hydration
    (B) Add benztropine to the medication regimen
    (C) Discontinue loperamide
    (D) Discontinue metoclopramide
    (E) Add a medication that is a known inducer of CYP2D6

4. The following should be avoided in patients taking HMG-CoA reductase inhibitors (lovastatin, etc.):

    (A) Bupropion
    (B) Citalopram
    (C) Fluvoxamine
    (D) Mirtazapine
    (E) All of the above

5. A patient, who is a heavy smoker, and has been stable on the medications listed below, decides to quit smoking. Which of these medications have to be closely monitored?

    (A) Bupropion 450 mg/day
    (B) Citalopram 40 mg/day
    (C) Clozapine 600 mg/day
    (D) Zolpidem 10 mg qhs, *prn* insomnia
    (E) None of the above

6. It is not advisable to take this medication with grapefruit juice:

    (A) Donepezil
    (B) Quetiapine
    (C) Sildenafil
    (D) Zolpidem
    (E) All of the above

7. What should be avoided in patients with renal disease?

    (A) Lithium
    (B) Memantine
    (C) Milnacipran
    (D) None of the above
    (E) All of the above

8. Which of the following may induce pregnancy in women taking oral contraceptive pills?

   (A) Carbamazepine
   (B) Lamotrigine
   (C) Topiramate
   (D) Carbamazepine and topiramate
   (E) All of the above

9. A patient with breast cancer and depression is taking prednisone, tramadol, tamoxifen, and metoclopramide (for nausea/vomiting). Which antidepressant is contraindicated in this instance?

   (A) Bupropion
   (B) Duloxetine
   (C) Fluoxetine
   (D) Paroxetine
   (E) None of the above
   (F) All of the above

10. A patient, a former opiate addict who is HIV-positive, is taking the medications listed below at the time of starting a new antiretroviral therapy. The patient develops significant sedation gradually. Which medication is likely responsible for this?

    (A) Alprazolam 0.5 mg tid *prn* anxiety attacks
    (B) Quetiapine 100 mg bid
    (C) Trazodone 300 mg 1 tablet qhs *prn* insomnia
    (D) Buprenorphin 8 mg bid
    (E) None of the above
    (F) All of the above

11. One should exercise care when starting a patient on valproate who is a regular user of the substance(s):

    (A) Alprazolam
    (B) Cocaine
    (C) Heroin
    (D) Marijuana
    (E) Phencyclidine
    (F) None of the above
    (G) All of the above

12. Which supplement should be avoided in a patient on (i) anticoagulant/antiplatelet therapy; (ii) lithium; (iii) antidepressants; and (iv) antipsychotics?

    (A) Ginkgo biloba
    (B) Kava
    (C) Melatonin
    (D) Psyllium
    (E) St. John's wort

Answers to DDI Review Questions

1. C. Ciprofloxacine (1A2 inhibitor).
2. B. Carbamazepine induces aripiprazole oxidation.
3. D. Pharmacodynamic interaction. Metoclopramide is an antipsychotic.
4. C. Fluvoxamine (3A4 inhibitor).
5. C. Clozapine (levels and effects may rebound as smoking induces 1A2).
6. E. All of them (3A4 substrates).
7. E. All of them (urinary excretion).
8. D. Inducers of estrogen elimination.
9. F. All of them (2D6 inhibitors may block conversion to active endoxifen).
10. F. All of them (3A4 substrates; elimination may be inhibited by anti-HIV medications).
11. C. Heroin (transformed in morphine, which is eliminated by glucuronidation).
12. (i). A. Ginkgo biloba (decreases platelet adhesion).
    (ii). D. Psyllium (impairs Li's absorption).
    (iii). E. St. John's wort (additive serotonin reuptake inhibition properties; induces several CYP450 enzymes).
    (iv). B. Kava (additive dopaminergic-blocking properties).

References

Chew ML, Mulsant BH, Pollock BG, *et al.* Anticholinergic activity of 107 medications commonly used in older adults. *J Am Geriatr Soc* 2008;56:1333–1341.

Doan J, Zakrzewski-Jakubiak H, Roy J, *et al.* Prevalence and risk of potential cytochrome P450-mediated drug–drug interactions in older hospitalized patients with polypharmacy. *Ann Pharmacother* 2013;47:324–332.

Flockhart DA. Cytochrome P450 Drug Interaction Table, web resource. Retrieved from http://medicine.iupui.edu/clinpharm/ddis/.rom

Gruber VA, McCance-Katz EF. Methadone, buprenorphine, and street drug interactions with antiretroviral medications. *Curr HIV/AIDS Rep* 2010;7:152–160.

Izzo AA, Ernst E. Interactions between herbal medicines and prescribed drugs: An updated systematic review. *Drugs* 2009;69(13):1777–1798.

Leucuta SE, Viase L. Pharmacokinetic and metabolic drug interactions. *Curr Clin Pharmacol* 2006;1:5–20.

Linnet K, Ejsing TB. A review of the impact of P-glycoprotein on the penetration of drugs into the brain. Focus on psychotropic drugs. *Eur Neuropsychopharmacol* 2008;18:157–169.

Mannheimer B, Wettermark B, Lundberg M, *et al.* Nationwide drug-dispensing data reveal important differences in adherence to drug label recommendations on CYP2D6-dependent drug interactions. *BJCP* 2009;69(4):411–417.

Marchetti S, Mazzanti R, Beijnen J, *et al.* Concise review: Clinical relevance of drug–drug and herb–drug interactions mediated by the ABC transporter ABCB2 (MDR1, P-glycoprotein). *Oncologist* 2007;19:927–941.

National Center for Health Statistics. Health, United States, 2011. Retrieved from www.cdc.gov/nchs/data/hus/hus11.pdf#099

Percha B, Altman RB. Informatics confronts drug–drug interactions. *Trends Pharmacol Sci* 2013;34(3):178–184.

Spina E, Santoro V, D'Arrigo C. Clinically relevant pharmacokinetic drug interactions with second-generation antidepressants: An update. *Clin Ther* 2008;30(7):1206–1227.

About the Authors

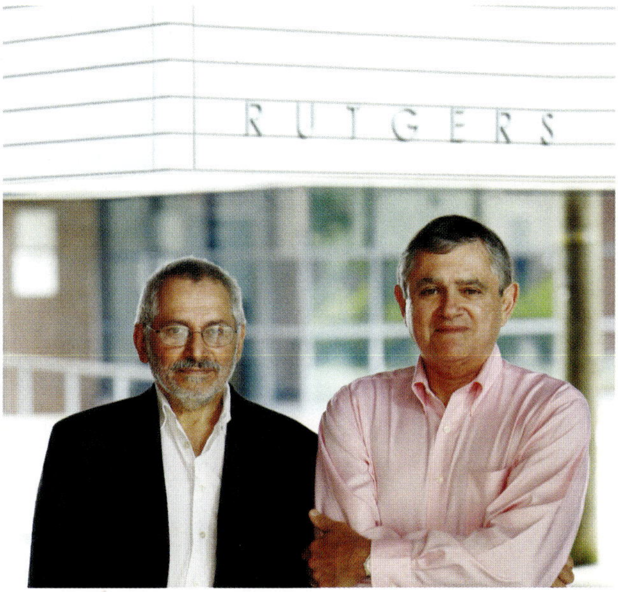

Humberto Marin (left) and Javier I. Escobar. Photo by Adam Olszewski.

Dr. Marin, an Associate Professor of Psychiatry at Rutgers University's Robert Wood Johnson Medical School (RWJMS), has been active in drug and cultural psychiatry research. Currently, besides conducting the Advanced Psychopharmacology Seminar for Psychiatry Residents and Fellows, and teaching Psychopharmacology to medical students, Dr. Marin continues to work with a large and multilingual group of patients with severe and persistent mental illness. He is also the psychiatrist at the Huntington's Disease Clinic at Rutgers University's RWJMS.

Dr. Escobar is Associate Dean for Global Health and Professor of Psychiatry and Family Medicine also at Rutgers University's RWJMS. He has been an active clinician, teacher, and researcher, and an advisor to the National Institute of Mental Health, the U.S. Food and Drug Administration, and the World Health Organization.

Index of Psychotropic Drugs, Substances, and Supplements